# the *Truant* *from* Medicine

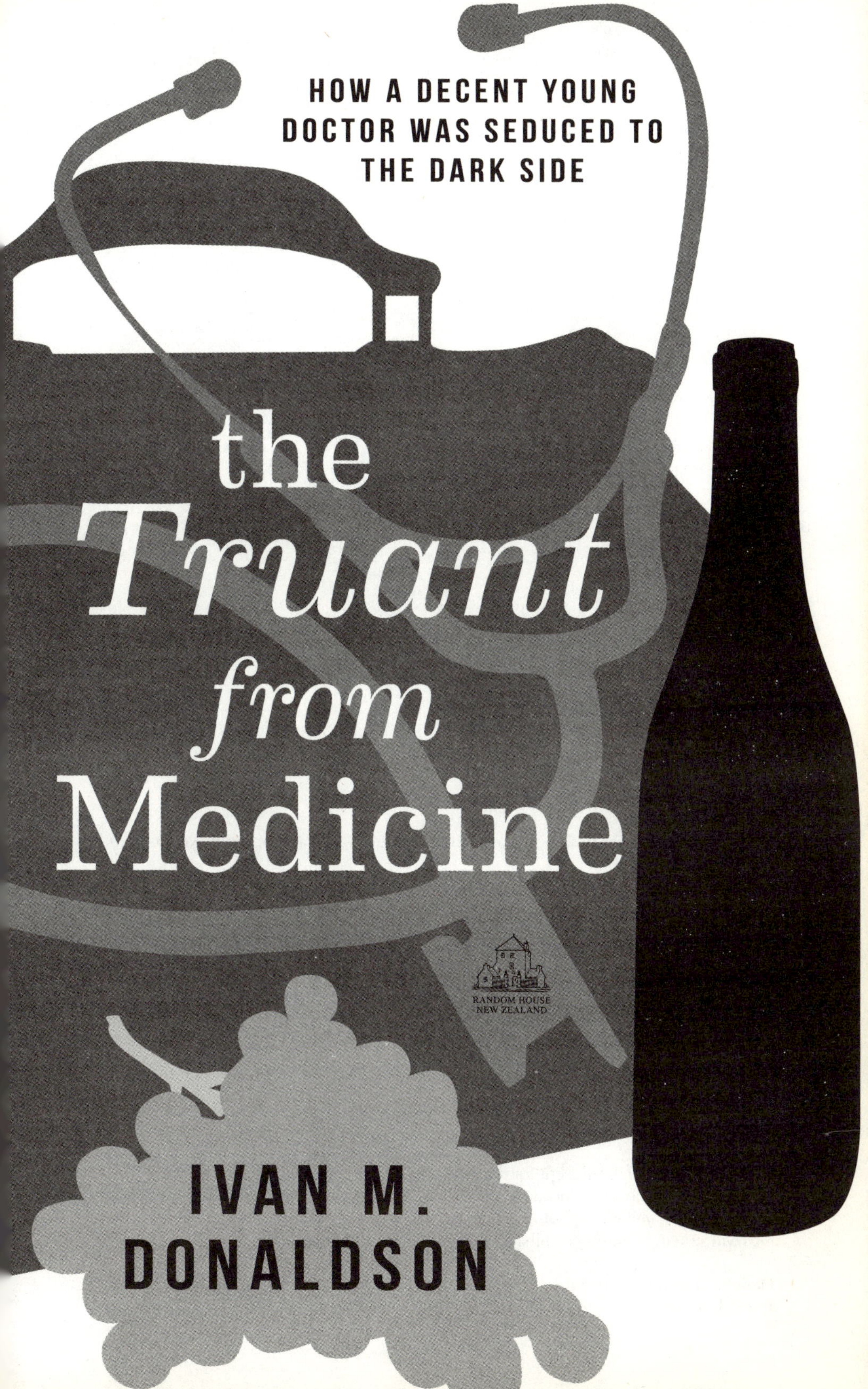

HOW A DECENT YOUNG DOCTOR WAS SEDUCED TO THE DARK SIDE

# the *Truant* *from* Medicine

IVAN M. DONALDSON

RANDOM HOUSE
NEW ZEALAND

A RANDOM HOUSE BOOK published by Random House New Zealand
18 Poland Road, Glenfield, Auckland, New Zealand

For more information about our titles go to www.randomhouse.co.nz

A catalogue record for this book is available from the National Library of New Zealand

Random House New Zealand is part of the Random House Group
New York London Sydney Auckland Delhi Johannesburg

First published 2014



ISBN 978 1 77553 735 9
eISBN 978 1 77553 736 6



Design: Megan van Staden
Printed in China by Everbest Printing Co. Ltd

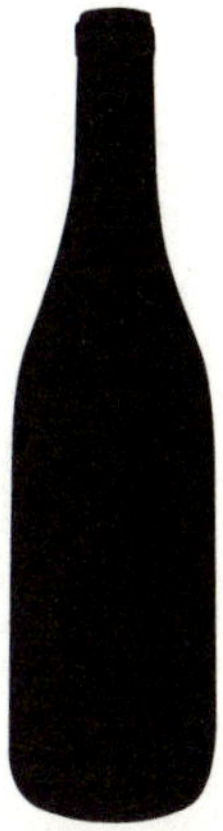

*This book is dedicated to Chris, my constant companion, guide and support over the last 48 years. Without your inspiration I would never have known the joy of the bondage and liberation of truancy.*

'All men dream, but not equally. Those who dream by night in the dusty recesses of their minds, wake in the day and find that it was vanity. But the dreamers of the day are dangerous men for they may act on their dreams with open eyes to make them possible.'

— *T.E. Lawrence*

# Contents

# Preface

**THE ROOM WAS ABUZZ WITH THE EXCITED** chirping of delegates who were pecking nibbles and sipping drinks at the Savour New Zealand conference. Both Chris and I had just finished giving presentations; hers on different styles of riesling and mine on wines to accompany a variety of dishes that had been prepared by a celebrity chef and just happened to include bull's testicles. How could I have been qualified to say what would be the perfect libation to accompany such a dish? A stranger eased her way through the crowd towards us. She introduced herself as being from a publishing company and asked if I would consider writing my autobiography. While flattered, I was also taken aback. It was something that I had never considered and thought would be pretentious.

That was 11 years ago; a year before I joined the board of what is now the New Zealand Brain Research Institute. After reflection I have decided to put pen to paper and tell you my little story, for what it's worth, and in doing so I am applying salve to my bleeding conscience by donating all of the author's royalties and profits to the aforesaid institute.

Neurological disorders are very common and blight the lives of many in the community. I firmly believe that it is only by understanding the causes, nature and effects of these conditions that we will be able to help those who suffer from them. Research into their origins, mechanisms and treatment is worthy of the support of all of us.

I urge you to reflect for a moment on everything that is near and dear to you; on who you, your family and friends really are. You might lose a limb, become paraplegic or have a heart transplant but you are still the same person. Should your brain suffer serious mischief then you are not, even though you may physically appear unaltered. The essence of who we are lies within our brains, and that is why we all have such a vital investment in neurology.

This is a true story and the events that I have outlined concern real people. Naturally, I have presented them as seen through my own eyes, and recognise that others' accounts would doubtless differ in some regards. I have changed the names of all of my patients, some of my colleagues and some of the other characters to protect their anonymity. In many instances, however, I have used their real names.

The dust of accumulated years lies on some parts of the tale and hence precise details may be blurred at the edges but my recall of the salient points remains bright and sharp. The same cannot be said of all of the dialogue. It would be impossible that all of the conversations were reported word-perfect. Nonetheless, their intentions and general flow is in line with my memory and verified by others.

In order to help the flow I have organised the narrative by subject rather than attempting to lay everything out chronologically. For example, chapter 4, 'Wine and Wine Country', is a compilation of a lot of different trips to European vineyards that occurred over many years. However, the order of the subjects in the different chapters, with the exception of chapter 1, more or less follows chronology. The order if the illustrations roughly follows their position in the text and are thus also not chronological.

I have been privileged to have two widely differing careers thanks to the indulgence of my wife Chris, our sons and my long-suffering professional colleagues, both those in medicine and those in wine. To all of them I owe an enormous debt of gratitude. Thank you from the bottom of my heart.

But I must not take myself too seriously, as all that I have learnt on the road of life shows that people matter more than things and that the voyage is as important as the destination. If you do not treasure the one then the other will be a bitter disappointment. Make sure that you revel in your journey, and enjoy the company on the road.

*Ivan MacGregor Donaldson*
*Christchurch*
*July 2014*

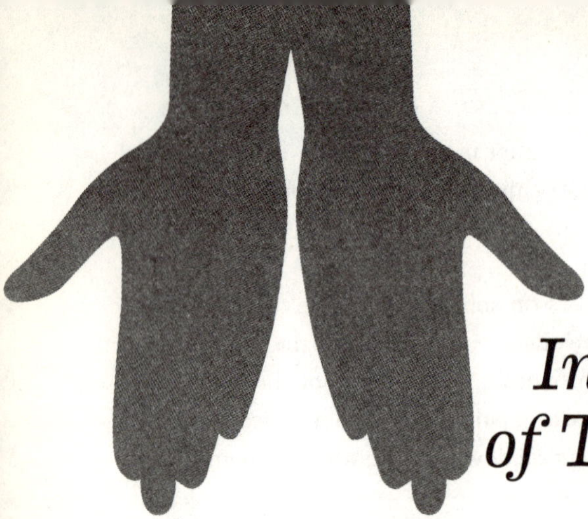

# CHAPTER 1
# *In the* Service *of Two* Masters

**AS I ENTERED THE WAITING ROOM** I was enveloped in a cloud of perfume: exotic, musky, spicy and sensuously alluring. The woman was striking; not ravishingly beautiful in the Hollywood sense, but more refined and classic. She was sitting very straight, her hands folded in her lap on a skirt of non-conservative length, her legs crossed. Her nose was aquiline, her cheekbones high, her lips full, and her teeth displayed a perfection that was clearly the proud trademark of an expert and expensive orthodontist. She had a generous but not excessive figure, and was dressed to show this to its full advantage, straining but not totally rending the bounds of social respectability. This blonde definitely exuded presence and she looked as though she knew it.

'Mrs Adams-Pinker?' I enquired. I took her smile as an affirmation, and added, 'I am Ivan Donaldson. Would you like to come through?'

Turning towards the pleasant-looking but nondescript little man sitting next to her, his hand protectively around her arm, I asked, as was my custom, 'Would you like to come through as well?'

As the couple rose in unison the woman turned to her husband, saying gently but firmly, 'I'll be all right by myself, dear.'

'But I'd like to come,' he protested weakly.

I didn't wish to get involved in a domestic, but two sets of ears are less likely to misinterpret what is being said during a consultation. In addition, the observations of a relative, friend or witness are often vital in unravelling a neurological problem and it can be time-wasting and painful to do separate interviews.

Hence, I came to the man's support by saying, 'It's up to you two to decide, and it's okay with me whatever you want to do, but I sometimes find it helpful to have someone else along.'

‘Oh, all right,’ the woman replied with an air of resignation, setting off a little alarm bell in my head.

It gave me a suspicion that she might have something she wanted to tell me alone, so I made a mental note to give her an opportunity to do this at some stage. As they preceded me towards the consulting room I noticed that the man was in fact neither little nor nondescript. He had only been made to look less significant by his wife’s appearance and poise.

Claire Adams-Pinker had introduced her companion as her husband, Richard. She entered the room first, and before he followed he turned towards me. ‘Call me Dick,’ he said cheerfully, but his general demeanour sabotaged his smile and he added in a whisper, ‘I’m very worried, doctor.’

Once in the consulting room she also seemed to be on edge, sitting forward in her chair and holding onto its arms. Although I could not recall having seen her before, she looked rather familiar. As I took her particulars it emerged that she was a real estate agent or, as the trendier of that set like to call themselves these days, a realtor. Being paid on a commission basis, our local realtors are generally only as successful as their advertising. Most promote themselves by way of flattering portrait photographs, which festoon their stationery, business cards and the ‘For Sale’ notices that are scattered around the city. Given the not-infrequent gap between glossy image and stark reality, I had a strong suspicion that many such photographs were airbrushed in order to rid them of inconvenient imperfections. Curious as I was, I judged that this was not the best time to pursue the truth of the matter, especially when it might seem that I was insinuating that Claire Adams-Pinker herself did not reach the impeccable standard of her portrait, which indeed she did.

When business gets a bit quiet the more enterprising of our local realtors attempt to drum up business by dropping letters in mail boxes. These inform the lucky homeowner that the realtor has a naïve client who has fallen in love with their property and simply must have it. The price is never mentioned but it is insinuated that it will be well above current market value and that this singular opportunity should not be missed. To find out more, the homeowner only needs to telephone the trustworthy face adorning the accompanying business card — and of course there is absolutely no obligation to take it further. I recalled having received such a mail-drop some months earlier, and the lady now sitting in front of me was the dazzling dropper. True to her photo she was still smiling, but now she seemed less confident.

Having read the referring letter from her family doctor I was aware that the confidence of this 42-year-old mother-of-three had probably taken a nosedive and that she may be feeling rather frightened. Her GP had referred her because he felt she may have suffered from a subarachnoid haemorrhage, which was a nasty piece of work at the best of times. He probably had not stressed the gloomy prognostic details such a diagnosis carried. About a third of patients would die within one month of their first bleed, and many survivors would be plagued by mental and physical disability. In Claire's case the presumed haemorrhage had occurred several weeks earlier and she appeared to be in very good physical shape and, so far as I could tell, reasonable mental health. This suggested that she was one of the lucky ones, if indeed there was anything lucky about having a subarachnoid haemorrhage.

The condition is caused by sudden bleeding into the subarachnoid space that contains the cerebrospinal fluid and separates the brain and spinal cord on the one hand from the membranes plastered against the inner surface of the skull and vertebral canal on the other. The bleeding usually comes from an aneurysm, a weak balloon-like swelling on one of the brain's arteries. Aneurysms are liable to rupture spontaneously, with disastrous symptoms. The most prominent of these is the instantaneous onset of overwhelmingly severe headache. The bleeding is brief and, should the patient survive without damage to the brain, the symptoms gradually resolve. He or she, however, is sitting on a time bomb, as rebleeding from the weakened aneurysm occurs in the majority of cases, with death and disability rates that are similar to those relating to the first event. Treatment is usually by surgery, which is aimed at obliterating this nasty little balloon.

The referring doctor would have known that confirming the diagnosis depended on showing the presence of blood in the subarachnoid space by means of a brain scan or lumbar puncture (spinal tap). The latter involves inserting a hollow needle into the lower spine and manoeuvring it between the vertebrae so that it enters the subarachnoid space, then withdrawing cerebrospinal fluid for analysis. If either a scan or a lumbar puncture confirmed that a subarachnoid haemorrhage had occurred, then Claire would need to undergo an angiography. In this procedure dye is injected into the neck arteries while x-rays are taken to outline the blood vessels in the head, hopefully showing the aneurysm or anything else that might have bled. Apart from the inconvenience and discomfort, lumbar puncture and angiography carry a small but not insignificant risk of complications, including stroke or even death. These days more reliance is placed on high-resolution brain scans, but when I saw Claire scans were not as sophisticated as they are now.

Clearly, the procedures I had available to me were not to be undertaken lightly. Normally, they would have been carried out urgently as the whole aim of the exercise was to prevent a further bleed. As Claire's suspected subarachnoid haemorrhage had occurred much earlier, evidence of bleeding may have disappeared, in the same way that a bruise slowly clears. A brain scan and lumbar puncture could now well be negative even if Claire had bled, and it might be necessary to proceed to angiography regardless of what they showed. Thus, a decision on whether or not to do any of these tests would depend entirely on our consultation. Looking at her I wondered why she had not sought help earlier for an event that usually causes excruciatingly severe symptoms.

After a few pleasantries I commenced by saying, 'Your doctor tells me that you had a very nasty attack of headache several weeks ago. Would you mind telling me exactly what occurred?'

'It was so dreadful I hardly know how to begin,' Claire replied, frowning. 'The pain was absolutely excruciating. I've had three children and none of my labour pains were nearly as severe. It just hit me instantaneously. One second I was fine and the next I was crippled over and in agony. I thought someone must have hit me on the back of the head with an axe, but there was only Dick there. I felt a searing pain at the top of my neck, just where it meets my head, and within a split second it seemed to explode right through my brain. I thought my head was going to blow apart! It was as though I had a thousand burning needles within my skull trying to force their way out. I just slumped over on my side, gripping my head and lying there with my eyes closed. I thought I was going to die and wished that I could, or at least lose consciousness so that I wouldn't feel the pain.'

'It sounds absolutely ghastly,' I commiserated. 'What happened then?'

'After a few minutes I began to feel nauseated and I thought I was going to vomit. I started to retch but nothing came up. Each time my stomach heaved I thought my head was going to fly apart as the pressure and pain intensified, although I don't know how they could have got any worse.'

'Did the light bother you?' I enquired.

'Did it ever! When I tried to open my eyes everything was such a glare and it made my head even worse.'

She looked very stressed and almost on the verge of tears as she relived the experience.

'I just lay there with my eyes screwed tightly shut.'

'I got her a cold wet flannel,' said a worried-looking Dick, 'and she just lay there holding it over her forehead and eyes. She was moaning loudly.'

'For how long did the pain go on?' I asked.

'It seemed to ease very slightly after what appeared to be an age, but it may have only been 15 or 30 minutes,' she replied. 'However, it remained very severe and it throbbed dreadfully for the next three or four hours. Then I drifted off to sleep. When I awoke about six hours later it had improved but I still had a dull ache. The following morning I felt muzzy, spaced-out and tired, but the pain had all but gone. The day after that I seemed to be back to normal.'

'She seemed so sick I was really worried she might die!' Dick exclaimed.

'Didn't you call a doctor or an ambulance?' I responded.

'I wanted to but Claire wouldn't let me. She just kept saying that she thought she would get over it and that I wasn't to bother anybody on Sunday.'

'But even so, didn't you go to see your doctor the next day? His referral letter is dated only a couple of days ago. You surely must have gone to see him before then?' I countered.

'I didn't go,' Claire responded somewhat defensively, 'because I felt so well, but then I had another strange attack which I thought may have been the start of a stroke. That was three days ago, and I then went to see him straight away.'

'Please tell me about that,' I requested.

'Well,' she explained, 'I was just getting ready to go to bed when my right thumb started to feel numb and tingly. After about five minutes this spread to the rest of my hand, and a little later it involved the whole of my right arm. During this time the right side of my face also began to feel the same way. I went to tell Dick what was happening but I couldn't talk properly.'

'Yes,' added Dick, 'it was hard to understand her. She seemed to be talking gibberish rather than proper words. I could make out one or two things but they didn't make sense. I thought she said the word "bum" several times.'

'I think I was trying to say "numb",' Claire cut in.

I then enquired how long this alarming attack had lasted.

'Less than an hour, perhaps about half an hour,' she replied. 'After about fifteen or twenty minutes the tingling and numbness seemed to slowly disappear, and shortly after this I found I could talk again.'

'At any stage did you get a headache?' I asked.

'No,' she said. 'I never suffer from headaches, although I did have a slightly thick feeling in my head for an hour or so until I managed to get off to sleep.'

I asked if she had experienced any similar episodes in the past, but she denied this. With further probing, however, she admitted to having had one or two attacks of visual disturbance several years earlier. These had consisted of an initial difficulty with focusing when reading, followed by a shimmering semicircle of zigzag light that gradually expanded from the centre of her vision outwards and then disappeared after about quarter to half an hour. She had been under considerable work stress at the time, she said, and had put it down to this. Otherwise she had kept good health and I could elicit no other symptoms or relevant details. I was just on the point of asking her to come through to the examination room when I realised I had omitted a vital detail.

'What were you doing when you developed that severe attack of head pain?' I asked.

'Well …,' she started, and then hesitated, looking somewhat embarrassed.

'We were having sex,' Dick said, coming to her aid.

'Making love,' Claire interjected, flushing slightly. 'Everything was going perfectly normally and I was just on the point of orgasm when suddenly everything exploded like I told you.'

Just for a moment, a story that I had been told not long before flickered into my mind, although I immediately suppressed it. It was as appropriate as a clown at an archbishop's funeral. The story involved a French salesman for a well-known brand of champagne, who was touring Australia promoting his company's ultra-fine product. He had been driving on a rather rough road and his wine samples had been badly shaken, and they had also become overheated as the car's air-conditioning was not working. With great aplomb, he was demonstrating to an admiring group of largely male wine aficionados how to open a bottle of champagne in the true French manner.

'You zee,' he said, 'ven you open zee bottle you muzt eez out zee cork gen'ly so zee gaz ezcapes zlowley and zounds like zee zigh of a zatisfied voman.'

Our risqué Frenchman had not counted on the power that was trapped inside that greatly deranged bottle of bubbly. The cork flew out of his hand and halfway across the room with a loud explosion, while the wine showered over the nearby guests.

'Hey!' shouted a dinkum Aussie male from the back of the room. 'I know that woman and she's a cracker sheila!'

Unfortunately for Claire, there had been nothing funny about her orgasmic explosion.

'Did you have your neck in an unusual position,' I queried, remembering that the pain had started at or near the top of her cervical spine, 'or were you putting undue stress or tension on it.'

'Well, not really, I guess. I was on top of Dick, but that is not unusual for us,' she said rather hesitantly. 'I think I was probably tilting my head back so perhaps I was holding my neck rather tensely. It's hard to relax when you're about to have an orgasm, you know.'

I assumed her last remark was a comment and not a question, or if it was a question then it was rhetorical, so I did not respond.

Having started down this track about their personal lives, Claire then continued by explaining that she and Dick had both been brought up within a strict religious sect but that lately they had been having doubts about its teachings and restrictive practices. They had been attending church less frequently and, in fact, they should have been there at the time she developed her excruciating head pain.

'You see,' Dick added guiltily, 'I know it's silly, but Claire said she thought the attack she had suffered that Sunday might have been a type of punishment and that we should just bear it out rather than seeking relief from a doctor.'

At that point I told them that I would like to examine Claire.

She then turned to Dick and said, 'Please go and sit in the waiting room, dear. I'll be all right.'

Dick left the room rather reluctantly, a little like a dog with its tail between its legs. I was starting to rise to usher Claire into the examination room when she said, 'I thought that attack of head pain would pass off by itself because it was exactly like the others.'

'Others!' I repeated in surprise, sitting back down.

'Yes,' she said determinedly. 'I had suffered three others before the last one hit me.'

It was now clear that she wanted to get something off her chest and I was certainly not going to impede this revelation. In fact, it seemed to me likely that this would provide an important clue. I had already mentally formulated a list of possible diagnoses from what she had told me.

The full physical neurological examination is a drawn-out and tedious affair. It occupies by far the longest part of any full medical consultation. Medical students hate learning to do a neurological examination and general physicians only carry out a much abbreviated version. To make matters worse, in the majority of patients it turns out to be completely negative. The most important part of any neurological consultation is the history. If a neurologist has not made a provisional diagnosis by the time the history has been taken, then the examination is unlikely to provide great enlightenment. This is unlike most other branches of medicine in which physical examination and laboratory tests frequently give the eager clinician more information than the history. I was thus very excited by this new information.

Claire continued, 'I had the first one about three months ago. I had shown a prospective buyer a house that I was trying to sell. He was a very charming, handsome young man and seemed particularly interested in the property. I became excited about the prospect of making a quick sale, especially as the market had been rather flat over the preceding months. He said he wanted to think about it and later phoned me, asking if he could re-inspect the house. On this second occasion we sat in the lounge and talked, first about property and then more generally. We really hit it off. Then he made a pass at me and I guess I was not thinking. I just fell for him. I knew the vendors were out of town so we used their master bedroom. Just as orgasm was on the point of occurring I had the same explosion of excruciating pain in the head. He thought he had injured me in some way and was terrified that I might die.

'Fortunately, that attack did not last so long and I was able to drive home after two or three hours. I felt very guilty and was concerned that God had punished me, especially as Carl was almost young enough to be my son. He telephoned me several times over the next few days to make sure I was all right. He was very understanding and concerned. Eventually we agreed to meet at a different vendor's property. Again I knew the owner was away. I was anxious to make certain that the same thing would not happen again. I felt that if it did then I would know I had been sent a message. I found I could make love and have orgasms without any problem. Carl and I kept seeing each other in this way. Five weeks ago and then again a month ago I had those same dreadful head pains at orgasm. We came to the conclusion that it must be some abnormal physical thing that we were doing and that we should stop seeing each other. We haven't been in contact since.'

'Hadn't you had any of these attacks with Dick over this period?' I asked.

'Not before three weeks ago,' she replied, 'but then his sexual needs are not as powerful as mine and he has been working extremely long hours in his legal practice. We have not made love all that many times during the past three months.'

**THIS STORY OF MULTIPLE IDENTICAL** attacks was vital in confirming my provisional diagnosis, and although I felt examination would be negative it was a necessary part of the consultation. What would you think of a cardiologist who didn't listen to your heart? I showed Claire into the examination room, where the nurse made her comfortable. Nothing untoward happened during the initial part of the examination, which involved testing the cranial nerves, in other words, those that supply the face and head. As I moved lower I suddenly felt Claire tense and saw her recoil slightly, with a look of surprise … or was it horror? Her eyes were bulging and she was staring at my hands. I had largely managed to keep them concealed up until then as I knew they were not my strong point. Even if she had glanced at them earlier she had probably been too distracted to pay any attention. Now there was no hiding my gruesome-looking paws.

These days we find it is not politically correct to lecture medical students on their appearance. One just accepts that students have a right to look dishevelled and have dubious personal hygiene, hoping that by osmosis they will gradually come to accept the standards of their teachers and senior medical staff. Generally it works. It was, however, not always thus. As I stood frozen in front of Claire, feeling rather like a naughty schoolboy caught in some unspeakable act, my mind momentarily flashed back to my days as a final-year medical student. No less a person than the Dean of our medical school had taken it upon himself to give us a good old talking-to regarding what was expected of students in these matters. Now that we were about to launch our glorious careers onto the great sea of unsuspecting and trusting patients, we must be aware that there were certain standards of etiquette that were expected of fully fledged members of the medical profession, no matter how junior. Central among these was the inviolate law of clean and beautifully manicured hands. Not mentioned, but well understood by all of us hopefuls, was that the Dean would be on the appointment committee when we came to apply for our jobs as junior medical officers at the local hospital. This was life-and-death stuff.

I have really only had one colleague whose standards of manual cleanliness and hygiene fell woefully short of the minimum standards that my dear Dean would have accepted. Russell, who had rotated as a general medical officer onto my medical team at the hospital, was good-natured but a wild and woolly looking chap who had a passion for old cars. He tinkered with their motors in his spare time and his hands bore proud witness to this. He usually looked as though a super-urgent call had brought him straight from the workshop to the bedside without a microsecond to spare.

I agonised over what I could say to Russell without hurting his feelings. I was just about to take him aside for a friendly chat, based on my Dean's splendid model, when he suddenly solved the problem himself. The clever lad had decided to train in psychiatry. In that specialty his rough-and-ready appearance would no doubt be seen as a positive, an idiosyncrasy, and would be of great value in promoting his career. Best of all, he would never have to examine anybody again, and when making notes and writing prescriptions he could probably hide his hands behind the impressive pile of books that would doubtless litter his desk. I was greatly relieved.

Unfortunately, the hands with which I was examining Claire would have made Russell's look positively glamorous. Their best parts could most accurately be described as being of a dark battleship-grey colour. These were interlaced with a network of black lines, looking rather like a prominent spider web. Under each of my nails was what appeared to be a thick layer of filth. This would no doubt have seemed strange to even the most hardened and indifferent of bushmen, and to a particular and exacting woman like Claire it must have appeared sinister. I suspect she imagined that I led a Jekyll-and-Hyde existence, playing the respectable Dr Jekyll by day and turning into a werewolf when the sun went down. Had I been working in the morgue after-hours? What should I do?

For a moment I froze, like a rabbit in the headlights of an approaching car. Should I say nothing and hope she was not going to comment? Even if she did not say something she was clearly surprised and dismayed by what she had seen. She would probably lose all confidence in me and my judgement, which was unlikely to do her or me any good. It occurred to me that frozen rabbits get run over. I decided to react positively to escape the looming disaster.

'Please forgive the state of my hands,' I stammered apologetically. Feeling a sense of rising panic, and uncertain what to say next, I feebly tried to make a joke of the situation by adding, 'but I have been trying to re-create the first miracle.'

'What do you mean?' she replied, now looking perplexed as well as worried.

'I have been making wine,' I said, 'and after all, grape juice is just flavoured water.'

Suddenly I realised that the sect to which she and Dick belonged was fervently anti-alcohol and vigorously promoted the evils of the demon drink. My heart sank. I had really blotted my copybook, and had done it with a great smudge of red wine!

From what Claire had told me it was readily apparent she was not a saint, but she turned out to be a more liberal-minded woman than I had given her credit for. She gave me a relieved and knowing smile, saying, 'I am glad they got that way by doing something so useful.'

She then went on to tell me that when she and Dick began to fall by the wayside and question the teachings of their church, they also braved an occasional sip of wine. They found it was 'not too bad', and they had even become quite partial to the odd glass. 'Just to help us relax at the end of a hard day's work,' she added by way of explanation.

I nodded approvingly. I explained that I had desperately tried to clean my hands before I started the day's consultations, but I had found that they were stained beyond repair. I then proceeded with the rest of the examination and, as I had suspected, it was entirely negative. I told her that I had not found anything abnormal.

Back in my office, Claire and Dick both still looked anxious. I tried to put their minds at rest. 'Although the head pain was very upsetting, these attacks … or rather the attack … was not due to any nasty disease or disorder,' I said. 'It was due to a condition called orgasmic cephalgia and not to bleeding in the head or subarachnoid haemorrhage, as your doctor suspected. "Cephalgia" just means a severe head pain, and this trouble is also sometimes called orgasmic headache. What you experienced, Claire, is entirely typical. These head pains always strike at the moment of sexual climax, they are extremely severe and they are totally incapacitating. They do not last as long as the severe head pain that is caused by subarachnoid haemorrhage and they are not likely to come on at any other time. They seem to happen more frequently in people who have a tendency to migraine.'

'But Claire has never had a migraine,' Dick interjected.

'Well, I think she has,' I explained. 'The attacks of shimmering vision that she experienced several years ago and the more recent bout of numbness and tingling in her hand and face, with the difficulty in talking, are really typical of migraine.'

'She never gets headaches!' he insisted, displaying his legal prowess for debate.

'Headache does not necessarily occur during attacks of migraine,' I continued. 'Migraine headache is thought to be caused by dilation of blood vessels in the scalp and skull. Other symptoms, like the upset in vision, numbness, tingling and disturbance of speech may be due to a lack of blood supply to the brain secondary to spasm of blood vessels inside the head. These symptoms are called the "aura". The aura starts as a localised disturbance in brain function. It commences in one spot and then gradually creeps across the surface of the surrounding brain tissue. The symptoms appear to be in the part of the body that is connected to the malfunctioning area of the brain. It is this slow spreading over the brain that leads to the way the symptoms gradually move and change during the attack, and they can vary from one episode to the next. Typically the aura starts 15 to 30 minutes before the headache and it disappears when the head pain starts. Some people with migraine, however, only get headaches, others only get auras, while many individuals suffer from a mixture of the two. They are all part of the same problem.'

'Does the severe attack of headache that I had mean that I might now be liable to get migraine headaches at other times?' Claire asked.

'Probably not,' I told her. 'As I mentioned, these types of head pains only occur at orgasm and do not really turn into anything else. They are harmless but dreadfully distressing. There are various treatments that have been suggested but none seems to be very successful. Abstinence from orgasm is the only guaranteed method of avoiding an attack. Unsurprisingly, this is not terribly popular. Fortunately, the trouble may disappear as mysteriously as it started. On the bright side, you have not had bleeding within your head nor have you suffered from a stroke. This will save you from having a lot of tests.'

They were both clearly very relieved, although concerned about what the problem meant for their future sex life. We discussed the various treatment options and lifestyle modifications that might help. Either because of or in spite of these recommendations, Claire's attacks of orgasmic cephalgia did settle. She had another two, which occurred over the following year, then they disappeared completely. Happily all this happened without their having to resort to celibacy.

**IN THE RESTAURANT BUSINESS** there is a saying that you should never trust a thin chef. I am sure it is equally valid that in the wine business you should never trust a winemaker with clean hands. If you are passionate about making a wine you cannot just stand back and let others do it. You need to be actively involved, and at the very minimum you will have to get your hands into it. This is not too bad, considering some of the alternative parts of your anatomy that could become stained beyond belief.

Traditionally, port has been made by treading grapes in stone troughs, called *lagares*, so that the berries are split and release their juice. This enables the grapes' yeasts to start off the fermentation. Images of merry and nubile young men and women dancing in *lagares* by candlelight are all part of the image of the port trade of yesteryear.

In Burgundy it has been customary to perform *pieage* on vats of fermenting red wine. In this process, winemakers immerse themselves in the wine to help break up a firm, nearly solid cap of grape berries and skins, which have become bloated with carbon dioxide and floated to the surface of the tank. The winemakers perform a type of wild dance in this deliciously warm mixture, no doubt encouraged by the enticing winey aroma. The thrashing of arms and legs also aids the extraction of colour and tannins from the grape skins. As red wine stains dreadfully and the discolouration is very difficult to remove from human skin, such winemakers are not a pretty sight for quite some time after the end of vintage. If I had been indulging in such wildly exotic and dubious practices, while sparing my hands, I can assure you that it would not have caused embarrassment in my consulting room. My problem arose because I was too conservative!

The obvious solution was to wear rubber gloves, and although I had tried this, no matter how resolute my intentions were, I always let myself down in practice. The gloves would leak, they were too insensitive, they became slippery, I misplaced them, I would mistakenly think that in doing a particular job I would not get my hands dirty ... In essence, gloves are not really practical for a working winemaker to use all of the time.

Many years later we had a charming gentleman working vintage at our winery who wore rubber gloves for all manual tasks. Gregory was from a prestigious winery in California's Napa Valley, and his aim was to get some real hands-on winemaking experience. Whether it was the gloves that impeded him or whether it was Gregory's fastidious nature I am not really sure, but he certainly would not have scored highly in a time-and-motion study. In fact, his work output would have brought tears to the eyes of a company accountant, but we did not have to fret as we were not paying him. His background was in wine marketing, and it is very fortunate that he did not end up wasting his well-honed marketing skills by becoming a mere craftsman of wine.

So, if gloves are impractical, can a passionate winemaker have respectable-looking hands? On the day of Claire's consultation I had scrubbed my hands until they were raw, but to no avail. A few months later I discovered a partial solution. I noted that my hands did not look particularly bad immediately after I had worked with grapes or wine. They only started to appear grubby after a number of hours had passed, and by the following day they looked really foul. What had happened? I suspected that the purple grape pigments must have oxidised to produce the disgusting black appearance. In other words, it was largely the result of a chemical reaction. Perhaps all that was needed was an antioxidant to get rid of the stains. I experimented and found that, hey presto, a cut lemon rubbed over my hands did the trick. The lemon's citric acid had made them brilliantly clean. A trial showed that other antioxidant-containing substances had the same effect. Grape juice and wine have antioxidant properties themselves, and these are touted as one of the reasons for the well-documented health benefits of a regular small to moderate intake of wine. When, however, the juice on your hands is exposed to the vast amount of oxygen in the air, it is simply overwhelmed and becomes black.

Antioxidants are also found in healthfoods other than grapes and lemons, and they are said to promote longevity. If antioxidants were perfect I guess we might all live forever, but we do not. Their effect is only partial and transient. Sadly, over a number of hours the atmospheric oxygen also fights back and the winemaker's brilliantly clean hands once again go over to the dark side; not as badly as before, but enough to be apparent.

When I told this to a friend of mine, he commented sagely, 'Lemon juice is somewhat like holy water. It sometimes takes several applications to obtain complete absolution and purity!'

The consultation with Claire gave me plenty of food for thought. It had been embarrassing.

An amateur winemaker for whom I have a lot of respect once said, 'A man cannot serve two masters', and I felt sure Claire and Dick would agree with his words. How had I got myself into this situation? Why was I trying to be both a neurologist and a winemaker, trying to serve the masters of both medicine and wine? I am not sure that I can really tell you, but if you care to bear with me I will try to explain.

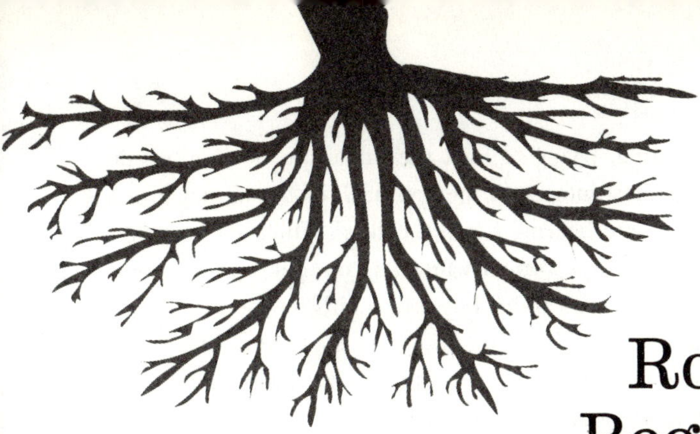

## CHAPTER 2

# Roots *and* Beginnings

**THE FLUORESCENT LIGHTING IN THE HALL** was functional and not exactly subdued. In fact, it was brighter than the noonday sun. I guess the grown-ups wanted to make sure everything was above board and that there was no hanky-panky going on. The combo — saxophonist, double-bass player and drummer — swung into a restrained, hesitant rhythm as the MC stepped up to make his eagerly awaited invitation. Short of stature, red of face, and with receding hair, he didn't seem an obvious fit with the title 'Master of Ceremonies'. He was also plump of body and sweating profusely. His dark suit may have fitted him at one time, but now his stomach challenged the strength of the one button that he had done up on the front of his jacket. His white shirt thrust itself out proudly both above and below this annoying restraint. The black bow around his bulging neck was of such perfection that it had clearly been tied in a distant factory and not by his own fair hands.

No one cared. It was what the MC said that was vital. It was the shot from the starter's gun that would enable the race to begin.

'Gentlemen, would you please take your partners for the first dance.'

None of us hopefuls thought of this as a question. To us it was an imperative command, and one that we were eager to obey.

I had been pressing myself back against the wall, trying to make myself look casual, or rather, inconspicuous. But now I had to act and move quickly or I might miss out.

'Oh God, I wish my heart would stop beating so hard! It seems to have swollen up inside my chest and is making me feel breathless. Surely she will hear the loud thumping and think I am an idiot. My face feels flushed but my armpits feel wet and cold. I think I must smell.'

I am not sure how I made it over to the other side of the hall, where a collection of girls was sitting, trying to look the other way so they would not appear to have the faintest interest in the approach of the motley group of spotty-faced lads who were bearing down on them. The girls' numbers were bolstered by a few married women who had come along to support the evening, as there were always more boys than girls at the Broad Bay community centre dancing class. The women were no doubt also there to see that we kids behaved ourselves. A smattering of husbands had graced us with their presence, possibly to see that their wives did likewise.

As was the ordained natural order of things, all the males had sat stiffly on benches on one side of the hall while the females had arranged themselves similarly against the opposite wall. There was a double sense of urgency as we boys rushed across the room. Not only were we eager to attain the favours of our particular chosen ones, but we were also all desperate to avoid the ignominious fate of having to ask one of the women onto the floor. While we might learn more about dancing, where was that daring sense of romance and intrigue in being wheeled around the room by the mother of your best friend?

Adair was sitting upright with her hands folded in her lap. She turned her head and smiled at me as I approached. She was a slightly built lass; some might even have called her skinny, but not me. She had been the object of my ardent attention for a few weeks. She had a pretty little face in an indescribable sort of way, except to say that it was all in perfect proportion. Her black hair was cut short; not like a boy's, but well above shoulder length. She was wearing an apricot-coloured cardigan, a white blouse and a knee-length brown skirt. While she could not be called well endowed, her blouse showed encouraging signs that puberty had kicked off, if not exactly gone for touch. And yes, she was wearing red lipstick.

'May I have the pleasure of this dance?' I asked hesitantly.

'Yes,' she replied, smiling again as she rose. 'Thank you.'

We stepped onto the floor, and while I held her right hand at shoulder-height with my left one, I gingerly put my right arm around her waist. To say that we glided across the floor would be an exaggeration, but we did not just shuffle and I only stood on her foot once. We were encapsulated in a magical world of our own: warm, rosy and intoxicatingly heady.

I had first met Adair about a month earlier. She was walking with her younger sister down a path towards the small bay where I kept my dinghy. I was coming back up from the beach, having just moored the boat. We had said 'hello', but nothing more than that. One evening the following week I saw her at the dancing class, plucked up my courage and asked her for a dance. In fact, we had several. I learned that she lived in the city and was staying for a fortnight with her aunt, who was a village postmistress. I must have had a surge of hormones to the brain because I asked her if she would like to come to the cinema with me a week or so later. I was overwhelmed with excitement and joy when she accepted. I can no longer remember the film or anything about it. What I recall quite vividly, however, is that I held her hand and even gave her a peck on the cheek when we parted. This was *true* love and I had found it! At 16, I was a year older than Adair.

Now, this was the second night we had danced together and it was so, so intimate. We did the two-step, the foxtrot and then a waltz. I was a thousand miles away, lost in a cloud of reverie, yet I was very aware of Adair's close presence. What was that enticing smell? Was she wearing perfume or was that just how young ladies actually smelt? I wanted this to last forever. Then the thought struck me that I needed to impress her. I needed to do something that would make her admire me; but how? A plan started to form in my mind.

'What do you want to do when you leave school?' I asked her.

'I'm not sure,' she said. 'I think I'd like to train to be a secretary. I'm good at typing and I feel I would enjoy an office job. What about you?'

'I think I'll train to become a schoolteacher,' I replied. 'I wouldn't mind teaching others, the pay is good and you get really long holidays.' Then I added as an afterthought, 'I would really like to become a doctor, but I think that would be impossible.'

'Why?' she asked in a surprised and somewhat scornful tone, stopping on the dance floor, dropping her arms to her sides and staring at me. 'Why do you say that?'

'Well …' I started hesitantly, 'you have to get very high marks to get into medical school and the course is very long. I don't think I could do it.'

I was becoming embarrassed — my face felt hot and I was starting to sweat. I wished I had never started this line of conversation.

Adair stared at me and said emphatically, 'If you want something, you shouldn't just talk about it. Do it! Just do it!'

She held her right hand up and her left a little outstretched at waist-height, in dancing stance. We continued to move around the floor in time with the music.

I had conveniently omitted to tell Adair that I had the lowest grades of any student in my entire year at school. The term before, we had all sat the state examination, School Certificate, a pass in which absolutely determined whether we moved up a grade and into the next class or languished below that bar for another year. A total of 200 out of 400 marks was required to make this quantum leap, and about six weeks before the examination the school principal had advised me that I had little if any chance of passing. I might as well withdraw and have a crack at the exam the following year, he told me. This had irritated me but also motivated me to do a little work. I had scraped through by the skin of my teeth with 201 marks, and boasted to my friends that I should not have wasted so much time swotting for the exam as I still had a mark to spare. In truth, three years before I had moved from a small country school to a large city one and I had felt totally out of my depth ever since.

Why had I not kept my big mouth shut and not said a word to Adair about medicine? There was also the inconvenient little matter of money. My widowed mother had none. Adair probably would not know that, but her aunt, the village postmistress and mistress of gossip, certainly would. Miss Bean was as thin as the pole that carried her name, and was surely an anorexic before the disorder became popularised by pouting catwalk tigresses. While she was a reasonably popular figure in our little local community, she was reputed to steam open envelopes in order to obtain extra ammunition to aim against its members. And it was none other than she who doled out my mother's pension every month.

And now here she was; she had just arrived to take Adair home from the dancing class. No chance of any parting little intimacy tonight!

All the same, I did not walk home alone in the moonlight that night; no, I flew on a cloud. Adair wanted me to be a doctor and that was what I was going to become, by hell or high water. If she believed in me then surely that was enough.

Adair had said, 'Just do it!' and by Jove I would. She had meant it as a challenge, and I would accept.

A few weeks later I was unceremoniously dumped by my true love. Perhaps the malicious postmistress was protecting her family's dubious honour. I was heartbroken for all of a week. The romance faded from my mind, but the dream did not — the dream of becoming a doctor. I have often found in life that the hardest part about doing something is making the decision to do it. I had made my decision. I would have to work like stink in order to achieve my goal, but I was now determined that I was going to get there!

It was 18 months later that the school principal whispered an apology for advising me not to sit School Certificate. The occasion was the final school assembly, where he pinned the school's Dux medal on my chest.

**THE SHARP BUT TANTALISING SCENT OF PINE** needles hung in the air, mingling with the delicious aromas that still wafted in from the kitchen, reminding us of the splendid meal we had just eaten. There had been roast lamb with mint sauce, roast chicken, new potatoes, fresh peas, and lashings of roast vegetables that were liberally doused with rich gravy. This had been followed by plum pudding with brandy sauce and fruit salad, plus the inevitable pavlova. It had been the best of Kiwi Christmas dinners. The afternoon sunlight filtered into the room, and coloured lights twinkled on the tree.

We should have been drowsy after our preprandial gin and tonic, followed by beer to accompany the meal, but we were alert and ready for action. It was time for the pressies and there was a great heap of them under the tree. Suddenly there was chaos. Everyone was talking at once and thrusting presents in every direction. Naturally, we all had to shout in order to be heard over everyone else.

'Happy Christmas, dear,' Chris said, giving me a kiss. 'I hope you like it.'

I held the present in my hands and turned it over. It was beautifully wrapped, complete with a red bow. I did not know it then, but I was holding a time bomb in my hands, one that would explode to hit me with such force that it would blow my life off-course — or, I should say, *our* lives. By contrast, what I had given Chris was a damp squib — a book that was really appreciated and a good read, but of no lasting consequence.

I had been introduced to Christine, or Chris as she liked to be called, some months earlier by her older brother Brent, a classmate at medical school. Not long before that I had moved from my hometown of Dunedin to Christchurch to complete my sixth and final year as a medical student. Chris and I had hit it off immediately and had been seeing each other regularly. I had been delighted to accept the invitation to spend Christmas Day with the Taylor family, not only because of the promised nosh-up but because my testosterone-soaked brain was quite insistent that I spend time close to Chris.

I pulled the ends of the bow and it undid easily. I was careful not to tear the wrapping paper. A smart-looking book lay in my hands. On its cover was a picture of a heavily moustachioed, portly, contented-looking old gent, who was wearing a beret and standing next to a wine barrel while nosing a glass of wine. It was the epitome of a French winemaker. The title of the book was simply *Wine*. The author's name meant nothing to me, as indeed there was no reason why it should. This was Hugh Johnson's first book, and he was known only to a few people in the wine trade prior to its publication. This was about to change, and he was soon to become arguably the most widely read and popular wine writer in the world.

After the ceremony of the presents had been thoroughly and noisily done and dusted in a way that I had never experienced before, I was unceremoniously introduced to another of the Taylor family's Christmas institutions. The assembled multitude, which seemed to include the most distant of relatives and friends, sang with great gusto a curious mixture of hymns, Christmas carols and bawdy songs while standing around a piano. It was supremely clear that they were a very musical family. I had hoped to make a good impression on them but, alas, it was immediately apparent to all that not only did I lack any formal vocal training but I also had a voice like a ruptured bullfrog and I could not even sing in tune. This was an embarrassment, but was that all it was? As I left that evening to return to my room at the single doctors' quarters at Christchurch Hospital, I wondered if it was of any real importance. Only time would tell.

It was dusk and the moon was starting to rise when I left the Taylors' house. Chris and I had lingered on the terrace, saying our fond farewells, before I drove back to my digs at the hospital. It was 1966 and I had recently passed my final medical exams and I had graduated as a bachelor of medicine and a bachelor of surgery (MB ChB). There was a remaining week of glorious summer freedom before I would commence my first real job, as a junior medical officer at the start of January. I was keen at the prospect of working in the thoracic surgery department, but first I was going to make the most of my remaining holiday. I would definitely spend it in outdoor activities, perhaps at the beach. Chris had a few days off from her job as a student nurse, and we intended to pass the time together.

Earlier in the evening I had felt very tired and I had intended to go straight off to sleep when I got back to my small room. Now, however, I was too excited by the events of the day and the thought of the week to come. 'Perhaps I should just have a quick flick through that wine book,' I thought to myself. 'It will take my mind off things and help settle me down.'

I got into bed, opened the book and began to read. It was three hours later when I reluctantly put *Wine* down and turned off the light. It was peculiar because the book had no plot, no characters, no real storyline and none of the things that usually make for a good read, but it was enticing, fascinating and absorbing, as well as being informative. I felt I had opened a secret door and peered into a hidden world — one in which the sun was shining and everything looked fresher and brighter than normal. I was an intruder but I felt strangely at home.

Over the following week I was completely seduced, not by Chris but by *Wine*. I did not spend my days at the beach or on open-air pursuits, not unless sitting in the shade of a tree reading can be considered an outdoor sport. I read and reread that wretched book, consulting and reconsulting different parts, looking at maps to locate various wine-growing areas, imagining their typical vineyards, wineries and people, but in particular I swirled, sniffed and sipped their wines inside my head, comparing one with another. I fell in love with wine — or rather with the concept of wine, given that I had had no real experience of the genuine article.

True, previously I had rather reluctantly sipped the occasional glass of cheap vinous plonk, but to all intents and purposes I was a wine virgin, and if it had not been for that book I might well have remained one. I'm not sure what inspired Chris to give me *Wine*, but if she had not I might now be contentedly growing cabbages in a little garden plot in suburbia rather than worrying about the weather, insects, birds, weeds, disorders of grapevines and all the other things that plague a vigneron's life. I might be able to sleep on a frosty night rather than getting up and driving 50 kilometres to make sure the vines do not come to harm. I might be able to enjoy the spectacle of a good thunderstorm without the anxiety that hail will destroy the crop. I might ... I might ... oh, there are a hundred and one annoying things that are now required of me that I would not have to do. In short, I would not have become a truant from basement of the brain, or indeed, a truant from medicine — but I would not have it any other way!

There had been many other wine writers before Hugh Johnson, but most books on the topic had been excessively technical, emphasising in minute detail the differences between the wines of one vineyard or vintage and the next and pontificating on the reasons for these. Johnson blew a breath of fresh air into this fusty little corner, and he did it with style. *Wine* starts with a description of a grapevine, and it outlines the vine's different parts. What could be more boring? Well, in fact it is not boring, it is exciting. And why is that?

It has been said that wine is liquid poetry. Hugh Johnson's book is poetic wine, or rather a poetic book written about wine. It would make a scientist or technocrat cringe. His description of a grapevine, although in prose, is written with a poetic flavour, and so is the rest of the book. This is what made *Wine* such a hit. It talks about wine regions and wine styles with lucidity and clarity, but in a way that fires up the imagination. It does not compare the wines of particular producers, nor does it attempt to award scores to any wine. When, however, you have read the descriptions of German rieslings from the Mosel and the Rheingau you can taste them and their differences without ever having put a glass of German riesling to your lips. Johnson's book had been written for the wine novice or rank amateur rather than the connoisseur. It was penned with flair and in language that the average person could easily relate to. *Wine* was at the forefront of the wave of popularisation of table wine that swept the English-speaking world in the 1960s and 1970s, thrusting cocktails, spirits and fortified wines unceremoniously to one side.

Perhaps the book just caught me unawares because it was written in a romantic style and I was in the middle of a romance. There is good scientific evidence that the brain places special importance on experiences that occur in emotionally charged situations. Memories of these experiences are stronger and more persistent than those that occur against a backdrop of the routine — hence your brain's enhanced ability to recall the aromas and tastes of the wine and the meal you had on a moonlit terrace during a *liaison dangereuse*.

It is the basis of the old story: 'I can't remember the night, I can't remember the place, I can't remember the woman, but the wine smelt of violets and truffles. It was Château Margaux.'

So, perhaps my fascination with wine would not have been so intense had I read the book under other circumstances. In the same way, perhaps I would not have really committed myself to medicine had I not made the decision after dancing with Adair. I will never know, but one thing was becoming very clear to me — I had not only fallen in love with wine, I had also fallen in love with Chris. The two had become inseparably intertwined.

*WINE* **STARTS WITH A DESCRIPTION** of the parts of a vine, which are basically those of any tree. The 'tree of life' is a mystical concept that has been used to describe the relationship between many things, including religious beliefs and scientific concepts. We all, however, have a tree of life: our own life. Its trunk is our self, our body and our mind. Its branches and leaves are the things that we have done: our thoughts, decisions and actions. These have responded to the external forces about us, just as a tree is shaped by the elements. But every tree has a part that is hidden — that part which supports and nourishes it. The roots are as old as the life of the tree itself and are vital in creating the form that our eye touches on. Is what we see attractive and healthy or is it malformed and stunted?

So our own tree of life rests on unseen roots, things that have happened to us in the past, happy and sad, thrilling and terrifying, all manner of events and emotions long forgotten. They lurk in the dark corners of our minds, untouched by the light of conscious thought but ready to spring into action and defend their territory. They influence our decisions, often pressuring us to act quite contrary to rational thought. We sometimes think we understand why we chose a particular path, but often the roots of our current behaviour lie obscured beneath the debris of bygone years; debris that has been solidly packed down from the outwardly calm and level surface of the present to the oldest and deepest crevices of childhood. So, my decision to study medicine and my sudden passion for all things vinous were indeed triggered as I have related, but they were no doubt influenced by what had gone before. And what were those things? Let me tell you what I know, although no doubt there is much more that is obscured by rubble.

The roots that grew in the medical part of me seem the easiest to trace. Their origin may have stemmed from the three admissions to hospital that I underwent prior to reaching the age of seven — two for surgery and the third for glomerulonephritis, an inflammation of the kidneys caused by an allergic response to a streptococcal infection of the throat. That incarceration, with its prolonged period of convalescence, seemed like a life sentence to a six-year-old brat whose main interest became tormenting his fellow inmates, who were suffering equal feelings of homesickness. One might have thought these experiences would have induced a severe lifelong allergy to all things medical.

We did not have a family history rooted in the medical profession, not unless frequently using a doctor's services counts. I have no memory of my father working. Henry (Harry) Te Hau Tepenui Otu Donaldson had been many things in his time: sheep-shearer, miner, soldier and stevedore, to mention but a few. By the time of my childhood he spent his time at home, gardening, pottering about his workshop and the like. I guess it was because he was always there when I came home that we formed a particularly close relationship. Being an afterthought, the youngest of five by a fair margin, I was his pet and no doubt spoiled rotten.

One overcast grey day, when I was playing in the garage, my brother Logan opened the door and said simply, 'Dad is dead.'

I felt numb, paralysed with grief, as we both sobbed our hearts out. I couldn't bear to see Dad's body or go to his funeral. He had died a few days before Christmas at the age of 52. I was 12. Dad had been a cardiac cripple for many years, but had always looked well and never complained. The piece of paper that officially recorded his passing simply said 'myocardial infarction', whatever that was. It had never occurred to me that he was sick, really, really sick, that is. Some time in the days or weeks that followed Dad's death, when I was feeling very low, I made a secret, soppy, sentimental childhood vow: I would become a doctor and save people from dying such nasty deaths. Over the ensuing months and years this ideal was jettisoned overboard and sank beneath the deep dark sea of hormonal poisoning, recalcitrance and dizzy excitement that we call teenhood. My promise disappeared, seemingly without a trace, but it must have become entangled in the roots of a piece of kelp that somehow became attached to those of my tree of life.

We did have a family history of teaching. This was definitely in our genes, on one of our family's respectable but unexciting chromosomes. It seemed as though this was a dominant gene and that it would definitely express itself in me, or that is what my widowed mother hoped. I guessed that she was correct, especially as my brother Don had followed this path. Admittedly my sisters, Heather and Fiona, had escaped, becoming a secretary and a florist, respectively, but I felt trapped. Resignedly, I plodded my way towards my inevitable fate. Then I discovered biology. Not the sort of biology you learn behind the school bike sheds when class is out, but the world of creepy crawlies and all those sorts of things. I became seriously interested in the whole spectrum of zoology.

'Perhaps I could become a zoologist,' I thought.

That idea really appealed to me, but were there really jobs for zoologists, especially in New Zealand? Then it occurred to me that humans were just another type of animal. Surely being a doctor of medicine would be just as interesting?

'It would be impossible,' my heart told me. 'With my school marks and my mother on a pension, I wouldn't stand a chance.'

And it was at this stage that I met Adair.

Just as a grapevine develops much deeper roots than those of mere medicinal herbs, I suspect that the *racines* that nourished the fruit of my wine passion lie concealed at a greater depth. My mother, Marjorie Cynthia Edith Donaldson, or Madge, as she liked to be known, came from a long line of self-righteous, God-fearing Protestants who eschewed any form of alcoholic drink, gambling or anything else that reeked of self-indulgence or just plain fun. They were solemn-faced toilers who strictly observed the Lord's Day. Shining from the brightest bough of the family tree was a branch of missionaries who had gone to China to save the souls of the unenlightened. This side of my family was most definitely stacked with dull teetotallers.

I suspect, however, that my father might have been partial to the odd drop, judging by the frosty reception that my mother sometimes gave him when he came home from one of his infrequent visits to the city. After his death my mother shamefully kept a bottle of whiskey hidden in a very high cupboard. She said it was only to be used in the Christmas cake. Sometimes I used to climb up on a high kitchen stool just to take a peek at it. It did not look very wicked, but then you just could not tell. The surface level of the firewater was recorded by a mark on the bottle. I never saw the level of the whiskey drop during the year, but I cannot guarantee that the bottle was not occasionally topped up with water. After all, I had two brothers and two sisters.

In spite of Madge's strict upbringing, she did occasionally succumb to temptation, but only with some higher motive in mind — like the time when she found that some juice she had prepared from surplus fruit had spontaneously fermented.

'We should drink this, Ivan,' she said; 'it would be wrong to let it go to waste. There are thirsty and starving people in the world who would be grateful to have this nourishing juice.'

We sipped it together but the 'juice' was so strong that we began to feel light-headed and giggly after only one glass. We were forced to come back evening after evening to drink a little more until we had finally done our duty to the indigent souls of this world and the 'fruit juice' was finished. I was uncertain whether the waifs and strays would be forever grateful. After this little mishap Mum started to make fruit juice on a more regular basis and, unfortunately, it happened to go off fairly frequently, no doubt because we did not have a refrigerator and we had to leave the juice in stoneware jars in the pantry. We did not shirk our duty. 'Wicked waste brings woeful want' was a strict motto in our house. This harmful little pursuit, however, remained only that. It did not morph into any other beast, and it was always with reluctance that my mother would accept a glass of 'wine' from a host. She only did it to be polite and would play with it for ages, never having a second one. I also followed in the family tradition and, like my siblings, drank very little alcohol, even as a student. I did not particularly enjoy wine — not, that is, until Chris gave me *Wine*.

**AFTER I GRADUATED, MY FIRST JOB** was that of house officer on the thoracic surgical unit at Princess Margaret Hospital in Christchurch. I thought I knew everything about it, because, after all, I had worked in the cardiothoracic surgical unit at Greenlane Hospital in Auckland. Well, to be honest, I had not actually worked there for dinkum, I had helped cover at nights when I was a medical student.

In those days, when Kiwi medical students finished their fifth year of study in November and before they started their sixth year in February, they were expected to work as surrogate house officers in hospitals throughout the country. This was a splendid scheme, as it gave them paid experience and allowed the real house officers to go on holiday. The only downside was that the frontline in many hospitals consisted of rank amateurs. It was a steep learning curve.

I had opted to leave Dunedin, the home of the country's only medical school at that time, and to spend this period at National Women's and Greenlane Hospitals in Auckland. It was while working in one of the crumbling old medical wards at the latter establishment that I found myself rostered on call at nights for the renowned cardiac surgical unit. This was the only one in New Zealand with facilities that allowed the heart to be stopped while the blood was circulated and aerated by machine. The place was made especially intimidating because I was an offsiding interloper and not at all familiar with the staff, the patients or the frightening equipment. In truth, I felt small and insignificant.

But now I was a big boy; a real doctor on my own ward, complete with a critical-care room where patients with respiratory difficulties or those who were immediately post-operative were connected to respirators. I loved the regular, reassuring hiss of those machines that did the breathing; I read their technical manuals and became competent at using them. We had two surgeons who were temperamentally and technically quite different from each other. For example, when operating on a lung, entry into the chest is usually gained through a long sloping incision between two ribs. These are then held apart by clamps, creating the hole through which the operation is performed. But a wide hole cannot be created while the ribs remain intact. One of my bosses would snip through the adjacent ribs to allow them to be spread, while the other would use his hands to pull the ribs apart, often to the accompaniment of gruesome cracking noises. For operations on the heart it was necessary to cut through the bony sternum in the midline of the anterior chest. Yes, my unit also did heart operations, but only those that did not require the heart to be stopped or the lungs bypassed. These were operations on the beating heart!

My boss, Heath Thompson, was an imposing figure, tallish, with a shining pate, save for a small, monkish rim of white hair. He always wore a bow tie. In his former life he had been a Quaker medical missionary in China. On one occasion I assisted Heath with an operation to help rescue a heart that had been ravaged by rheumatic fever. This allergic response to a childhood streptococcal throat infection is best known for its acute fever, rheumatic joint symptoms and skin rash, but the brain and heart commonly become inflamed as well. Involvement of the brain produces brief involuntary jerky movements that can come to involve all muscles and can occasionally be extremely severe. Years later, I looked after a girl in whom this chorea, which is what these movements are called, would probably have flailed her to death had she not been padded like a mummy and given medication to still the agitation. While all symptoms seem to settle after weeks or months, damage to heart and brain can persist.

Alison was a 38-year-old who, contrary to medical advice, had become the mother of three fine children. She had contracted rheumatic fever when she was six and she now had heart failure due to mitral stenosis. The damage that the rheumatic fever had inflicted on the mitral valve, which separated the two chambers of the left side of her heart, had caused its opening to slowly narrow over the years. Now, the opening was so small that the blood was dammed back in her lungs and she was heading towards certain death if she did not have surgery. She was forced to sleep sitting up and even then she struggled to get her breath at night, coughing up bottles of frothy sputum. Heath had cut a hole in her atrium, the upper of the two chambers on the left side of the heart, and while strictly controlling any blood loss he had split the delicate leaves of the beating mitral valve to widen and re-form its orifice. She had done well and a few days later was making a good post-operative recovery.

'Good afternoon, Alison. How do you feel today?' I enquired as I pulled back the bedclothes to take a routine listen to her lungs and heart.

'Great, thank you, doctor,' she replied, smiling.

Suddenly it was my heart that felt sick. The dressing covering Alison's central chest wound had become undone on one side and the padding was hanging limply downwards by the adhesive tape on the other. The ends of the detached sticking plaster were nowhere to be seen because they had disappeared into a great hole in the centre of her chest and there, in the bright light of day, was her beating heart. I felt rising panic as I knew that Heath Thompson was not in the hospital, and I also had a strong sense of *déjà vu*.

On a Saturday evening a year earlier, I had been checking up on the patients in the recovery area of the cardiac surgery unit at Greenlane Hospital when I had come across a nurse changing a patient's dressing. She was busy dabbing antiseptic around the wound, seemingly oblivious to the fact that the wires and sutures had come undone and the wound had completely split apart. That was the first time I had seen a beating human heart, and, while there is no doubt that it is a magnificent piece of equipment and a testament to the great pump-maker's art, it was not a sight that filled me with joy. On that occasion I had been rescued from ongoing responsibility by a senior surgical registrar who happened to be in the vicinity and rapidly arranged for the patient to go back to theatre. There was going to be no such luck this time.

'It's Mr Thompson on the phone for you, Dr Donaldson. He says he's somewhere in the centre of the city,' a staff nurse called out from the neighbouring office.

Those were the days before cellphones, but Heath had been carrying his pager and he had been able to use a nearby telephone to respond to my urgent bleeping. I explained what had happened.

'Call an anaesthetist and have the patient transferred to theatre. I will leave immediately and be there as soon as possible,' he said calmly and reassuringly.

'I've already called the anaesthetist and theatre, and will now organise the transfer,' I told him.

It seemed an age until Heath arrived to reclose the wound, but in reality it could not have been much more than half an hour. As for Alison, she took it completely in her stride and made an uncomplicated recovery, returning home free of symptoms to care for her family. I think I was the only one spooked by this harmless little post-operative complication.

It was a week or two later that I was introduced to one of Heath's more adventurous procedures. He worked closely with his wife, Bunny, who was a thoracic physiotherapist and spent much of her time pummelling the chests of asthmatic patients, trying to get them to bring up the phlegm that was clogging their airways. Heath reasoned that this thick mucus might more easily be dislodged with the aid of a little fluid, just as a dirty sponge or grubby handkerchief might be cleansed by washing. Hence, he hit on the idea of bronchial lavage. Asthma is not a surgical disorder, but the only respirators at Princess Margaret Hospital were in the thoracic surgical unit and that is where patients with severe asthma attacks ended up; just in case they needed assisted respiration. Heath worked closely with the respiratory physicians, but when patients were in dire straits in spite of the best medical treatment he might step into the fray with a bit of dribble and slurp.

Ross had suffered from rotten asthma since early childhood, and on at least one occasion annually for most of his 18 years he had ended up in hospital in *status asthmaticus*. During these extremely severe and prolonged episodes his blood oxygen levels would become dangerously low, and each struggling breath seemed as though it might be his last. The attack could last hours, days, or even a week. Then he would bounce back and be seemingly normal. The current bout had been going for two days, and it was probably his most severe to date. His bronchial tubes were constricted by severe spasm of their muscular walls although he was receiving maximal medical therapy. Listening to his lungs with a stethoscope was like hearing an orchestra playing the 'Bubble and Squeak Symphony' at full tilt. In spite of this evidence that his lungs were clogged with phlegm he could not cough anything up.

'Nothing else for it, I'm afraid. We will have to do a bronchial lavage,' pronounced Heath, apparently talking to himself but perhaps addressing me. Then he turned, adding, 'Book the theatre, Ivan. I'll call the anaesthetist.'

While not a technically challenging procedure, bronchial lavage under these circumstances is definitely white-knuckle material. Through a rigid tube called a bronchoscope Heath flushed a saline solution into a part of Ross's lungs and then sucked it back out, which made a greedy slurping sound. Slowly, the large glass jar that collected the aspirate, as this returning fluid was innocuously called, began to fill with gelatinous strands and lumps of yellow mucus. Heath worked methodically, cleaning one section of lung before moving on to the next. While breathing oxygen, even before the laundromat was let loose on his lungs, Ross had been a cyanosed, dusky blue-grey. This was a sure sign that his body was being starved of this life-sustaining gas. Now, however, as the salt water was poured down his bronchial tubes, he became obscenely dark in colour. I became mesmerised by watching the amount of fluid going in and that being sucked out. There was something radically wrong. It dawned on me that there was a huge discrepancy. It seemed that many litres were being poured into the young man's lungs but probably less than 50 per cent of the volume was being removed. We were drowning him and surely he couldn't survive much longer. I had to say something!

'Mr Thompson, we are going to have to stop,' I quavered.

'Why is that, Ivan?' came the assured reply of a man who knew what he was doing, or at least thought he knew what he was doing. But I knew better.

'We are not sucking nearly as much out as we are putting in! His lungs must be full of saline. Ross looks as though he's going to die and I'm sure we are drowning him.'

'Don't worry, that's normal. A lot of the fluid gets absorbed into the bloodstream from the lungs. So as we remove the mucus that is clogging his bronchial tubes he will start to improve.'

Rather than being reassured, I became increasingly anxious. But after what seemed an eternity, we finally finished and Ross was still alive. He roused from the anaesthetic not long afterwards but he seemed as breathless and wheezy as he had been prior to the procedure. But who had said that recovery from drowning, or near-drowning, was instantaneous? Over the next two or three days Ross showed gradual improvement, and by the end of the week he was well enough to be discharged.

Whether that or any of the other bronchial lavages that we performed during my stint on the thoracic attachment were of any use I do not know. However, all the patients survived to tell the tale and were discharged to continue their ongoing battles with their nasty illness. I guess that nobody else knows either, as this pioneering therapy was overtaken by improved medical treatment for asthma and it ended up in the dustbin of therapeutic curiosities. As house officers, we were also overtaken by new happenings as we were moved to other medical or surgical firms every three months in order to give us a broad experience. Only too soon my stint in the thoracic surgical unit came to an end.

'DO YOU THINK HE'S DEEP ENOUGH?'

I peered down at Max's body, which was stretched out full-length on the operating table. He now looked pathetically runty and fragile, although he was an adult. It was hard to believe that he had once terrorised the town. But Max was now completely defenceless and vulnerable.

'He's out for the count and probably much longer,' I replied, feeling both guilty and satisfied. It was the first anaesthetic I had given since graduating, and I felt proud of my new-found skills.

'Adjust the operating light please, nurse,' the surgeon said. 'I want it centred right on the pubic region. In fact, right there!' he said, pointing with his gloved finger towards a sensitive part of the patient's anatomy.

As the light was moved it briefly flickered over John's face and I caught a glimpse of his eyes. His face was almost obscured but in the small gap between the surgical cap and the mask I thought I saw a gleam of delight — the maniacal delight of revenge — or was it just my anxious imagination? Heaven knows, John had every reason to crave revenge. Max had put him through hell, but was not this crossing a bridge too far? If we were caught there would undoubtedly be serious consequences; consequences that might irreparably tarnish the vision of the brilliant medical careers that glinted so alluringly ahead of us.

'Sometime, somewhere in your medical career you may be asked to help a young lady in distress,' said a voice in my head. 'Don't be swayed by your emotions or succumb to the glint of gold, for they will destroy you. No matter what your personal views are regarding the termination of pregnancy, it remains a fact that abortion is illegal except under highly specified exceptional circumstances. Society, your medical colleagues and the Church will condemn you, even if you believe you have acted in good faith. You will end up on the medical rubbish heap!' The fleeting image of one of our obstetric teachers flashed through my mind, complete with flashing smile, slicked-down oily hair and black pinstripe suit.

'But surely this little procedure wouldn't remotely equate to that,' I said to myself as I began to have grave doubts about the wisdom of what we were doing.

John had said that if Max did not have surgery he would be as good as dead. 'We will be saving Max's life. I know he has got a deadly infection and that it's poisoning his whole system. He can't settle, you can see that he is unhappy, and he's as skinny as a rake. We'll be doing him one enormous favour.'

'I'm not so sure,' I had countered, trying to voice my underlying resistance. 'It's not as though we'll get signed consent from Max himself.'

'We don't need to. Leave it to me. I'll get permission from his nearest and dearest,' John had replied, and I now realised that I had glimpsed the same nasty look in his eye then.

I was on the verge of saying that we should call off the whole escapade when 'Scalpel please, nurse' brought me out of my lugubrious reverie.

Max was largely obscured by drapes, but the offending anatomical specimens protruded proudly. They did seem swollen, but were they really the source of a deadly infection? Could not their size just be the result of hypertrophy? Was Max not just the equivalent of some muscle-bound weightlifter? Surely most organs will enlarge if they are overused.

Then, in rapid succession, came the requests: 'Artery forceps … scissors … sutures please, nurse,' and before I could utter a word it was all over.

But there, in the kidney dish, they looked lonely, pathetically small and innocent. Were those the testicles that had launched a thousand loves and burned the topless towers of sexual desire?

'That's put an end to Max's hormonal rages,' John said with an overt smile as he removed his mask. 'No longer will he terrorise the neighbourhood at night and keep me awake with his caterwauling. The Ginger Tom is no longer cock of the walk!'

We hurriedly cleaned up the equipment while Max was left to sleep it off on a suitably orange cushion in an overnight bag. John then pulled back the curtains and, having ascertained that the coast was clear, we scuttled off, John to his surgical ward while the nurse and I headed to the Casualty Department's office. John had a bright surgical future ahead of him once he had completed his training. Unfortunately it was not to be, as several years later he died suddenly as a result of a skiing accident. I never did ask him whether the cat was his or a neighbour's.

That had been during my second week as a house officer attached to the Christchurch Hospital Casualty Department, and I am sure that the hospital hierarchy would not have been amused by our little exercise in combined anaesthetic and surgical training. My immediate boss, Duncan Scott, however, would have been quite relaxed. He was a sage, elderly ex-general practitioner who was the sole permanent medical presence in the city's only Casualty Department. He worked from 9 a.m. until 6 p.m. five days a week, and he had two house officers to assist him. We alternated, and each worked 24 hours every second day so that Duncan always had one of us at hand, but we covered the nights unassisted.

Whoever invented this type of rostering had never heard of the diurnal rhythm, that very orderly and highly regulated cycle of hormonal release and brain function that controls our normal patterns of sleep and waking activity. It takes about a week for this diurnal clock to adapt to any change in the normal sleep/wake cycle, which is why a house officer in Casualty felt continually jetlagged, with a brain made of diurnal rhythm soup. Quite simply, in the timeframe that was allowed, the body and mind could never adjust. In addition, the job was busy, very busy. Over the following decades, casualty departments were to morph into accident and emergency departments and finally, in line with the American trend, were to call themselves simply emergency departments. Accompanying this was an enormous increase in trained staff and facilities, but the type of patients and problems that come through the front door have remained much the same.

There are all sorts of medical and surgical emergencies that need to be dealt with and many require admission to hospital without further ado. Some, however, need more thorough evaluation, tests or treatment before going further. Such were the 'overdoses', those who had intentionally or unintentionally consumed potentially harmful substances, most frequently excessive amounts of their own prescription medication. It was on these unfortunates that I learned all that I ever want to know and more about gastric lavage, which was never a pretty sight. After a tube was passed down the throat and into the stomach, large volumes of fluid were flushed down to cause distension and to induce profuse vomiting. I regretted having to add to these patients' already profound misery.

Less sympathy was evoked by the abusive and violent louts who had unintentionally injured themselves, often while intentionally injuring others. Usually, they were drunk or drugged and turned up on our doorstep around the witching hour or later. Fortunately, I was often protected by the nursing staff. It is surprising how many bogans will see sense when confronted by an attractive woman, although some of the fairer sex, who had become battle-hardened, could give just as good as they received.

The Casualty Department was the best place to learn about the gentle art of suturing, and it was while using the needle and catgut that I stumbled upon one of life's profound truths: macho males are most often cowards at heart. While the majority of little girls will let you stitch them up without turning a hair, there is many a toughened rugby player who will turn pale and swoon at the sight of a hypodermic needle. Some thugs are so afraid that they will even try to fight you for trying to administer the treatment for which they have come.

'You're looking glum,' I said to Ben at lunch one day.

'I think I'm angry rather than glum.'

'Why? What's the matter?'

'I just received a bloody letter from a lawyer telling me that I'm going to be taken to court,' Ben replied exasperatedly.

'What on earth has happened?'

'An orthopaedic surgeon has said that I was negligent because I missed the damage to an ulnar nerve in a patient with a lacerated wrist.'

'And did you?'

'I guess so … but it was hardly my fault. It happened about three months ago when I was working in the Casualty Department.'

Ben had been a classmate and we had graduated together. I knew he was conscientious and careful — there had to be extenuating circumstances.

'What happened?'

'It was during my first week working as a real doctor. I happened to draw the short straw, ending up in Casualty for the first three months. In the early hours of the morning this cretin was brought to the hospital drunk. He had smashed a window and cut his wrist while breaking into a house. The nurse and I were the only ones in the department and we had difficulty controlling him. I explored the wound as best I could, and I didn't think that any of the nerves or tendons had been injured. There was blood everywhere, and as he was fighting us I had no option but to sew the wound up. A few weeks later his GP noticed the problem with the hand and sent him to see the orthopod. Now I'm in a fix.'

'Surely you could argue inexperience, battle fatigue and other extenuating circumstances?'

'I intend to do that. I felt shattered by the stupid 24-hours on-off routine that I had just started. I have gone back and counted up the patients that went through Casualty that shift. Before that chump turned up I had personally attended to 120! How dare he say that I was negligent without knowing the circumstances!'

'Praise be for medical insurance,' I commented.

Ben argued his case in court and fortunately the judge was a man of reason. My classmate was discharged without a conviction.

Things have changed in hospitals, and the junior medical staff now have much better training, guidance and working conditions. Looking back on it, we were frequently asked to do things that were well beyond our level of training, things that exposed both the patients and us to risks that would today be seen as unacceptable, but at that time it all seemed normal. In those days life for young doctors involved a steep learning curve and the slope was very slippery!

**RENAL MEDICINE WAS A CINDERELLA** of the medical specialties, and in fact it emerged as a specialty rather late in the piece. I was still a house officer at Christchurch Hospital when the first kidney doctor, Peter Little, was appointed and it was not long before I was attached to the newly established renal unit. To increase our understanding of this marvellous filtering system junior staff were shown a film on the subject by a certain Dr B. Dryer. Thereafter, our own consultant became known as P. Little, which, given the fact that these doctors' names indicated a major symptom of kidney failure, seemed very appropriate.

I had only been on the renal firm for about a week when the unfortunate Terry was admitted. His luck had started to run out when he had won the state lottery. This was still the era of compulsory military training, although the politicians' enthusiasm for it was on the wane. Immediately after the Second World War all young Kiwi males had to do military training for a couple of months each year, but in the 1950s the paranoia about invasion started to fade. Our masters decided that we did not need so many gun-toting men in the community. We still, however, had to have a fair portion of our blokes gun-savvy, so that they could be called up at a moment's notice should the need arise. After all, the wounds from the Korean War were still raw. But how to choose the potential fodder? Then some bright spark hit upon the idea of a lottery. Only those whose names were pulled out of the hat would have the privilege of being conscripted. That was the beginning of Terry's woes. This 19-year-old had been sent to Burnham military camp, along with hundreds of other young bucks, and it was there that he caught the meningococcus.

Meningococcus is a double-crossing little bacterium that can live quite happily in your throat and not cause you any trouble. In fact, up to 15 per cent of us are probably providing it with a comfortable home right now. Without us it has nowhere to go because it does not infect other animals. It jumps from one person to the next by spit or sneeze, as it is only by sharing the secretions of our noses and throats that we infect others. Then, just when we are being so kind to it, this little bug can turn nasty and attack us. Fortunately, this is uncommon, but when it decides to go on the rampage it really does it in style. This is particularly likely to occur when people live in close quarters, such as boarding schools, summer camps and army barracks. Then there may be an epidemic.

Meningococcus can cause the mildest or the most devastatingly deadly disease and covers all points of the compass in between. I had first been introduced to it a month or two before I met Terry, when I was working on paediatrics. Stephen, a five-year-old, had been well when he was put to bed in the evening, but the following morning his father had found him in a delirious state. He was also covered in the tell-tale patchy red rash that was the result of bleeding from microscopic blood vessels in the skin. He had meningococcal meningitis and blood poisoning. In spite of immediate admission to hospital, the best antibiotics and all of the other supportive treatments available, Stephen died before midnight.

The onset of Terry's illness had been just as dramatic and, like Stephen, he had suffered from a severe drop in blood pressure. Unlike Stephen, he had responded to treatment and had been cured of his meningococcal septicaemia. The prolonged period of hypotension, however, had caused his kidneys to shut down. He had gone into renal failure and his urine had dried up. Whether his kidneys would ever recover from this was uncertain, but one thing was definite: he would die within the next few days unless this kidney failure could be treated. The only therapy available was peritoneal dialysis. Dialysis machines were a thing of the future.

'It's really quite a simple technique and easy to perform, Donaldson,' said P. Little, as though I was the only ignoramus, although the registrar alongside me, George Abbott, was also a dialysis virgin. This was one of the early, if not the first, such procedures carried out in Christchurch.

'Firstly, you inject local anaesthetic into the abdominal wall,' P. said with a flourish of his well-loaded syringe, 'and then you make a little nick in the skin before you push this plastic tube through the muscles and inside the peritoneal cavity.'

The boss performed this manoeuvre adroitly and Donaldson was mightily impressed, although Terry looked as though he was having second thoughts about having given his consent to such an assault.

'Then you just trickle in the dialysis solution. See, there is nothing to it. Naturally, it's going to make Terry's stomach swell up and he will feel just a teeny weeny bit uncomfortable,' P. explained with a smile, turning to pat the patient's shoulder reassuringly. 'The peritoneum, the inner lining of the abdominal cavity that also covers the surface of the bowel,' he added for Terry's benefit, 'is very large and permeable to small molecules. This means that all the toxins that the kidney would normally remove can just diffuse from the blood vessels through this lining and into the dialysis fluid. We have to wait for a period and then drain the fluid off. By repeating this procedure many times we can cleanse the blood and do the work of your kidneys, Terry, until they start to function again.' P. nodded confidently, as though affirming that the recovery he had predicted was assured.

Abbott and Donaldson stood mesmerised, watching the dialysis fluid disappear into Terry's insides as they gradually started to swell. This was simple. Surely they could do it themselves.

Suddenly, an agitated look appeared on Terry's face and he cried out, 'Quick! Quick! I need a pan urgently!'

At this, Donaldson's two companions immediately turned towards him and Donaldson felt compelled to race from the room, returning moments later in triumph, waving the requested equipment. Terry was with difficulty helped onto the throne, and moments later his expression of relief turned to one of dire concern. The contents of the pan consisted of a large amount of watery bloodstained fluid. It was clear to all of us, even Terry and Donaldson, that all was not well.

'Damn! I must have made a hole in the bowel,' said an embarrassed P. 'I'm terribly sorry, Terry. It is a rare complication of peritoneal dialysis. It's really just chance where the tube goes. It will almost certainly heal itself up without any bother.'

But the perforated bowel did not heal, and the hole in the abdominal wall through which the dialysis tube had been inserted began to leak a smelly brown semi-fluid material. As the peritoneal dialysis had to be repeated every few days, and as the insertion site of the tube had to be moved regularly, Terry's tummy became covered with small holes that leaked similar material and looked like multiple miniature colostomies. He was euphemistically said to have developed a 'watering-can abdomen'.

In spite of this minor complication, which would have dampened a lesser spirit, Terry remained cheerful and optimistic. Perhaps he was grateful for being freed from the army. After many weeks of sulking his kidneys perked up, and a month or two later surgery dried up the well-manured garden and the can watered no more. Terry's renal treatment had become an unqualified success and Peter Little went on to establish an excellent renal unit at Christchurch Hospital, complete with haemodialysis, renal transplantation and all the other trimmings. Time heals most things, including wounded pride.

**'IVAN, I'M NEEDEN Y'ER HELP OORGENTLY,'** said the small voice on the other end of the line.

I recognised the caller immediately. It was the medical superintendent of Burwood Hospital, an institution that specialised in spinal injuries, plastic surgery, and ear, nose and throat surgery, as well as having obstetric, general medical and general surgical facilities.

'What's the matter, Dr McIntyre?' I enquired.

I had got to know Archie McIntyre reasonably well as a final-year medical student when I was seconded to Burwood to fill in for a house officer who had become ill. Archie was a friendly, undemanding little Scotch physician who was nearing retirement. He had been helpful when I was called upon to deal with a problem that was well beyond my capabilities as a mere student. One Saturday morning I had received a call from the Christchurch Hospital Casualty Department about Ian MacPherson, a young farmer who had been caught in a fire. He was being dispatched to the burns unit, aka the plastic surgery unit, of which I was acting house officer.

'He's in a bad way,' the doctor in Casualty said.

'What does that mean?' I enquired.

'Eighty per cent burnt,' was the grim reply. 'Almost certainly won't survive.'

Ian had got up early to avoid the heat of the day and to take advantage of the calm morning. He had started lighting fires, systematically working his way through a large patch of gorse that he was trying to get rid of. All was going well until a wind sprang up. Perhaps the crackling noise, flames and smoke diverted his attention. By the time he was aware of any danger he was completely surrounded by a raging wall of fire. Frantically, he tried to find a way out, but in vain. Instead, he stumbled across a small ditch, in the bottom of which was a little water. He lay down, praying that the water would protect him and that the fire might somehow jump over him. They did not. Ian lay there in a daze for what seemed like eternity as the inferno raged above and around him. When he finally came to his senses the worst had passed and he had survived! He had been snatched from the jaws of Hell, or so it seemed.

Everywhere about him were the twisted, blackened remains of smouldering bushes. Here, they were lying on the ground in a smoking heap; there, they were upright, with flaming branches that resembled the limbs of tortured runners caught in the act of fleeing from Vesuvius. With the superhuman effort that is born from the will to survive Ian managed to get himself to his feet and stagger in the direction of home. He was a gruesome sight, and completely covered in the charred remains of blackened skin. Completely, except for where he had been protected by his boots and short pants. These were all he had been wearing that fateful morning and they had soaked up a little bit of water from the ditch; just enough to save the skin in those areas. Elsewhere he had suffered full-thickness burns, which meant that this skin was dead. His eyes had been saved by his lids but they had been incinerated in the process.

The Casualty Department officer had managed to put a needle into a vein in the surviving skin on Ian's right foot and he was receiving copious quantities of saline through this as he had lost a large amount of fluid. He was conscious and lucid, although his ability to talk was restricted. Having admitted him to Burwood and prescribed the regimen of fluid and medication ordered by the plastic surgeon, I settled down for what promised to be a long and difficult weekend on duty, especially given the lack of other junior medical staff.

'It's the charge nurse on the burns unit here,' said the voice on the other end of the line. 'Please come immediately; the new burns patient has become delirious and has got out of bed, pulled out his intravenous drip and says he's going home.'

I glanced at the bedside clock as I leapt out of bed, muttering unprintable expletives. It was 1 a.m. Ian had seemed settled when I checked him at 10.30 p.m. His drip was vital as his burns had started to ooze, and if he survived long enough they would soon flow copiously from all over his body, causing the loss of vital body and blood proteins as well as fluid and electrolytes. His blood pressure had already dropped due to the fluid loss that we were trying to replace. This had caused his veins to collapse, which would make reinsertion of venous cannula difficult. The only surviving skin veins were a few in his feet, and each of these was precious.

When I arrived at Ian's room I was confronted by a raving black patient wearing white shorts and boots. We had been unable to clothe him so he had been lying naked beneath a large frame that was covered with blankets. Ian thought that he was in Hell and that the nurses were the Devil's assistants. He was determined to walk out into the night and would fight anybody who tried to stop him. No amount of pleading would make him heed common sense. There was only one thing for it and that was sedation: a sedative that would act very quickly, but what and by what means? He had pulled out his intravenous line and he was in no mood to allow me to insert another, or to agree to take a tablet.

As Ian turned to look towards the door he had a moment of inattention, during which I was able to give an injection directly into a muscle. With the combination of agitation, dead skin and background pain Ian was quite unaware of the jab. Now all I had to do was to wait for a short while until the jungle juice kicked in. Ian had to be humoured and diverted. As it turned out, this did not exactly tax my acting skills because before long he was sleeping soundly. A short while later the reinsertion of an intravenous cannula was greatly facilitated by complete lack of patient movement. His intravenous pain relief and sedation, which had clearly been inadequate, were increased and I retired to bed once more.

Amazingly, Ian survived, thanks to the skill of the plastic surgery team at Burwood Hospital. The skin that eventually came to cover his whole body, his head, face, neck, trunk, arms and legs, had to be painstakingly shaved from his surviving shorts and boots, reapplied and regrown in these other areas. New Zealand was at the forefront of plastic surgery as many of our finest exponents had worked with Sir Archibald McIndoe. This Kiwi had pioneered the specialty in Britain while working with Allied servicemen who had been badly burnt in the Second World War.

My part in Ian's recovery had been trivial but had not gone unnoticed by the nursing supervisors, or 'snoops', who patrolled the hospital at night, checking on misdemeanours and the like. They had reported the episode to the medical superintendent, including the fact that Ian had been constrained and had been given medication against his will. I had only dealt with the situation to the best of my very limited ability, never giving a moment's thought to the possibility of medico-legal implications.

Archie had given his stamp of approval, but not without toeing the official line by adding, 'I'm oolways 'appy to be consulted on sooch matters, day 'n' night, m' boy. Thart's whoot we medical sup'rintendents are foor.'

I had always been mystified about a medical superintendent's functions, but I retained a sneaking suspicion that fielding calls in the dead of night did not rank high on their list of duties, either in popularity or in frequency.

'We goot this wee lad 'ere, Ivan, und e's coullapsed through 'eavy bloud loss,' I heard Archie's desperate voice, bringing me back to the present with a jolt. 'Thair's oonly me un a medical student 'ere art Burwoud. The lad's 'ad a toons'llectomy this arfternoon. He voom'ted a 'uge armoont of blood 'arf un hoor bark. I canna g't soorgeon nor aneath'tist. There moost be other dooctors 'ere but I carn't find eeny orf them. The student 'n' I canna poot a dreep een t' geeve the lad blud. Wee'v treed 'n' treed. His circulation has shoot doon 'n' I canna geet a blud preessure. He's semicoonscious 'n' I'm scairred we'll loose 'im.'

'But why did you call me, Dr McIntyre?' I asked rather selfishly, wondering who else might take over this responsibility.

'I spooke t'ooperator art Christchoorch Hospital 'n' she toold me you were 'ouse oofficer orn call fuor anaesth'tics. All th' oother anaesth'tists are boosy.'

I did not stop to clarify if my colleagues in the anaesthetic department were engaged in the gentle art of gassing people or were at the pub. The buck clearly stopped with me, and I had better do something about it fast if I was to be of any use.

'I'll be as fast as I can, Dr McIntyre.'

It was not very far, the distance between the two hospitals being a mere ten or eleven kilometres, but it seemed to take an age even though I drove like a maniac. I did not jump any red lights but I think I broke most of the other rules in the traffic book.

Rangi Turangi was a big boy for nine years of age, and although I could not truthfully say he looked as white as a ghost, his dull slate-grey complexion, lack of pulse, cold clammy skin, faltering respirations and semi-conscious state strongly suggested that he might soon join his ancestors. Rangi was slumped on his side and a stainless-steel bowl containing a copious quantity of vomited blood was sitting on his bedside locker. His arms showed the evidence of many desperate attempts to obtain venous access. Crowded around the head of his bed were Archie McIntyre, a final-year medical student and two nurses, all of whom looked extremely pale and worried.

After warming the right elbow, forearm and hand in a bowl of hot water, applying a tourniquet and slapping the skin vigorously, I could see just the faintest hint of a vein.

'No chance to insert a cannula. It will have to be a needle … one big enough to allow a reasonable flow of blood but small enough to fit inside this excuse for a vein.'

I chose a size-20 Butterfly, so-called because of two flat plastic tabs or butterfly wings that could be pinched together with the thumb and first finger while sliding the needle, which lay in the position of the butterfly's body, through the skin. And then it was in the vein, as confirmed by the sluggish flow of dark-blueish-looking blood back along the thin clear plastic tube that was attached to the blunt end of the needle. Five nearly simultaneous sighs were audible, and in the twinkling of an eye the blood was flowing, not rapidly but fast enough. The flat open wings of the butterfly were now taped down to the skin. In 15 to 20 minutes it was clear that the worst had passed and that even if Rangi continued to bleed we could control the situation. He was conscious and his blood pressure was close to normal.

A short time later Archie McIntyre came back into the room and announced that the ENT surgeon was on his way. He had been travelling between his private consulting rooms and his home when Burwood Hospital had tried to contact him. Rangi's bleeding stopped spontaneously and he rapidly made a full recovery, although he was kept in hospital a day or two longer than usual for such an operation.

There was nothing remarkable in putting an intravenous drip into a flat patient like Rangi. It is something that occurs routinely in any big hospital and is performed daily all over the country by paramedics attending call-outs. However, it made an impression on me during my first week as a house officer on the anaesthetic attachment and I am sure it probably coloured my view of that specialty.

Proficiency in anaesthetics requires a number of technical skills but perhaps the most vital is that of intubation, the placing of a tube through the mouth and into the windpipe (the trachea) via the voice-box (the larynx). Once the tube is in position, a little collar near its tip needs to be inflated to seal off the trachea. Then everything that enters or leaves the lungs must do so by way of this endotracheal tube, giving the anaesthetist full control over the patient's airway.

This little inconvenience has been made necessary by a nasty design fault in each and every one of us, namely the necessity to poke our food and beverage down the same tube through which we breathe. Admittedly, this conjunction of vital functions only occurs over a very short distance, but it is sufficient to be quite a nuisance. This small space of dual function is the throat (the pharynx). When the passage of solids or fluids between the pharynx and the gullet (oesophagus) is in the downward direction it most commonly gives us pleasure, but when it comes back up it is usually nasty. While we are conscious, coughing or spluttering protects our airways from any misdirected traffic, but when we are anaesthetised our lungs are utterly vulnerable, especially to the vagaries of a nutrient-enriched belch or full-throated vomit. Hence the need for the anaesthetist to have full control of the airways of the unconscious patient and to separate the shared respiratory and gastrointestinal functions of this poorly conceived piece of anatomy. Would not it be much more sensible if we breathed through the backs of our heads, rather like whales?

Having an empty stomach is good for anaesthetics as well as the diet. Hence anaesthetists wisely try to protect their medical insurance premiums by ensuring that their clients have fasted for several hours and preferably overnight prior to putting them to sleep. Unfortunately, in urgent medical situations this generally held dictum sometimes has to be put aside.

A couple of months into my anaesthetics job I received a call from my boss. 'Hello, Ivan. I have just been telephoned by Colin Gibbs. He has got a two-year-old girl who has been admitted with acute appendicitis. They think that the appendix may well rupture and they want to take her to theatre tonight to try to prevent her from developing peritonitis. All the rest of the anaesthetic staff are tied up in theatres, both at Christchurch and over here at Princess Margaret. Colin will be ready at 10 p.m. That will be six hours after the kid last had anything to eat or drink. I'm sure you will be able to do it okay. If there is any problem, just give me a call.'

I had a feeling of apprehension. By now I was reasonable at gassing adults and I had also assisted in anaesthetising children, but I had never really done it alone, especially to someone so young. But I knew that Colin, the surgical registrar, was very competent, and if he said it was urgent then who was I to question him? If my boss thought I was up to it, then perhaps I was. Maybe I just lacked confidence. I did not like to say no.

'Okay, Bill,' I responded. 'What size tube would you recommend?'

So here I was all 'alone', peering down the tiny throat of an anaesthetised and paralysed sweet little kid, surrounded by surgical and theatre staff who all seemed to be anxiously peering at me — or was that just my imagination. I was trying to poke a rubber tube, which seemed about the size of a drinking straw, through the narrow black V-shaped gap that was outlined between her brightly illuminated, but tiny, vocal cords. Then it was over and I had done it. I had intubated her. I felt a bead of sweat trickle down my forehead and disappear somewhere under my mask.

'From here on in it should only be a piece of nerve-racking cake,' I told myself.

And it was. Before I knew it, the diagnosis was confirmed, the operation was over and the patient was awake, none the worse for wear. It might have been just another day in the anaesthetic department but it was one that I was glad was over.

**'IVAN, I WONDER IF YOU WOULD MIND** giving an anaesthetic for me. I've got a young woman with a badly displaced fracture of her forearm. It would be best if I could manipulate it back into position and set it in plaster tonight.' The speaker was Alistair Hester, a young orthopaedic consultant.

'No problem,' I replied. 'Shall I give the axillary block in the orthopaedic outpatient department?'

'I really want to do this one under GA. I don't think she would tolerate an axillary block,' Alistair said. 'She hasn't eaten for a few hours and by my calculation it would be safe for her to have a general anaesthetic in three-quarters of an hour.'

Having been a house officer in the orthopaedic surgery department I was proficient at axillary blocks, in which a local is injected into the armpit, anaesthetising the nerves as they pass downward into the arm. Like most local anaesthetics, they are generally very safe, although a mishap had occurred when one of my classmates was administering an axillary block a month earlier. The young patient had suffered a convulsion, no doubt due to the local anaesthetic getting into a vein by mistake, but he had recovered rapidly and within an hour was back to normal.

But who was I to argue with Alistair Hester? After all, he had come back into the hospital at 9 p.m. to manipulate the fracture himself, so it had to be important.

'All right,' I acquiesced. 'I'll see her in the prep room outside theatre in three-quarters of an hour.'

Judy was a pleasant, 30-year-old blonde who had tripped coming out of a grill after finishing a meal of fish and chips, washed down by an unknown quantity of beer. And no, she had had nothing to eat since then, and yes, the meal was sufficiently long ago that it could be considered safe to give her an anaesthetic for an urgent procedure. And yes, Alistair Hester thought there was sufficient urgency to proceed. All was in order, or at least I thought it was.

I gave the intravenous anaesthetic, followed by the muscle relaxant that was necessary to allow intubation. Both medications were short-acting, allowing me only a few minutes to have Judy's airway secured against a possible invasion by her evening meal and also to have her established on breathing an anaesthetic gas. This would keep her unconscious while the fracture was set. I then picked up the laryngoscope, the curved instrument that was essential to allow me to put the endotracheal tube into her larynx, and pulled down the sheet that was covering her lower jaw. I froze momentarily. Judy had a minute lower jaw, a shrivelled-up excuse for a mandible that medics call a 'shrew's jaw'. It then occurred to me that while I had been taking a brief history and examining her in the preparation room she had held a handkerchief over her chin, as though she was dabbing something around her mouth. I had not thought anything about it at the time. Now I realised that she was clearly embarrassed by her jaw and had skilfully kept it concealed from my unsuspecting gaze.

During intubation it is normal to have a patient lying on his or her back, just as Judy was positioned, and while standing behind her head I had to fully extend her neck so that her unconscious face was 'looking' back towards me. I then had to open the mouth fully, pulling the jaw as far upwards as it would come, while also holding the tongue up and out of the way with the laryngoscope. In this way it should have been possible to look directly at her paralysed vocal cords. But Judy's jaw was so small and short that it and its attached tongue could not be swung out of the way, and I was probably not experienced enough to be able to pass the tube by feel alone. I tried once, I tried twice, and I tried thrice, each time becoming more desperate. Then I heard the noise of a freight train coming towards me as I desperately tried to back out of the tunnel; the tunnel that had an obstructing curve in it, around which light would not penetrate. The freight it was delivering was a full load of fish, chips and beer and it was heading straight for me! I flung Judy's head over the edge of the theatre table, turning her body onto its side at the same time. An acrid jet of Friday night's fine fare splashed off the tiled floor and dribbled down my theatre garb. The sucker was already roaring in her mouth and throat, greedily gobbling up the remains of her dinner.

With a mixture of embarrassment, shame and terror, I looked down at the stunned Alistair Hester and said in a shaky voice, 'I'm afraid I'm going to call this off, Mr Hester. I'm just going to wake the patient up. If you want to do this tonight you're going to have to get another anaesthetist … a real anaesthetist!'

'It's okay, Ivan,' he replied. 'It would have been better to do it tonight but it's not essential. We'll let her have a good night's sleep and do it in the morning.'

'Why didn't you tell me that before?' I thought to myself, but I heard my voice say, 'Sorry, but I think it would be best.'

I stayed with Judy until she woke, then I explained to her what had happened and why she needed to wait until the morning. She was very understanding and looked none the worse for wear.

I knew early on that the gentle art of anaesthetics was not for me. It seemed to consist of periods of routine punctuated by episodes of sheer terror. I envisaged that being an anaesthetist and an international pilot would be somewhat similar; the interesting parts being largely restricted to the start and finish of each mission. A few anaesthetists took books or magazines into theatre, and I occasionally spotted a *Turf Digest* or *Financial News* being sneaked out from under a theatre gown. One senior colleague livened up his life by talking incessantly, which drove the surgeons to distraction. He was frequently asked to limit this gaseous exchange, which he could manage for 10 to 15 minutes before exploding in an outburst of chattering.

In those days anaesthetics was virtually the only discipline in which GPs participated in city hospital medicine. A good number of anaesthetics were given by people who spent most of their week as family doctors, and they thus had a professional life outside of the operating theatre. These days many anaesthetists have expanded into areas such as intensive care and pain medicine, which has given them extra clinical interests. In addition, anaesthetics itself has come a long way since a chloroform rag was the order of the day, and it is now an interesting and vibrant specialty.

But if anaesthetics was not my cup of tea then what was? In addition to the specialties I have already mentioned, I also rotated through cardiology, respiratory medicine, gastroenterology, rheumatology, endocrinology, ophthalmology, ear, nose and throat surgery, general surgery and, of course, neurology. This was providing me with a good general grounding in medicine, but sooner or later I would have to decide what I wanted to do with my life. I knew that I wanted to specialise, but in what? I told myself that I had plenty of time to make up my mind. As far as I could see, all of my hospital bosses were totally wedded to medicine, largely excluding other interests, with the exception of family life, the share market and the occasional game of golf. I was happy with this prospect. I needed nothing other than medicine to fulfil me. It would become my mistress, my 'magnificent obsession'. I only needed to decide what medical discipline I wanted to train in and to apply myself to this — or so I thought. But let us backtrack slightly to see how subtly a decent young doctor was already starting to be led astray.

**'WE DON'T WANT ANY OF YOU GIRLS** to eat any of those grapes growing on the pergola,' Chris said in her most commanding voice.

'Who's *we*?' demanded her younger sister Kate. 'And why not?'

'It's Ivan and me. We want to use them to try to make wine,' Chris replied in a more conciliatory tone, adding as an afterthought, '... and you girls will be able to have some of that.'

Surprisingly, Kate and her friends apparently succumbed without a struggle. Chris, who was something of a natural leader, was also the eldest of the little group. Although only 20 years of age, she had become their mother figure ever since her parents had departed on a six-month tour to 'see the world', leaving Chris, Kate and three teenage girlfriends 'flatting' in the family house. It was March, and the grapes had only started to show a faint tinge of purple on their skins. They were hard, bitingly bitter and acidic, and about as inviting as raw onion and garlic ice cream. As March flowed into April, however, the berries swelled dramatically, becoming tantalisingly soft, black and delicious.

Without a doubt, the genes of Eve are firmly imprinted in each female chromosome, or that is what we males would like to believe, but to their credit the girls held fast. They did not succumb to temptation and sin, or if they did they only took the teeniest of bites of the fruit. It is true that these were grapes, but even if they had been apples, Chris, who sat on the judgement throne, would not have counted this minor loss of crop sufficient to warrant their expulsion from Eden. Yes, we did notice that the odd especially plump and succulent grape had disappeared, and here and there an occasional bunch seemed to have gone missing, but, as her flatmates pointed out, there were quite a lot of birds in the garden. This we accepted, although secretly we thought it would have taken a vegetarian eagle to have nicked a whole bunch. Finally, near the end of April, we deemed the flavour-rating of the grapes to have topped 100 per cent and we were ready for the big harvest.

Only four months had passed since Chris had given me *Wine*, but we had not been idle. We had read up on winemaking and considered ourselves experts. We had even done the most important winemaking task. We had named the unborn wine 'Saint Martin', after the suburb where the grapes had been grown. This wine was going to be made in the very best of French traditions.

We might have lacked the berets and striped T-shirts, but we were ready to go. We each had a weekend's leave from hospital to devote to the task.

We felt somewhat deflated when the two of us picked the entire crop in about half an hour; nonetheless, the mound of fruit looked impressive. We had read that the grapes had to be crushed up, wine yeast added, and then the mixture left in a cool place to ferment. All this we did. We put the fruit into large plastic bags, trod on them, then emptied the contents into the bowl of a defunct washing machine. Two days later we were enraptured to find bubbles gently plopping on the surface of the liquid. A distinct, delicious winey smell filled the wash-house where we had stashed our brew. Over the ensuing few days we became firstly fascinated and then alarmed by the fermentation. The whole house reeked of wine, and the other girls began to complain about this and the swarms of fruit flies. Fortunately, we had put the lid on our makeshift fermenting vat and this kept the flirtatious little beastiols out. Worse, however, was the agitation of the imprisoned monster trapped underneath the lid. It seethed and writhed, threatening to break loose and throw itself over the edge and onto the floor. It was also clearly exuding heat.

'What should we do?' asked a worried-looking Chris.

Sounding superior, because I had read the procedure in a book, I replied, 'Just what any desperate nurse would do to a delirious patient who was trying to get out of bed. Punch him back down, subdue him, take his temperature, and then formulate a management plan! But what can we use to force him back into his cot?'

We looked around, and after rejecting the broom, the garden rake and a large suction cup that was meant for unblocking drains, Chris hit upon the vegetable masher. By breaking up the nearly solid, floating 'cap' of grape skins and pushing it back down into the rapidly forming wine we were able to release much of the natural carbon dioxide gas that had built up. Thus deflated, the patient relaxed back and perfectly refitted the washing-machine bowl. We took his temperature, which turned out to be 33°C. While he would be hypothermic if he were human, this young fellow might suddenly kick the bucket on us because he had a fever. We had read that wine yeasts die much above this temperature, and if this happens the remaining natural grape sugars will leave the wine sweet. *Quel horreur!* The last thing we wanted was for our first growth, Saint Martin, to be a soppy sweet wine.

'What should we do about this high temperature?' I asked.

After a moment's thought Chris replied excitedly, 'Why don't we do what we would with any very hot patient? Apply ice.'

'But it will dilute the wine. We can't have that. Not with our very first wine,' I complained.

'I've got some unopened plastic bags of frozen peas in the freezer,' Chris retorted briskly; 'let's use those.'

Her brilliant suggestion worked a treat, and within a quarter of an hour St Martin was a comfortable 29°C. His prognosis looked excellent.

'We'll need to do this regularly to stop it from happening again,' Chris said.

'Great idea,' I agreed, 'and according to what I've read this "punching", which is what it's called, also helps to extract the purple colour out of the skins and transfer it into the wine. I think it probably needs to be done twice during the day and twice during the night. What a pity I don't live here and can't take responsibility for it. Do you know a reliable nurse who is used to night duty?' I enquired, trying to look vague.

I received a vigorous shove and a grin.

'You bastard!' Chris said. 'Don't think you're going to pass off this winemaking to me. You're the one who has become obsessed by it.'

She was joking, of course, but then many a true word has been spoken in jest. The significance of her words has come back to haunt us many times over the subsequent years.

As well as working during the day I was also on duty every third night, and the night after we had resuscitated Saint Martin was one such. The following day I was called to admit a patient to a ward that was not my home base. As was common in those days, it was a single large room, rather like a hall, which housed 30 patients. These were separated only by curtains around their beds. The curtains were normally closed only if a patient was being examined or doing something private. I was sitting at the bedside of a cheerful, plump, middle-aged woman who was soon to have gallbladder surgery, taking her medical history, when I spied out of the corner of my eye a curvaceous form sail by. It had shoulder-length blonde hair, a fringe, a blue skirt, starched white apron and black stockings.

'Hello, Nurse Taylor,' I called out. 'How is that patient that I had to help you with a couple of nights ago?'

After a momentary look of perplexity the nurse asked sweetly, 'Do you mean Mr Martin?'

'Yes, that's him. How is he getting on?'

'Oh, doctor,' she said innocently, 'he's doing very well. He is no longer delirious or struggling and his temperature is normal. Not surprisingly he seems quite tired and is resting, but he's gone quite red.'

'That's not unexpected, nurse,' I responded. 'I think he probably has scarlet fever. I will check his condition tonight and give a professional opinion.'

'Thank you, doctor, but make sure you take preventative measures. There must be a risk attached to the visit,' she said with a knowing smile.

A couple of days later we came to the conclusion that Saint Martin had given up the ghost and died, as there was absolutely no sign of life. We removed his outer garments, gave them a good squeezing in a makeshift press and then we threw them away. We put the additional liquid that we had obtained by pressing, along with the rest of his remains, into a large carboy and let them settle for a few months. We then bottled the clear supernatant portion into wine bottles, while the sludge we callously threw out.

With commendable restraint we refrained from opening the first bottle of the Saint's relics for several months.

'He's not very dark, is he?' Chris commented as I ceremoniously poured the first glass and held it up to the light.

In fact, it was no more than a pale rosé.

'It is clear that we cured his scarlet fever,' I quipped; 'he must have died of something else.'

Although our Saint was a fairly colourless character, he made up for it with his other heavenly ways. This was undoubtedly the best wine that we had ever tasted and clearly a masterpiece of the vintner's fine art. It had a bouquet and flavour of rose petals, violets, blackberries, cherries and almost every other desirable thing that we could think of. In the mouth it was beautifully balanced, if not exactly rich, with an exciting lightness on the tongue that gave way to zingy acidity. We served most of our St Martin up to our unsuspecting friends over the next year or so. We were surprised they did not rave about it, and we could tell by their faces and comments that they were not as impressed as we were.

'Jolly good effort,' Peter commented, before adding, 'for a first attempt, I mean.'

'Very creditable,' said Mark, 'it's really quite drinkable. Thank you, but I won't have a second glass. I am assisting in the operating theatre tomorrow afternoon.'

While their lack of the expected orgasmic enthusiasm or near-delirium was disappointing, it did not really bother us; after all, what did they know? They weren't wine experts like us, merely beer swillers. They were so rough and undiscerning they would probably end up as surgeons!

Some years later, Chris whooped excitedly, 'Look what I've found — three bottles of our old Saint!'

She held them up to show me. They looked impressive and were covered in dust, just as bottles of venerable old wine should be. We had just returned from living in Britain and she had come across them amongst the small collection of motley items that formed the sum total of the worldly goods we had left behind in New Zealand.

'Let's save them for when we have special guests around for a meal,' I suggested proudly.

'Don't you think we should try one first when we are just by ourselves?' Chris responded.

'I don't see why,' I said. 'Good wine may lose some fruitiness as it ages, but it should not really go off.'

'But the old boy is nine years old! He's bound to be a bit tired.'

'Well, Mrs Pessimist, let's open one up when your mother is here. She'll drink anything and then look around for a second glass!' I retorted unkindly.

It was duly agreed, and the next time we had Norma around for a meal I opened a bottle, with all the reverence and ceremony accorded to a saint's relics that were being paraded around a French village on his or her special yearly day out on the town.

'It looks rather muddy,' said my mother-in-law, peering at it suspiciously. 'In fact, it looks just like muddy water.'

'Think of it as a grand old Burgundy,' I enthused. 'They are always pale and they can go a bit brownish.'

'Brickish-looking,' my wife corrected me.

'Here's to us and our good old patron Saint Martin,' I said.

I did not know then that the patron saint of vintners is really Saint Vincent. Perhaps old Vincent felt a bit snubbed by our ignoring him. If so, he must have been enjoying himself knowing that payback time was just around the corner. We swirled the wine and sniffed it before putting the glasses to our lips for a very tentative sip.

'It smells and tastes like compost!' Chris complained.

'More like manure, I would say,' said Norma, screwing up her nose.

'Now, girls, aged fine Burgundy can be redolent with all the complex and fascinating smells of a French farmyard,' I said rather lamely.

'You drink it then,' said my mother-in-law sarcastically. 'Go on, let's see you!'

Chris nodded in assent. It was with difficulty that I managed to finish the small amount in my glass.

'It's probably just a bad bottle,' I said hopefully. 'It may be corked. I'll open another.'

It proved to be exactly the same, as did the third bottle, at which point I had to admit defeat.

'Let us get the taste out of our mouths with a good old glass of sherry,' said Norma, in an imperious tone.

Reluctantly I had to obey.

Why did the wine seem so terrible? Had our palates become more sophisticated while we were overseas? Undoubtedly, as we had supped on the wines of all the major European viticultural areas and had become used to drinking a glass or two of decent, if not exactly high-class, wine every day; but it was more than just that. We had not become too fussy. We were still happy to have a fairly rough wine if there was nothing better at hand, but our old Saint had become actively evil.

It was then that we realised that the garden vine we had jealously guarded was an American vine and not a member of the *Vitis vinifera* or European winemaking grape family. American native grapes are resistant to the microscopic root-sucking insect phylloxera, and to fungal diseases that damage the leaves of *Vitis vinifera*. American vines are thus ideal for the home garden as they require little care. Unfortunately, they are inferior for winemaking because the grapes contain a natural chemical substance, methyl anthranilate, which gives wine a peculiar and unpleasant smell and taste that is described as 'foxy'. These new world interlopers are banned from vineyards in Europe, apart from being permitted as grafting material. They form the roots of each vine, while the upper parts that proudly carry the leaves and fruit are *Vitis vinifera*. Ironically, these American cousins saved Europe's vineyards from extinction when they were ravaged by phylloxera about a century ago, but now they are relegated to spend their miserable lives in servitude below ground.

Unregretfully, neither Chris nor I has ever had the opportunity to be downwind of a fox, but if its aroma is anything like that of our wine, it must be generated very close to the base of the crafty animal's tail. But why had the wine been so acceptable initially? Perhaps the natural fruitiness in the young wine covered its foxy nature, which only became apparent as the fruit characters faded.

I now know that the most likely scientific explanation of our Saint's unfortunate decomposition was a grubby little bug called brettanomyces. This hangs like the sword of Damocles over the head of any winemaker who does not filter it out of the wine at the time of bottling. Many people believe that if wine is aged in the bottle for too long it will turn into vinegar. This is nonsense. The microorganism that is capable of changing wine into vinegar, acetobacter, needs oxygen to survive, and once the wine is bottled oxygen is effectively excluded. If you open a bottle of wine and it is vinegary, then it was this way before it was bottled. Brettanomyces, on the other hand, can lurk like a hidden assassin within the sealed bottle. It does not need oxygen to do its dirty work. The wine can appear splendid for a year or two and then brettanomyces blooms, growing throughout the wine. The tell-tale dirty footprints it leaves behind reek of vomit, a sumo wrestler's loincloth, what the French call *merde*, and many other things of a similar ilk. A refined version was characteristic of some Australian red wines many years ago, when it went under the imaginative descriptor 'sweaty saddle'. The good old Aussies long ago cleaned up their act, thoroughly scrubbing their saddles with disinfectant.

There is, however, yet another explanation, and this is the one I prefer to believe. The bodies of some martyred saints have been said to remain fresh long after the time when they should have putrefied. The fact that our wine remained fresh for several years before finally rotting is to me a clear indication of its heavenly nature.

Whatever the explanation, we had learnt several hard lessons from this unfortunate episode. Firstly, we vowed that we would never again make wine from an American vine. Secondly, our winemaking hygiene would in future make an operating theatre look like a cesspool. Thirdly, perhaps — just perhaps — we might place more weight on the opinions of our budding surgical colleagues.

**I HESITATED, MY FINGER POISED** over the button, before I finally gave it a determined push. The door chime sounded loudly and then repeated itself, but in a decrescendo. We had no idea who were to be our hosts and we both felt somewhat apprehensive. The door swung open and there standing before us was a mature gent of indeterminate age and generous, if not bountiful, girth. In former times he might have attracted the descriptor 'stout'. There were flecks of grey in his black hair, and he was dressed in a dark suit. He had a welcoming air and a beaming smile on his jowly face.

'I'm John,' he said warmly. 'Please come in.'

Chris and I entered the lounge to find about 10 strangers sitting around chatting, clearly getting to know one another. There was a lull as the diverse group gave us the once-over. We were obviously the last people who were expected, as John immediately launched into a general preamble about our intentions.

'A very warm welcome to everyone,' he began. 'You all know why we are here and we might as well get on with it without any fuss or delay. I and my wife would like this evening to be as informal and relaxed as possible. I know that some of us will have had more experience than others and we might have some complete novices amongst us; so much the better. Those of us who know the ropes will enjoy teaching them. Perhaps the best way to break the ice is for each of us to introduce ourselves and give some indication of our experience and personal preferences. Shall we just go around in a circle starting from my left?'

Ron, a plumpish, happy-looking man, kicked off. He appeared to be in his late twenties and had a twinkle in his eye. His chins wobbled during his frequent chuckles.

'Call me a simple soul,' he giggled, 'but I like nothing better than a simple root: none of this fancy stuff for me. You can be too intricate. The more you try to put into it, with a bit of this and a bit of that, the longer the whole process takes and it is never as satisfying in the end. It should be natural, not like something you have dragged up out of a recipe book.'

We were all sitting around the periphery of the room facing towards the centre, and Chris and I were opposite Ron. I gave Chris a nudge with my elbow and she eased herself back in her chair, effectively pulling the hem of her trendy 'sixties miniskirt down towards her knees.

'You might be right, Ron, but give me a fruit anytime,' interrupted Ted, a slightly built man of about 40 with a meticulous central parting in his wavy fair hair, a pale blue button-up cardigan and red slacks. 'Everyone to their own tastes, but I have a definite leaning toward fruits. On the whole they are sweeter, more refined and not as coarse.'

Chris and I had been married for less than a year. It was not as though we were unhappy with things. Our first experiences and experiments had gone well. It was just that we wanted to broaden our horizons, to learn more of what the world had to offer. Perhaps, waiting out there were exciting things to be discovered; other ways and methods that could give us satisfaction beyond that which we had known, or at least a different perspective. Christchurch was a small city, but unless you were prepared to look around with a completely open mind you would never know what talent lay hidden within its apparently sleepy centre and respectable-looking suburbs.

A slightly built woman, who had introduced herself as Tessa, appeared excited and her eyes were bulging slightly. A few flecks of grey were starting to show in her black hair, and I noted with clinical precision that one side of her nose was slightly browner than the other. At first glance it looked as if it was more suntanned than its companion — a sure sign of a heavy cigarette-smoker who habitually held her fag on one side of her mouth. Her upper lip sported a growth that would have kept a depilation therapist happy for hours, if not days.

She was looking straight at Ron with her head turned away from me, but I thought I heard her say in a low, gravelly voice, 'You can't … ah …' she hesitated, 'well … beetroot?' She shrugged her shoulders and spread her semi-flexed arms apart.

'No,' Ron replied, 'I'm not at all comfortable with beetroot. As far as I'm concerned you can't go past a good parsnip, so long as you clean it and prepare it properly. I've brought some of my own with me and I'll show you later.'

Things were going along very well at the inaugural meeting of what we all agreed would be called the Canterbury Amateur Winemakers' Club. Ted waxed lyrical about the superiority of stone fruit, especially peaches, plums and cherries. Others preferred the lighter, more aromatic touch that flowers gave, while pipfruits, including apples, pears and quinces, also had their advocates. John, our host, was clearly an expert with raspberries, blackberries and the like. Finally, it was our turn to reveal our innermost secrets.

'Most of our experience has been with grapes,' I announced, feeling rather superior.

'What!' exclaimed Harry, a thickset, red-faced young bloke in a leather jacket. 'That's not real winemaking. That's just like cheating.'

'Yes, that's far too easy. Grape wine just makes itself. Where's the skill in that?' Tessa chipped in.

The more experienced amongst the group nodded sagely in assent.

'We've got open minds and we are here to learn,' Chris explained hastily, adding with a smile, 'we are prepared to mend our wicked ways.'

The heads nodded again, this time in approbation, and there were friendly smiles all around. We had been cleansed of our incipient leper status.

Before long the formal part of the evening was over and a few prized bottles of wine were produced. We had to agree that Ron was a wizard with roots and that his parsnip brew would match any of the fine Kiwi 'Sauternes' that we had tasted. We had never tried the real thing. John's raspberry wine was also a winner with the members of our newly established club. When it came time to leave we were all in high spirits and we felt as though we had achieved something very important that night. I did not know it then, but the lessons that Chris and I were to learn and the technical expertise we were to gain with this little group would be vital for us in coming years.

**AS I GLANCED UP I HAD A VISION** of an inverted straw-coloured mop slowly rising into view from behind the bushes, then a pair of blue eyes swam into focus.

'Get down,' I whispered. 'It's not safe yet.'

The mop and eyes disappeared again.

'I'll give a loud cough when the coast is clear.'

A couple of minutes later I coughed and Chris stood up.

'We shouldn't be doing this,' she said, looking worried.

'Why not? We are only helping the gardeners. I'm sure they will be delighted with our work.'

'It's not that. I'm not worried about what we are doing. It's just that I shouldn't be doing this in my nurse's uniform.'

'Then let's finish it quickly so I can go home and you can go back to work.'

We were in the Botanic Gardens, which were situated just a short distance from the hospital, across a little footbridge over the River Avon. It was Chris's meal break and she had chosen to join me in the rose garden. Her nurse's hat had been removed and she had put on a jacket over the top part of her uniform. The blue dress and black stockings remained clearly visible. I, on the other hand, having just finished my ward rounds, was off-duty and in my street clothes. One of the senior staff in the nursing hierarchy had just walked past, but fortunately Chris had spotted her from a distance and swiftly taken evasive action. Her fearsome superior had now toddled off on her happy way.

Standing in the middle of the rose garden, I was gazing at Chris over the top of a sea of flowers. Under normal circumstances this would have been a delightfully romantic scene, but we were now feeling a little guilty and a trifle panicked. When we had been disturbed we had been in the process of deadheading roses, removing any dead or dying flowers and putting them in plastic bags. The thought had flashed through my mind that it might have been less stressful and just as profitable to have carried out our little harvest in the local crematorium rose garden, but no doubt that would also have had its own problems. There was the possibility that some narrow-minded relatives might object, not appreciating that we would be raising the memories of their dear departed to higher things.

Too late for that now; now was the time for action. We quickly went about our business, choosing the blooms that were overblown, fully open and with their petals starting to fall off. It was delicate work. Just touching the stems inadvertently was enough to send all the beautiful red, pink, yellow and primrose coloured petals tumbling wastefully onto the dark brown earth. We had to pluck each bloom by pinching it closed, then all the petals would come away in our hands. We were saving them from oblivion and giving their delicious scent a place in posterity.

Our task quickly completed, I was about to head off to our small hospital flat with my sacks full of loot when Chris said, 'No you don't!'

She tapped her cheek and pouted her lips, making a smacking noise.

'You won't have the opportunity to kiss me in a more romantic situation than this, surrounded by the best roses in Christchurch. And surely I deserve it after giving up my mealtime to help.'

I guiltily obliged before slinking away with our aromatic prize.

**OVER THE PRECEDING YEAR** we had come to sympathise with our clubmates' view that making grape wine is akin to cheating. Undoubtedly, the grape is the perfect fruit from which to make wine. Its yummy constituents are all in the right proportions and it is capable of making wine of a quality that cannot be matched by other fruits. The best grapes can make themselves into wine with only minimal intervention from the human hand. Not so with wine made from other things, so-called 'country wines'. Few other fruits or roots contain enough sugar to produce the alcohol content required to keep the wine stable. We found the addition of crystals of 'white death' was almost inevitable, and thus we had to buy large amounts of sugar. Then there was the problem of body or fullness in the mouth, that sensation of richness or unctuousness which, if lacking, results in a wine tasting watery.

Some fruits that had good flavours simply made wishy-washy wine. We learned that banana added to the ferment increased body, as did a small amount of glycerine. The latter also gave smoothness and a touch of sweetness without the risk of the wine refermenting in the bottle. Aroma or bouquet can be lacking in country wines, and there is nothing better than flowers to remedy this; hence, our expedition to the rose garden. As you might expect, flowers in the full flush of youth have more perfume than the dead and dying rose heads that we had collected. Ours, however, still retained enough of this vital essence to be useful. Elderflowers were a favourite of ours; they have a delightful sweet smell, very akin to some sauvignon blanc wines. Some harvesters of tall poppies refer to this as cat's pee.

We learned a myriad of tricks that enabled us to patch up the various deficits that can beset country wines, but there is one very recalcitrant flaw that afflicts many, particularly the whites. This is a degree of hardness or coarseness in their finish. It is for this reason that most country wines are made sweet or medium-sweet. The remaining sugar conceals what would otherwise be a disagreeably bitter or astringent aftertaste. As the song says, 'A little bit of sugar helps the medicine go down . . . in the most delightful way!'

It was in this alchemist's secret cave, this apothecary's workshop of country wine, that we first learned the mysteries of real winemaking. We taught ourselves how to measure and adjust the levels of sugar, acid and many other things in 'must' (i.e. fruit juice or pulp) and wine, as well as how to increase or lower alcohol levels. We found out how to add millionths of a part per litre of antioxidant before testing to see how much of it remained active, unravaged by that great, all-destroying demon of wine, oxygen. Being of a medical bent, we also learnt how to avoid, diagnose and treat the maladies or so-called *casses* of wine. These dastardly sicknesses can result from widely differing causes, such as infection, contact with some metals, excess protein and so forth. They can cause a wine that is crystal-clear just after it has been bottled to become a disgusting-looking cloudy mess some months later, even though the taste may be unaffected. We knew that they were of only trivial annoyance to amateurs like us, but to real winemakers any one of these sneaky diseases could prove economically fatal.

But during this Country and Wild Western period, as we like to call it, we did have an occasional shameful indiscretion; a temporary relapse in an otherwise exemplary record. Perhaps these foretold our eventual return to the easy, dark side of the street. There was the time we acquired a small load of palomino grapes, the ones that are used to make sherry. After we had made them into wine, we managed to acquire a special culture of *flor*, the yeast that is used to make the real McCoy in Spain. We were even able to get this to grow on the surface of our precious 'sherry', as we wanted it to do. We thought the result was pretty creditable, although we did not dare tell our clubmates.

At this time our cramped little hospital flat was crammed with merrily bubbling containers, mainly one-gallon plastic cubes that we had scrounged from our local Mr Whippy ice-cream van, guessing these had to be made of food-grade material. The place reeked like a winery, but oh, what a beautiful smell, or at least we thought so, although some of our neighbours were not so enthusiastic. We made wine out of almost every available type of flower and fruit, and we even took up Ron's suggestion of exploring the world of diverse roots. It was into this chaotic but happy little household that the first of our four sons, Matthew, was born. Perhaps it was the sweet-smelling spirits wafting through into his bedroom that eventually drove him to become a winemaker.

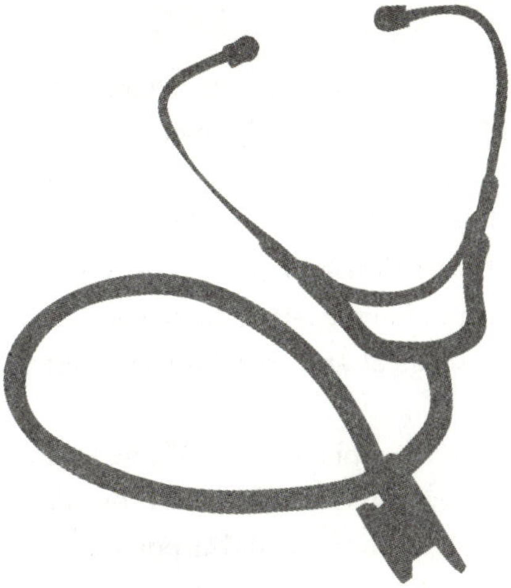

## CHAPTER 3

# Restarting *at* *the* Bottom

### London, 1972–1975

**THERE WAS A SUDDEN BURST** of disorientating bright light as the underground train emerged and rushed headlong into the midday sunshine of dreary suburban south London. Everything looked the way I felt — wretched to the core. Why was I subjecting myself to this? Surely it was not really necessary.

I disembarked unenthusiastically at Tooting Bec station. Was it prophetic that the station was on the Northern Line, the so-called 'misery line'? My feet slowly dragged themselves towards the local hospital. I was sweating and I could feel that my armpits were very damp, but it was an unhealthy, cold sweat. An unnaturally pleasant and cheerful porter, with a peculiarly wide-based gait that I desperately and unsuccessfully tried to diagnose, showed me into a dimly lit room lined with a number of unfortunates who looked exactly the way I felt — terrified and miserable. The enclosed space reeked of body odour. Not any old body odour, but an international, or should I say multicultural, body odour, to which I was no doubt adding my own disagreeable tuppence-worth. I waited restlessly to hear my name. I did not mind whether it was whispered or shouted, so long as it came soon, but it did not.

For the umpteenth time I thought, 'Why the bloody hell am I putting myself through this?'

I had put my foot on this fateful path when, while developing my skills as an amateur winemaker, I had decided to become a neurologist. To do so I would have to complete my neurological studies overseas, and there were two accepted paths: one led to the US, the other to the UK. I really did not have a choice. The allure of Europe's vineyards had decided it for me. Knowing of my neurological aspirations, the consultant in charge of the medical unit in Christchurch, Dr Don Beaven, had kindly invited Chris and me to his house to have dinner with a visiting London neurologist, Ian McDonald. Dr McDonald was a suave and urbane Kiwi who had made it in the big smoke. An olive-skinned Adonis, with sleek dark hair, black pinstriped, double-breasted suit, and matching floral tie and handkerchief, he regaled us with amazing tales of his international neurological and social adventures; nay, successes.

On his way back to London he had to make a couple of stop-offs, he told us, one in Southeast Asia and the other in the Arabian Gulf. He would consult on the neurological difficulties afflicting a prime minister and a potentate, respectively and respectfully.

'A bit of a fag really, as I have a research project on multiple sclerosis that I should get back to. However, the fees will no doubt be something of a consolation.'

To say we were riveted by his every word would be an understatement. We were bewitched.

Dr McDonald was a consultant at the National Hospital for Nervous Diseases in Queen Square, the only hospital in Britain dedicated solely to neurology and neurosurgery. It had been my dream to train there, but how should I proceed? Dr McDonald strongly advised me to spend the next year getting more experience in the excellent neurology unit at Auckland Hospital, before chancing my hand at Queen Square. He explained that the pressure to get a registrar's training post was such that I would have to restart at the bottom and work my way up. I would need to work unpaid at 'The Square' as a junior medical officer for an indefinite period until one of the incumbent registrars resigned. This way, the consultants on the selection committee would be familiar with my strengths and weaknesses and would be able to weigh up the merits of my case against those of the many other applicants. There were no places reserved for 'colonials'.

A puff of wind blew out one of the candles on the table and the euphoria that I had felt earlier in the evening trailed off through the open window after the vanishing smoke. Chris and I had just become parents. How would we support ourselves? We did not have any cushy family money we could lean on, let alone fall back on.

**'I'M SORRY TO TELL YOU** that eight new clinical neurology registrars were appointed last month, but I'm equally pleased to tell you that I was one of them.'

I had, just by chance, met the likeable, larger-than-life Lindsay Haas in a street neighbouring Queen Square. Also an aspiring Kiwi neurologist, he was a year ahead of me in his training.

'Reg Kelly, my boss at the neurology unit of St Georges Hospital, was on the appointments committee at The Square as he also works there. He told me afterwards that the standard of applicants was so dreadful that they were forced to appoint me,' Lindsay said, bursting out laughing. He always liked to tell stories against himself but it was clear that he had hit it off very well with his boss.

Suddenly my heart felt like a lead balloon. I had just arrived for my first day at The Square, but the dreadful significance of Lindsay's words was not lost on me. There were only 10 such registrar positions and they were each for a duration of two years. This meant that, failing disgrace, madness, some other wretched affliction or even death, there probably would only be two new registrar appointments made during the next 24 months. Lindsay commiserated, wished me well and went on his merry way.

This was the reason I was now standing in this funereal little room, surrounded by the most dejected and grieving specimens of humanity. I had decided to try to become a Member of the Royal College of Physicians (MRCP UK), as I felt membership would increase my chances of getting the posting I so desperately wanted. Theoretically, I did not really need it, as I had passed the examinations and become a Member of the Royal Australasian College of Physicians a few years earlier. The two qualifications were regarded as being equivalent, at least by Australasians. I was not quite so sure about the perfidious Albions, hence I felt it would be better to have two strings to my bow.

I had sat my oral examination the previous week at University College Hospital, where I had been grilled by the medical Gestapo and asked to interpret all sorts of laboratory test results, x-rays, cardiographs and even an electroencephalogram (EEG) or brainwave recording. Fortunately, my unsympathetic torturers did not know I was training in neurology and they seemed mildly surprised when I 'helpfully' turned the EEG graph through 180° and handed it back the correct way up before enlightening them on what it showed. They had just been looking at it upside down! It was a stroke of luck that was unlikely to be repeated today.

Finally I heard my name. 'Dr Donaldson, would you please come this way?' It was the same unpleasantly jovial, unsympathetic porter who had shown me into the waiting room. I followed him, racking my brains. Was his problem neurological, rheumatological, orthopaedic or was it just that he had a problem with continence? Before I could decide I found myself standing in front of a small, swarthy man in a dark pinstripe suit. He had a full thatch of black hair on his lower head but a shiny pate above, bushy black eyebrows, a nose like a sickle and small piggish eyes behind thick lenses — he was clearly extremely myopic, with eyeballs that were made to look tiny by his spectacles. Before I could complete my nightmarish reverie, he held out his hand and gave me a kindly smile.

'Pleased to meet you, Dr Donaldson,' he said graciously, introducing himself and the two similarly uniformed colleagues who were standing beside him. 'And where are you working at present?' he asked.

'At the National, Queen Square,' I responded, as my cold, clammy hand was vigorously pumped up and down by what seemed an unnaturally hot one.

'Excellent. And why are you there?'

'It is part of my neurological training,' I replied.

My questioner turned to his colleagues with a broad grin and said, 'We must make certain we do not give Dr Donaldson any neurological cases. He might show us up!'

I inwardly cursed myself for being so stupid as to fall into this little trap. Admittedly, this was a general medical examination, one for a physician who had expertise in all branches of medicine, and I had four years of such training under my belt. Daily, however, some of the cutting edge of my general medicine was being blunted by my focus on the brain and its many bodily outposts. Examinations are always a bit of a lottery. I had prayed that the dice would roll impartially and that I would get an unselected spread of patients with various medical disorders, which might include neurology. No such luck! I knew the format of this clinical examination would be the same as the Australasian one and that it would comprise one long case and multiple short cases. In the long case, I would have an hour to interview and examine a patient unobserved; a patient who would probably have multiple disorders and present complicated problems. I would subsequently have to discuss the patient's history and my findings, conclusions and management plan with the examiners. In the short cases I would be taken around a series of patients and directed to examine particular body systems and report my findings while being observed by the examiners.

During the impossibly short few minutes that remained to me before I was served up to the patient who was lying in wait, I thought of the coaching session Dr Don Beaven had given to a small group of candidates not long before we sat the Australasian examination. He had explained that he was not there to teach us medical theory or the art of clinical medicine, but solely the art of sitting a medical examination. He told us what was expected of us, the pitfalls that might ensnare us, and how to steer around them without being afraid to use cunning and guile when needed. He explained that while usually it is the doctor who feels sorry for the patient, in the examination setting it is vital that the patient feels sorry for the doctor and tries to help him or her.

Little did I know then that this slightly built, boyish-looking but inspirational figure, with his impish, somewhat quixotic approach to life in general and the establishment in particular, would one day become not only my boss and a very close friend but also a 'partner in crime' — in the crime of winemaking.

'Getting the full cooperation of the patient is the secret of success,' Don had said.

Pretending to be the exam candidate and sitting himself in front of a surprised patient who had volunteered to take part in a mock long-case examination, Don went out of his way to gain Mr Barnett's confidence and sympathy. He told the patient a story of long, hard hours spent in preparation for the examination, and how tired he was because he had risen early to see his sick patients before coming along to the exam. His poor wife and children were depending on him passing the exam, he said. He would try to be as gentle as he could, but if he in any way upset Mr Barnett during the examination the patient should tell him immediately. By the time Don had finished introducing himself to Mr Barnett our small group had tears in our eyes: partly in sympathy for the poor 'junior' doctor, and partly from suppressed laughter.

'The few minutes you spend doing this are the most valuable part of your hour,' Don advised, smiling encouragingly and patting Mr Barnett's hand.

'As for the short cases, these are for the examiners to see your examination technique. Examine quickly and surely, but not so fast that the examiners might miss seeing exactly what you are doing. The aim is to expertly examine as many patients as you can and correctly report their clinical signs in the allotted time.'

I was grateful for Don's open, enlightened and mature approach to gaining admission to the medical hierarchy's apparently invincible fortress. Many a crusader has died on the battlements.

'Just think of it as a game that has to be played for a day,' I now recalled.

While skill is needed in such situations, it also helps to have a bit of luck. As I boarded the underground to return home after the examination I felt the black dog of depression snapping at my heels. Examiners were undoubtedly unsympathetic torturers who were out to get you. It was only after I received my exam results several weeks later that I underwent an epiphany and then I knew, without a shadow of a doubt, that all medical examiners were only there to help you through the gate, kind, sympathetic, forgiving and helpful folk that they are.

Even then I never dreamt that in the dim and distant future, after I had returned to New Zealand, I would become the chairman of the Royal Australasian College of Physicians examination committee and chair of the College's board of censors.

**'AND WHAT DO YOU THINK** is the diagnosis, Dr Richards?' asked Professor Gilliatt. The professor cut a handsome and imperious figure, tall and lean, with a time-etched rather than wrinkled face. He had a full head of well-oiled black hair and imposing, spiky eyebrows of the same colour.

'I think Mr Shepherd has Parkinson's disease,' the unfortunate Stephen Richards proffered hesitantly.

'Has he been given a good trial of L-dopa?'

'Yes, sir. He is on that now.'

'He hasn't had much of a response to it then, has he? Has there been any improvement at all?'

'Not so far as I can tell, sir.'

'How often does that happen in Parkinson's disease? Having no response at all?'

'I'm not certain, sir.'

'And what about his incontinence? How often is that an early symptom of Parkinson's disease?'

'I thought it was probably due to his prostate, sir.'

'Mr Shepherd is a bit young for prostatism, isn't he?'

'I suppose he is.'

'What does the literature say about these things and Mr Shepherd's other unusual symptoms, Dr Richards?'

'I'm sorry, sir, but I haven't yet had time to go to the library and review the literature.'

'What do you mean, "haven't had time"? This patient has been in hospital two days. How long is he supposed to spend here before you find time?'

'I will do it straight after the ward round, Professor Gilliatt. Could I please be excused for just a moment?' Stephen asked breathlessly.

There was a parting shot as he made for the door. 'Do not bother to hurry back, Dr Richards.'

I heard a hissing sound outside the door, once, twice and even thrice. Stephen came back into the ward still looking flustered. His wheezing remained audible, but at least he had managed to use his asthma inhaler and its effect would probably kick in before long. His chubby red face and generous figure gave him a somewhat comical Billy Bunterish look, but they were probably the result of the steroids he took. He was a kind, gentle person and well liked by the patients.

A few days earlier I had been attached to Professor Roger Gilliatt's ward as my first posting at The Square — my mentor, Ian McDonald, had described it as a baptism by fire. 'It's important to emerge from your time there unscathed, or relatively unscathed,' he had added sagely.

I was on my first ward round with the professor and his team, which consisted of his lecturer, senior registrar (Stephen Richards), registrar, house physician, unpaid clerks (including me) and his invaluable ward sister. Quite an intimidating little entourage for Mr Shepherd and the other patients. As I was to discover over the ensuing weeks, Stephen's asthma regularly peaked during these ward rounds, in which the junior medical staff, and in particular the senior registrar, were put through an inquisition. Roger Gilliatt had a reputation for being a hard taskmaster and ruling the roost with an iron claw. If you got on the wrong side of him, then look out! Stephen had somehow ended up in this position, although nobody knew how it had happened.

Roger Gilliatt's parents were medical people; his mother had been an anaesthetist and his father the Queen's obstetrician, as well as the president of the Royal College of Obstetricians and Gynaecologists. Roger had gone to the best schools, had done well at university, and had emerged from army service during the Second World War with distinction, and he knew it. When, in 1960, the Queen's sister, Princess Margaret, married Antony Armstrong-Jones, Roger had been pressed into service at the last moment as the best man — the first choice had just been convicted of 'importuning'.

'Importuning? What's that supposed to mean?' I asked the registrar who had been filling me in about the matter.

'I think it means he was had up for pestering young boys.'

I didn't know whether or not to believe him, but I subsequently noted that a newspaper report implied that 'the strongly heterosexual' Gilliatt was a suitable choice for the role. Whatever the truth of the matter, it was for this reason that Roger was known by the junior medical staff at The Square as 'the second best man', although the title had not rubbed itself onto his personality. Six months before going to Queen Square I had had dinner with an eminent neurologist from the Mayo Clinic who, like Roger, specialised in disorders of the peripheral nerve.

'When you meet Roger Gilliatt,' he had told me, 'just remember that the sun does not shine from a particular part of his anatomy, and that from the other side of the toilet seat he looks just the same as anybody else.'

I was naïvely shocked by this crude remark from a colleague, even one who was potentially Roger's rival, and I tried to forget it. Nonetheless, when I was confronted by the professor a nasty little cherub-like souvenir of that evening would sometimes worm its way into my consciousness and it would take an effort to suppress an amused smile, or worse, a fatal giggle. I found him to be exacting but fair, in spite of his reputation. I suspect that being a 'colonial' antipodean was an advantage as it provided a cloak of anonymity. This was not allowed to his fellow countrymen, whose pedigree was known, or would be as soon as they opened their mouths.

I had been working at my unpaid clerking job for Roger Gilliatt for six weeks when one day he said to me in a commanding tone: 'I would like to see you in my office at the end of the ward round, Dr Donaldson.' I felt a gripping sensation in my abdomen, accompanied by mild nausea. What had I done? I had done my very best during my time with him, or so I thought. The ward round dragged on interminably, and my symptoms became more marked. I tried to concentrate on each patient and the problems that I was presenting to the entourage. Finally the round came to an end and I followed my boss back to his little office. He sat down behind his desk and eyed me.

'I don't need your services any longer, Dr Donaldson,' he said gruffly. 'Don't come back on Monday.'

I knew that I looked pale and I felt ready to collapse. There was no cherub image to mock me at this meeting.

'I want you to go to the Dean's office and speak to his secretary, Pat Harris. Tell her I said that from now on I want you to do the locum jobs for any registrars who go on leave,' the professor continued, breaking into a smile. A wave of joyful warmth spread upwards from my feet to my head, enveloping me — surely it must show.

'Oh, and by the way,' he added, almost as an afterthought, 'my wife and I are having a little party at home on the night of Saturday the twenty-fourth. We would like you and your wife to join us if you are free.'

When I left for home that night I found that the 'misery line' had closed and the Northern Line had been reopened as the 'happiness line'. The underground no longer dragged itself along the rails but fairly flew. Chris would be excited beyond belief at the prospect of my rejoining the working class and getting paid, even if it was only on an intermittent locum basis.

I had been lucky enough to be awarded a Commonwealth Medical Fellowship to study neurology in London, and this had provided us with a small income, enough to enable us to survive. In addition, we had found a basement flat in Hampstead that had proved to be a lifesaver. We paid no rent on the basis that Chris cleaned the upper four floors, did the washing, the ironing and the like, and looked after the owners' three children when they came home from school.

It was great except for a few trivial details. Our landlord had that obsessive-compulsive streak that is the hallmark of a good solicitor, and his wife had the dreamy temperament of a professional musician. The corners of the handkerchiefs had to meet with legal precision in case they caused embarrassment should they be revealed in front of one's colleagues or clients. Shoes had to shine so that not only could one see one's face, but one could also use them as shaving mirrors. Light switches and door handles needed to be swabbed with antiseptic, as one never knew who might have touched them. Chris had always been a broad-brush type of person and not so good at minor details — more 'Let's get it done efficiently and move on to the next thing'. But she was fantastic with kids, so the 'upstairs, downstairs' arrangement of the house worked.

That night we had a celebratory bottle of bubbles — not champagne, which was well beyond our budget, but a pleasant middle-of-the-road Vouvray. Life was again full of exciting prospects and expectations.

**'I CAN'T GET IT TO CHANGE** from third into second gear!' Chris shouted.

'Look out!' I screamed as a car passed dangerously close on the left and another honked loudly on our right. 'Just let the van slow down and see if you can get it into first gear,' I suggested.

There was a loud graunching noise as she succeeded in engaging first gear, but we had almost slowed to a stop and now there was frantic honking from behind. We had stupidly decided to drive our clapped-out 1964 Bedford campervan through central London to the Gilliatts' party, which was in the most fashionable area of Knightsbridge. We had only bought the vehicle that day, and this was our first experience of driving in London. Speeding around the five-lane racetrack that surrounded Hyde Park at 7.30 on a Saturday night was not the ideal place or time to discover the vagaries of our new old beast.

'Now see if you can change up to third or fourth again, Chris.'

It worked and we extricated ourselves from the raging sea of vehicles that seemed intent on destroying themselves and us. Chris parked well away from our hosts' house to avoid embarrassment. Our transport looked jaunty, but out of place among the Jags and Rollers.

The house was thronging with the neurological élite as well as its odds and sods, like us. Most of Roger Gilliatt's junior medical staff were there, as well as many of his colleagues. The Inquisitor had not come along tonight. He had been replaced by Roger the charming host, the life and soul of the party. He and his wife, Penelope, mixed freely and talked animatedly to all, even the humblest and most gaffe-prone of his junior staff. It was a generous thing to do and it showed him in a completely different light. I talked to Ian McDonald and asked him how often the Gilliatts held these parties.

'I don't know,' he said. 'I have been at Queen Square for quite a number of years now and I have never heard of one before.'

As Chris and I made our merry way home we felt ourselves lucky to have had a glimpse behind the scenes and to know that there was another side to the master of our fates. We also felt lucky not to have further trouble with our gears that night, but the fight between two and three was still lurking there, and it was not long before the aggression became apparent again.

'Sorry, but it's a big job,' the thickset man in the dirty blue overalls commiserated with us as he dropped the bonnet. 'We'll need to take out the motor in order to get to the gearbox. It'll be over 40 quid.'

'We haven't really got much option,' I said to Chris, shrugging hopelessly.

It was a lot of money and we really did not have much to spare.

'Let's think about it over the weekend,' she replied. 'We may have to live with it.'

And that's how we left it.

'Oi know the problem, Guv,' chipped in a bright-faced little old man in a dirty back street behind St Pancras station. 'U see there's a gear rod from the column change what has t' fit int' a litle 'ole, an' th'oles got worn den, aint it? So when rod pokes thru 'ole it don't line up proper. All't needs is washer t'old rod in centa an' job's dun.'

I looked at him suspiciously. 'How long will it take and what will it cost?'

'Two min'tes an' 50p,' he answered, smiling. Suddenly he looked like an angel.

'Do it!' I almost shouted excitedly.

We had the van for another four years and drove it many thousands of miles over Europe. Not once did we experience an angry gear again. That little angel taught us a valuable lesson: always get more than one opinion if you are not happy — and that applies to medical opinions as well!

**THE NATIONAL HOSPITAL** at Queen Square had an outpost in the fashionable London suburb of Maida Vale, not far from Marble Arch, and it was there that I was sent to do one of my early locum registrar's jobs, the incumbent having flitted off to take a holiday in Scotland. When I alighted from the bus and made my way up the street in the direction the helpful driver had indicated, it was clear that I had been let off at the wrong stop or that I had been misdirected. There was no hospital in sight and I had surely walked much more than the hundred yards the driver had suggested. I turned around and retraced my steps, but to no avail. I then made enquiries from what looked like a local, a stooped, elderly woman who was slowly tottering by. Her basket was so heavily laden with groceries that I marvelled she did not pitch forward and end up sprawled on the pavement.

'Why! You must need glasses,' she said. 'We are standing right outside it. That's the Maida Vale Hospital.'

I turned to look where she was pointing. There was an undistinguished-looking old house of three or four storeys, little different from the other dwellings in the street. It was not actually dilapidated, but it looked decidedly tatty and as though it had seen better days. Was this really a hospital? I had walked right past it, failing to look for the sign that announced its presence, simply because I had automatically discounted such a preposterous possibility. Did they really perform brain operations in there? I knocked at the door hesitantly, and when there was no response I turned the handle and walked in.

There was an old — no, ancient — nurse sitting in a chair in a dimly lit hallway. Could she really be a nurse? She was wearing a blue-and-white uniform so she clearly had some official position.

'Who are you looking for?' the crumpled form enquired in a trembling whisper.

'I don't really know,' I replied. 'Perhaps you can help me? I'm a new locum registrar. I've come to do Dr Peter's work while he is on holiday. Who should I see?'

'I'll get you a white coat,' the apparition volunteered as she shakily defied both gravity and her age, hoisting herself into a semi-upright position before shuffling off.

Returning 10 minutes later she handed me a white coat, saying, 'You can have another one in a week. Take care not to get it dirty. Lord Brain allows the young doctors to have a clean white coat once a week, but only once a week, so make sure you don't get it dirty.'

She then returned to her chair and closed her eyes, which suggested to me that she was sleeping, praying, having a minor epileptic seizure or just wanting to get rid of me. As I knew that Lord Brain, an eminent neurologist who had previously worked at Maida Vale Hospital, had been dead for some years, it was clear that I was going to get little further with her, so I wandered off to find somebody else. Later, I learned that in earlier days she had been Lord Brain's devoted nurse/secretary/assistant, and that when her employment was at an end it was apparent that dementia had set in and the lady had nowhere else to go. She had compassionately been kept on the staff, and now her sole job was to supervise the distribution of the doctors' white coats.

The unprepossessing appearance of the Maida Vale Hospital for Nervous Diseases belied its illustrious past and the high standard of neurology and neurosurgery that was practised within its cramped confines. There are only a handful of medicos who are elevated to the peerage, but this little hospital could boast two. There have been studies of meaningful surnames and it turns out that there is a distinct tendency for occupations to be linked to people's names. Thus, even these days, Carpenters, Butchers, Bakers and so forth have a greater chance of ending up in those particular jobs than someone who is called Fletcher, Brown, or Richards.

I do not know if Russell Brain's occupation was predetermined, but his fame and that of his book was surely assured when he could legitimately call the latter *Brain's Diseases of the Nervous System*. It is still a 'must have' for all budding neurologists and physicians. Lord Brain became Winston Churchill's neurologist, but he fell out with the other Maida Vale peer, Charles Wilson, who rose to become Lord Moran by dint of being Winston Churchill's personal physician. The latter's book on his famous patient became mired in controversy because, among other things, it broke the taboo of doctor–patient confidentiality. Lord Brain added his voice to the criticisms, pointing out multiple mistakes and inaccuracies.

'Dr Blunt, the radiologist in charge, will be ready to perform the myelogram on Mrs Pettit in half an hour. It is time for you to insert the Myodil into her spine,' Staff Nurse Buck informed me in an authoritarian tone. I had made her acquaintance when I had started on the ward that morning. She was a formidable Irish colleen from County Cork who had ended up being an unclaimed treasure and had found her solace in food. Even the largest of nurses' uniforms was strained to breaking point. No one could remember when she had started at Maida Vale, but judging by her greying, bristly moustache she had been around for quite some time. In spite of her domineering manner I did not want to cross her, as she was clearly a mine of information regarding the workings of Maida Vale Hospital and I would be reliant on her assistance during my time there.

'I've never had to put Myodil into a patient's spine before. Everywhere else that I have worked, the radiologist has always injected it under x-ray control in the department.'

'Dr Blunt doesn't work that way. He thinks it's a waste of his time and he prefers the registrars to insert the Myodil on the ward and then transfer the patient up to the radiology department to have the x-rays. It's more efficient because they can x-ray more patients that way,' Nurse Buck assured me.

I had a distinct feeling of uneasiness. Mrs Pettit was slowly developing paraplegia and difficulties with her bladder, and, although it was suspected that this was due to an inflammation in the spinal cord secondary to multiple sclerosis, we wanted to make certain she did not have a tumour of her spine. The latter, but not the former, would require an operation. Myodil (Pantopaque) was an oily, heavy substance that is injected into spinal fluid in the lumbar subarachnoid space and then run up the spinal canal by gradually tilting the patient downwards while x-rays are taken. Being opaque to x-rays, the Myodil's silhouette would be deformed by a tumour, but not by multiple sclerosis. Although it was not technically difficult to insert the Myodil, the procedure was normally done by the radiologist under x-ray to make absolutely certain the needle was in the correct place. However, I did not want to upset Dr Blunt, who had the reputation of living up to his name and being quite bad-tempered. In the back of my mind I also had a lurking suspicion that if I crossed him it might adversely affect my chance of getting the full-time registrar's job that I wanted.

'I just have to attend to an urgent matter in the next ward,' I told Nurse Buck. 'I'll be back in a few minutes.'

I quickly located a registrar and asked his advice.

'I'd be very careful if I were you,' Stuart advised. 'Blunt asked me to do the same thing three weeks ago. I knew that I was in the right place because cerebrospinal fluid came back out of the needle and I was very careful not to move it during the procedure. When I came to inject the Myodil I seemed to feel quite a resistance, but then it's an oily viscous substance so I thought that was probably normal. When the x-rays were taken the Myodil was in the wrong place. It was in the epidural space rather than the subarachnoid one. Blunt was annoyed and I was upset. The patient was very good about it, but her examination was hopeless and needed to be repeated.'

I returned to the ward, where Nurse Buck urged, 'You had better hurry. You don't have much time left and the hospital orderly will be here any moment to take Mrs Pettit to x-ray.'

'You can ring Dr Blunt and tell him that I am not happy to inject the Myodil down here in the ward,' I told her. 'If he wants me to do it I will put it in under x-ray control up in his department but I will not do it down here.'

I moved on to another patient, and a minute or so later Nurse Buck poked her head around the bedside curtains.

'I don't think he was very happy but he said he will do it himself, so I have sent the patient off to the x-ray department,' she said with a grin, and then, by way of an afterthought, she added, 'He always tries that one on with the new boys.'

'Thanks very much for letting me in on the secret!' was my exasperated reply.

A few days later I walked into the cramped little ward office to be greeted by Staff Nurse Buck: 'You have three new patients that have to be admitted to hospital this morning; I would suggest that you see the one in Room A first. I have put all the necessary files and papers on the locker by his bed.'

'Why should I see him first?' I asked. 'Is he urgent?'

'Not urgent, dear — important,' she replied with a wink.

I was taken aback when I opened the door to Room A. There, lying on the bed, looking completely relaxed, at home and as suave as usual, was Ian McDonald.

'What are you doing here, Ian?' I enquired, feeling rather embarrassed at the prospect of having to examine my mentor and the supervisor of my Commonwealth Medical Fellowship.

'I've got sciatica. I was stretching up to a suitcase on the overhead rack of a train a month ago when I suddenly developed a prolapsed intervertebral disc. I felt an acute pain in my lower back that then spread down the back of my right leg to the ankle and the foot. That ankle reflex is depressed and I've got an area of decreased skin sensation that corresponds to the first sacral nerve on that side. The pain is still very troublesome.'

I suppressed a sigh of relief. At least I did not have to try to diagnose some devilishly difficult neurological problem and my boss was not about to croak with some dreadful neurological disease.

'Are you going to have surgery?'

'No fear! I have seen Professor Valentine Logue. He recommends complete bed rest for four to six weeks, and that means *complete* rest, lying flat on my back. I have tried, but I just can't do that at home as I have to get up to get meals, etc. So here I am. Valentine says there is a 95 per cent chance that it will get better without operating if I do this. He says that if I had an operation I would still have to rest up for a similar period of time, so I might as well try this first. I'm keen to avoid the knife if I can.'

I was familiar with Professor Logue's views on prolapsed discs and sciatica. Although he was an excellent neurosurgeon he was very conservative and he tried to avoid operating, whereas others would resort to surgery at an earlier stage.

'And just treat me as you would any other patient, Ivan. Put me through a full medical and order any other tests you think may be necessary,' Ian said reassuringly. 'I wouldn't have it any other way.'

So began the patient's enforced rest, aided by regular analgesics and a great pile of books. The good professor's treatment regimen was successful and, as the pain gradually settled, Ian was able to be mobilised and eventually discharged. Few people would opt for such conservative management these days, particularly given the enormous cost of providing hospital beds and the trend towards early postsurgical mobilisation. But it was a convincing demonstration of the old adage 'Time heals'.

There were two neurosurgeons at Maida Vale Hospital during my time there. The senior, Valentine Logue, sported a beautifully coiffured shock of white hair and was every inch the quiet-mannered, deliberate, cautious academic gentleman. His colleague, Lindsey Symon, a quick-moving, charming Scotsman, was the slickest of operators and a consummate technician. They were like chalk and cheese. A neurosurgical registrar told me that if he was ever to have neurosurgery he would like Valentine Logue to diagnose and decide on the operation and Lindsey Symon to operate. One of these two surgeons loved nothing better than to watch motor racing — the Le Mans or Formula One Grand Prix type. And can you guess which one it was? I found it surprising, but it was none other than the pensive professor. This perhaps explains why neurologists and neurosurgeons frequently work closely with their psychological colleagues!

I enjoyed my sojourn at the Maida Vale Hospital for Nervous Diseases. It was like a glimpse into a bygone era, but I was not unhappy when the time came to go back to The Square.

**I FOUND THAT ONE ADVANTAGE** of doing short-term locum registrar positions was that I rotated around most medical firms and thus became known by most of the neurologists at The Square. Another was that I rubbed shoulders with the registrars, sleeping in their quarters when on night duty and eating in their dining room. The junior medical staff had their own dining room, which was rather dingy but sported two chefs. It was said that on the eve of the contentious and much-contested birth of the National Health Service in 1949 there was a hush-hush last-minute agreement. All of the staff on the payrolls of nationalised hospitals would be retained on their same conditions and pay. Having got wind of this, a senior administrator at Queen Square rushed out and lured chefs from top London restaurants with the promise of a feather bed made from the golden goose. Whatever the truth of this rumour, the food at The Square was a cut above that in most hospitals. The standard had no doubt dropped as the infant darling of the National Health Service had matured into a less than charming adult. However, we still had a pretty decent choice, and if we turned our noses up at the meat or fish dish of the day then a chef would always whip us up a tasty omelette or something similar.

One evening I was having dinner in our little dining room at The Square when I found myself sitting next to Erik Claveria, a charming and urbane Englishman whom I liked and admired; a colourful, larger-than-life character. I had mainly seen him from a distance, and I had never really had a chance for a good chat. He looked somewhat like a plumper, sandy-haired version of King George V, complete with the same beard. I guessed he had been to one of England's top private schools, given his self-assurance and tell-tale accent.

'They tell me that you are hoping to get on The House, old chap,' he said affably. 'The House' was in-speak for being a registrar.

'Yes, I am, but I don't like my chances very much.'

'Why not? I can't see any problem,' he said encouragingly.

'As far as I can see there are only two jobs that will become available during the next two years, and I know there are a lot of people waiting around, hoping to get one of them.'

'A couple of years is not long. It will fly by in no time.'

'That's what I'm afraid of, and at the end of it I might have nothing. How long did it take you to get on The House?'

'About seven years, I suppose. I worked at just about every junior medical job there is at The Square, but I had a speech problem which held me back.'

I knew that King George VI had suffered from a bad stutter, but to my knowledge it had not afflicted his father, whose image I was now gazing at.

'A speech problem?' I echoed in surprise. 'You don't seem to have a speech problem. There are times when I would like to have your voice instead of my rough antipodean one. I only have to open my mouth and I get asked which part of Australia I come from. Did you have a speech impediment like the late King George VI, a stutter?'

'Worse than that, old chap. I had a real handicap in the form of my accent. I had a "Spanish handicap".'

'Do you mean you're not English?' I was stunned.

'Not a bit English. I am Spanish. I could speak English quite well. My father was a university professor and he made certain I was fully fluent. But I had a dreadful accent, which included a type of American twang. After being here a while I got the feeling that my accent was holding me back so I began to practise speaking English in front of a mirror every night. I worked at it really hard and I think it helped me in the end. They say that imitation is the sincerest form of flattery, so perhaps the powers that be felt flattered that I had gone to so much trouble. Those who didn't know me before just think this is my normal voice.'

I admired Erik all the more after this revelation, but I knew I didn't have that type of sticking power or the time to spend on this quest. I had a wife and child to support, and yes, another one on the way — child, that is, not wife.

Erik — or as he turned out to be — Lois Erik Claveria Soria, returned to his native Spain to work after he left Queen Square, and there, among the many other things he achieved, he became the mayor of his town.

And me? I did eventually get onto The House. I did not get the first job, which came up only four months after I had arrived in the UK, although I applied. I was shocked to see about 20 candidates at the interview, most of whom just seemed to have emerged out of the woodwork. That job went to a South African, who had been waiting around for longer than me. I was lucky on my next try, however, so that I only had to wait a total of 10 months. One of the good things about being a pessimist is that you get more than your fair share of pleasant surprises in this life.

**THERE WAS A BREATH OF SPRING** in the air, with occasional buds tentatively extending tiny green fingers and a few brave crocuses and snowdrops showing their welcome faces above the firmly packed cold black earth. Pretty little Queen Square was very unusual in that it was home to three separate hospitals. One of these was the picturesque Italian Hospital, which was, like the National, situated on a corner of The Square. As a registrar I was expected to look after any Italian Hospital private patients who were under the care of the neurologists for whom I was then working at the National. Unsurprisingly, this private hospital had been established in bygone days to care for errant Italians who happened to find themselves in the cooler climes of London or who had gone there for treatment. In my day it was largely stacked with ladies and gentlemen in long flowing black or white Arabian robes, who no doubt found the climate even less to their liking. In the 1970s the Middle East had 'discovered' British medicine and, even if the sufferer was not cured, an associated course of retail therapy in London would no doubt provide some relief.

I was overseeing the work of an Iranian neurologist at the time, and he was able to fill me in on some of the quaint little customs that his friends used to ease their distress. They would go to Harrods, Selfridges or some other emporium of note, one that would have fashionable and acceptable brands. Wandering around the establishment, trailed by shop assistants, they would wave at this and that, demanding that multiple items be put onto the ever-mounting heap. When each piece of the vast assemblage had been individually gift-wrapped, they would demand, in the best eastern market fashion, a 40 per cent discount. The apoplectic shop assistants would at first refuse, explaining politely that this was not a bazaar but a 'Maison' of standing and high repute. The department head would then be called, and eventually it might go as far as the manager of the whole store, but always — *always*, I was assured — a compromise would be reached. The discount would usually be 30 per cent, but never less than 25 per cent. We all like a bargain, and this is what is called the 'opiate' way of shopping, as it not only soothes the pain but also gives the spirits quite a lift.

I was impressed that the oil, which lubricated the political cogs, allowed not only princes, sheiks, potentates and the like to seek relief from their ailments but also some of the less well-heeled, including the odd poor villager. I was now on my way to see one of the last-mentioned in order to admit her to hospital and to make sure she was ready for investigations that were scheduled for the next day. I also had to make sure that she was fit for an anaesthetic. I rang the bell at the door of the Italian Hospital and waited somewhat impatiently to be admitted myself. With ward rounds, an x-ray session and outpatients, I was in for a busy day back at the other corner of The Square, and I did not have time to waste. Eventually I heard the door being unlocked, and it swung back to reveal a sweet little nun in habit. She recognised me and beckoned me to enter. I did not really understand why they kept the door locked, but mused that it was probably to stop the likes of her from escaping. I showed her the name of the patient I had come to see. The nun did not speak English, I did not know any Italian, and the patient would not have a clue about either language, so in this *ménage à trois* there was plenty of room for tripartite confusion. Language difficulties, however, were par for the course around here.

The patient, a young Iraqi mother-of-two, who had recently developed epileptic seizures and headaches, was suspected of having a brain tumour. She was lying in her bed talking to her concerned-looking husband. Sitting next to them was a woman I recognised. It was my lucky day. They had brought a translator, and a good one at that, so this little job might not take me as long as I had feared. Even so, allowing for questions and responses going back and forth via the translator, it took a good three-quarters of an hour before I managed to extract an adequate medical history. I closed the hospital case notes and opened my little black bag of tricks, signalling that we were now moving on to the next phase.

'I would now like to examine the patient,' I told the translator, who passed this information down the line to Almas and her husband, Ma'bood. This provoked a stunned look on Almas's face and one of extreme agitation on that of Ma'bood. They conversed volubly in machine-gun Arabic, and then Ma'bood rose to his feet, his arms flailing like those of a drowning man. His swarthy face had darkened with what I took to be either embarrassment or anger, I was not sure which.

'Ma'bood says he doesn't want you to examine his wife,' the translator explained. 'Almas has uncovered her face for you, and they feel that this has been embarrassment enough. They have been told that the problem is in her brain and they will agree to you examining her head, but nothing else.'

'Could you please explain to them that I need to examine Almas's body and her arms and legs to make certain that she does not have a problem anywhere else? Perhaps an illness or sickness is concealed there, which has spread to her head and has caused the epileptic attacks that she has had. In addition, I need to make certain that she is well enough to undergo the tests that are booked for her. I also need to see if there are any other tests that she might require and to be sure that she is fit to have an anaesthetic, should this become necessary.'

After more rapid Arabic a relieved look spread across the couple's faces, Almas spread out her hands towards Ma'bood and he put his right hand to his chest, smiling as he did so.

'He says that it is now perfectly all right and they are happy. He knows that she is fit for an anaesthetic, or anything else for that matter. He is willing for you to examine him instead.'

I shrugged my shoulders and looked skywards. 'Ask Ma'bood if Almas's pulse is regular, what is her blood pressure, whether she has any heart murmurs, or whether a kidney is enlarged. These are the sorts of things that I need to know and that he cannot tell me. Nor can I find these out by examining Ma'bood. You will be with me to translate for her, and naturally he is welcome to stay if he wants to be here.'

After further good work by the translator the couple acquiesced to my request, but only on the condition that I kept my eyes averted while examining Almas's chest and palpating her abdomen. This I readily agreed to and the whole examination went off uneventfully, although the husband looked relieved when I had finished. I was able to inform them that, happily, Ma'bood had been absolutely correct and that the problem seemed confined to Almas's head. Everything else was perfectly normal. I thanked them profusely for being so helpful and cooperative when I knew that they must be feeling very stressed and worried.

Hurrying back to the National through The Square, across which Almas would come the following day on a stretcher for her angiogram and other tests, I glanced up at the threatening clouds that were now blowing in on a cold northwest wind. Her trip would not be a lot of fun if it was raining heavily. Meanwhile the delay caused by their reluctance to agree to her examination had cost me dearly. I was late for the outpatient clinic and I had not had a chance to write up Almas's hospital records. It was late in the evening and raining heavily when I again rang the bell to gain admission to the Italian Hospital to finish my job.

Fortunately, Almas was found to have a large but benign tumour, a meningioma, pressing on her brain and it was able to be removed successfully. The happy couple returned to their little Middle Eastern village where no doubt they regaled their neighbours with tales of their adventures in a foreign land, but I suspect they would have omitted the part about the cheeky young doctor who insisted on examining Almas. They were lucky to have such an apparently benevolent government.

**THE TRAFFIC IN MEDICAL OPINIONS** was not all one-way, and on occasions even busy Harley Street consultants were generous enough to donate their valuable time and expertise by flying to the Middle East where they would make difficult diagnoses, initiate daring new treatments and enlighten the locals. Jay, my astute, swarthy, good-looking Iranian house officer, had trained in neurology in Teheran, where he had worked with some of the best specialists in the country. I am sure that Jay was not his real name, but I am ashamed to say that I never found out what this nickname stood for. He was a mine of information on all things Middle Eastern, and was prepared to freely share his opinions and experiences with me, possibly because Chris, Matthew and I had travelled through the Middle East on our way to London and had spent some time in Iran.

'One thing that I dislike about home is the fact that it takes so long to get anything done,' he complained exasperatedly over a luncheon bowl of soup.

'What do you mean?' I asked.

'It's all this bargaining. It's so time-consuming.'

'I thought it was only the tourists who had to bargain.'

'Not a bit of it. When my wife and I were living in Teheran we had to bargain for absolutely everything. We had to bargain for every vegetable and piece of meat in the market. We even had to bargain for our bread each day, although we had been buying it from the same baker for years. We all knew what it was worth, but he would try to overcharge us and we would have to go through this charade every morning. He would tell us the price of flour and wood and how he had to support his elderly parents, his wife and four children. We would have to say that we knew the real price of bread and that we could not afford any more. You couldn't do any shopping quickly.'

'And what about medical practice in Iran?' I asked. 'Is there any bargaining in that?'

'Not so much bargaining, more discussion of fees, which can be somewhat flexible, depending on circumstances. But I'm talking about the local doctors, not overseas specialists. You can't quibble with them. It is not often that the patients really need the opinion of an overseas consultant, but sometimes the rich insist because they think the locals aren't good enough.'

'Oh,' I said, trying to sound more interested than I was, 'what do you mean?'

'To give an example,' Jay continued, 'just before I left Teheran we had an elderly but important government minister who developed weakness of the right side and confusion. He had had poorly controlled hypertension for many years, and it was thought that he may have suffered a stroke due to hardening and blockage of the arteries. A well-known neurologist was flown out from London. He agreed that the diagnosis was typical of a blockage of the middle cerebral artery. It was his opinion that, apart from rehabilitation and lowering the patient's high blood pressure, there was nothing else that could be done. Part of the deal was that the consultant had to be paid in cash. He arrived in the morning and left for Zurich that night, carrying a case full of Swiss francs.'

'Really!' I exclaimed. 'But I suppose it was worth it just to satisfy the patient's family and colleagues that you had got the best opinion and done everything that was possible,' I added, trying to be conciliatory and to justify the apparently mercenary attitude of a member of the profession that we were aspiring to join.

'But wait, there's more to the tale,' Jay replied with a bitter edge to his voice. 'During the following days the patient continued to worsen, so in spite of his age and fragile condition we decided to ignore the advice and we performed an angiogram.'

'Well?' I enquired, now sitting forward expectantly.

'It showed a large subdural haematoma!' Jay exclaimed triumphantly.

The subdural (epidural) space lies immediately beneath the dura mata, a leathery membrane that separates the inside of the skull and spinal canal from the delicate arachnoid membrane that covers the surface of the brain and spinal cord. Normally this space is empty, except for a few delicate veins that cross it, passing between the skull and the brain. This is why it is called a 'potential space'. A blow on the head can cause one or more of these veins to bleed and this is particularly likely to occur in the elderly, in whom the precipitation can be a trivial knock. The slow build-up of blood compresses the underlying brain and, if left untreated, may squeeze it to death.

'And what happened?'

'A local neurosurgeon operated and released the blood. The old man made a rapid and complete recovery, much to the delight of all.'

'One to the home side and 0 to the visiting team?' I suggested.

'Definitely!' Jay agreed with a satisfied grin. 'But the "visitors" were a team of one, and I have to admit that usually the score is the other way around.'

**THERE WERE TWO OR THREE** younger consultant neurologists at The Square who were fluent in Arabic, but the older brigade, who had done most of the consulting in the Middle Eastern countries and the Maghreb up until that point, did not speak the language. Amongst the latter was Dennis Williams, a charming little man who was a great raconteur with an impish sense of humour. He had been a consultant to the rich and famous and, given that international statistics show one in six people can be expected to develop a neurological disorder, he had been kept very busy. Dennis was one of the more senior neurologists and liked nothing better than to talk of his experiences when we stopped the ward round for a tea break in the office.

'There is a difficulty in knowing what to charge the excessively rich,' he said one afternoon, sipping his cuppa and happily munching a biscuit. 'You must not charge them too little or they will be insulted and they will certainly believe that you are not much good at your job. On the other hand, to ask for a large amount of money may seem rather mercenary and inappropriate.'

'How do you manage to get the right balance, Dr Williams?' I asked. At that moment I had a very definite feeling that I would not mind seeming mercenary and inappropriate if it significantly increased my modest National Health Service salary.

'Well, take the case of King Idris,' he mused.

I started sieving through the nerve cells in my grey matter, trying to recollect the regal gent, and I was just about to ask who he was when Dennis, who was starting to warm to his subject, continued.

'I happened to do a little job for him. He was extremely grateful and I was asked what I would like in return for my services. Not by the king himself, you understand, but by one of his minions, a minister of this and that. We discussed what might be right and proper given the circumstances. We agreed that it would be rude to ask for money and that a gift of some sort would be more appropriate. Kings are used to giving and receiving gifts from all sorts of visitors. You see, it's much more personal than just doling out money.'

I did see, and indicated as much by nodding my head enthusiastically. This was starting to get interesting.

'I had been giving it some thought, even before I was approached by the minister, so when he asked me if I had anything in particular that I would like I said that I was a simple man at heart and I had a love of nature. Some little living and growing thing would provide me with great satisfaction and be a constant reminder of the generosity and nobility of His Highness.'

'But a plant would seem such a tiny, inconsequential gift,' the minister objected, in a way that Dennis had already foreseen. 'Surely, we must do more than that?'

'Well,' acquiesced Dennis, 'perhaps you are correct. I will accept the King's generous offer to be more bountiful. Perhaps I could have my little garden in London landscaped. Would that be suitable?'

And so it was decided. Dennis would have his not insubstantial 'little' garden landscaped, and he would organise it himself as he knew someone personally who would do a decent job. It would be paid for by the embassy in London.

A top landscape artist was employed and the work was progressing very satisfactorily when one morning, while Dennis was having an early breakfast, a little news item on the radio caught his attention. King Idris had just been overthrown in a bloodless coup and a little-known colonel, Muammar Gaddafi, had taken control of Libya. Dennis seized the telephone and called the landscape artist.

'I need the invoice, the total invoice for the landscape work that is to be completed in my garden, and I need it immediately!' he commanded.

'But the work is not finished and there may be additional expenses that we haven't thought of,' the artist spluttered.

'Make allowance for them and have the invoice ready within 30 minutes, when somebody will be calling for it. Have it ready or you won't be paid!'

Dennis then called his private medical secretary, who had just arrived at work in central London, and instructed her to leave straight away, go and get the invoice and take it to the Libyan Embassy. She was not to leave without a cheque for the total amount, which she was then to take directly to Dennis's bank, insisting that it be cleared immediately. In the meantime, he tried desperately to speak to his bank manager and to the diplomat with whom he had been dealing at the embassy.

'Did it work?' I asked excitedly, having become quite caught up in this little saga.

'It did. It was the first and last cheque that the embassy wrote after the coup. You see, there was confusion in Tripoli that morning, resulting in a delay in the embassy receiving instructions. A little later all financial transactions were suspended.'

Dennis paused a moment and then continued. 'But perhaps most of all I enjoyed going to Ethiopia. They always used to send one of Haile Selassie's own limousines to the airport to pick me up. It would be flying the Emperor's own standard. The people regarded him, the so-called Lion of Judah, as being next to God. All the way from the airport at Addis Ababa to the palace, everyone in the street would prostrate themselves in the dust as the car went past and it would only be little old me sitting in the back seat. Naturally, I would always give them a cheery wave,' he said, smiling, a faraway look in his eyes. I suspected that his pale visage would not have fooled anybody if they had dared to look up from their terrestrial position.

'Well,' he said, 'I guess we had better get back to work. There are still patients to be seen.'

**'I HAD TO GO TO ETHIOPIA** at the weekend,' said a pleased-looking Peter, a wide grin on his face, 'and you need to know about it, Ivan Donaldson.'

I liked Peter. He was a plump, larger-than-life character with a booming voice, tousled black hair, a commanding presence and a generosity of spirit, and he brimmed with self-assurance. It was a Monday morning and I had just met him on my way into the hospital. Being a senior registrar he was a notch up in rank on me.

'Why was that, Peter?' I asked, full of curiosity tinged with envy. This sounded like a real adventure.

'Your boss asked me to accompany him out there. We flew over and back in a private jet. He had been asked to go and see a leading politician who had collapsed suddenly. He had suffered an apoplexy. This man had virtually run Ethiopia single-handedly for Haile Selassie at one stage after there had been political unrest. We thought we would need to bring him back, and we took an anaesthetist with us in case his airway became obstructed or he needed resuscitating. He has a dense right hemiplegia and is aphasic. We suspect he has had a left cerebral hemisphere haemorrhage. It seems to be very common out there and, like him, a lot of people in Ethiopia have hypertension. He's in the private ward. You had better go and see him before the ward round.'

Our Ethiopian patient was indeed completely paralysed on his right side and was unable to talk, although he did seem to understand a little of what was said to him. Investigations proved the diagnosis to be correct. He made very slow progress and it was clear he would be left severely disabled.

A little before this, Haile Selassie's son, the Crown Prince and heir to be, had suffered an almost identical stroke and had been left with severe right-sided weakness and a major speech problem. He could say 'yes' and 'no' but often got these words around the wrong way. This was not a promising situation for a future head of state, particularly in a country with a history of insurrection and a rebellious army. It may have been a little unkind and disrespectful, but the junior medical staff referred to him as 'the half-crown Prince'.

Such tragic neurological events become even more poignant when they affect a loved one, as I was to experience many years later when one of my brothers had a similar, but right-sided haemorrhage in his brain when he was in his fifties and suffered severe left-sided paralysis. Fortunately, as in his case, right-sided brain haemorrhage usually spares speech.

These haemorrhages had all occurred deep within the cerebral hemispheres, those two massive lobes of the brain, one on the left and one on the right. These are responsible for consciousness, thinking, behaviour, memory, voluntary movement and appreciation of sensation, among other things. The deep areas, where the bleeding had occurred, connect the cerebral hemispheres to the brain stem and spinal cord, and they are also vital for motor activity and sensation as well as a variety of other functions. As we will see, these deep structures are part of what has been called the 'basement of the brain'.

**IT WAS DURING OUR FIRST YEAR IN LONDON** and we were still ensconced in our basement flat in Hampstead when I arrived home one night to find Chris bubbling with excitement.

'Great news! We've just received a letter from Larry and Prue. They want to come and stay with us. Larry is looking for an O and G job in London, and they need a base for a week or so after they arrive so that they can find a flat and get themselves established. We could move Matthew into our bedroom and they could have the other one.'

'Fine,' I replied. 'It'll be great to see them again. We'll need to check it out with Mr and Mrs Upstairs, but I don't think there will be any problem.'

Larry had been in my class at medical school and we had been in adjacent rooms when we lived in at Christchurch Hospital during our sixth and final year. He was a charming, outgoing, generous person and we had been good friends. Even at that time, when most in our class had no professional ambition beyond graduating, he had declared his inclination and intention to become an obstetrician and gynaecologist. Then we had been single and fancy-free. Now things were serious. We were married men with families to support and career paths to climb. Larry had already done a good deal of obstetrics and gynaecology training as a registrar, and he would no doubt be trying to land a plum job. It would be great to catch up and renew our friendship.

Putting up new arrivals was common amongst the expat Kiwi community in London. Chris, Matthew and I, in our turn, had earlier dossed down in a small flat with Chris's brother Brent and his wife, Moira, until we got ourselves on our feet. Conveniently, Brent was doing paediatric training at The Hospital for Sick Children in Great Ormond Street, which backed directly onto the National and he lived only two blocks from Queen Square.

Larry was a man of action, but he allowed himself one day of rest after he and his family arrived on our doorstep, having flown directly from the other side of the world. Like us, he did not seem to believe in jetlag and immediately started to comb the medical journals and to telephone agencies looking for a suitable job, in between searching for a flat.

'Look at this,' he shouted excitedly one evening, waving the latest copy of the *British Medical Journal* above his head. 'It looks just the thing for me.'

We all crowded around for a look.

'There!' he said triumphantly, jabbing at the page with his finger. 'Doesn't it sound perfect? It's too late to apply today, so I'll get onto it first thing tomorrow morning.'

*VACANT*
*TOP LONDON OBSTETRIC CLINIC*
*Registrars wanted.*
*Previous experience required*
*but training will be provided.*
*Excellent salary and conditions.*
*Apply ........................*

We all agreed that it sounded promising. That issue of the *British Medical Journal* had only come out that day, but surely there would be a rush of applicants. If he was quick, however, Larry might stand a chance. We retired to bed that night with high hopes for our friend's rapid ascent up the O and G training ladder. It all seemed too good to be true.

I was eager to get home the following evening to find out how Larry had got on with his enquiries and doubtless application. I knew he would interview well, so that if he was shortlisted he would make a good impression. I had bought a special bottle of wine in anticipation of a celebration. When I entered our small lounge Larry and Prue were slumped on the couch, gazing out of the French doors onto the small garden with its neatly trimmed lawn encased by bright flower beds. All was quiet. The children were already in bed, and Chris was sitting opposite Larry and Prue reading.

Sensing that the mood was not entirely festive, I asked hesitantly, 'How did it go? Was there still a vacant position?'

'Yes, and it may stay vacant for some time,' Larry replied dispiritedly.

'Why? Are they particularly fussy? I suppose that if they are one of the top O and G clinics in London they can afford to pick and choose, but with your background I would have thought they would have snapped you up.'

'Top clinic, my foot … TOP clinic! Yes, Termination Of Pregnancy. That's what it meant. That's all they do there: abortions. They were keen for me to apply, but I have not come to London just to do abortions. I intend to round out my training by getting broad experience of obstetrics and gynaecology and not get stuck doing terminations.'

We stared at each other for a few seconds, and then we all burst out laughing.

'Don't worry, Larry,' Prue said gently, patting her husband's hand. 'We have really only just arrived in London. I'm sure you will get a good job quite easily.'

And that is what he did.

**'MAD DOGS AND ENGLISHMEN** go out in the midday sun', Noel Coward wrote in his 1931 hit tune. He should have known, because he is said to have composed the words and music to the song in his head, without the aid of pen, paper or piano, while driving from Hanoi to Saigon. While he may have had a roof over his head, he must surely have been in a lather of sweat as the steamy jungle passed by, given that it was before the era of air-conditioning. Doubtless Coward had accurately diagnosed the state of mind of any stray dogs that he saw wandering in the sunlight and was regretting the stubborn cultural attitudes of his countrymen, who did not partake of that most delightful of hot-climate rituals, the siesta.

You would think that when the mercury soared and he could cook an egg in his pith helmet the English gent would relent, but no, it was just not the done thing to retreat. Perhaps it was the prospect of a midday meal with one's wife or mistress, washed down with a glass or two of wine, followed by the inevitable retirement to bed that was so frightfully un-British. Whatever the reason, any native of hot climes knows that he has a God-given right to the siesta and, like the dog that totters down the noonday street, anyone who does not take it is clearly crazy. Such a mad dog is not only unpredictable, but is so aggressive that it may even bite the beloved hand that feeds it.

Ronald Reagan once referred to Libya's Colonel Gaddafi as the 'Mad Dog of the Middle East'. Given the latter's behaviour, this epithet seems deadly accurate, for we are not talking about a pampered poodle that gets the huff because it cannot sit on its mistress's lap at its favourite restaurant, a schizophrenic schnauzer with both smiling and snarling sides to its personality, or even a neurotic nipper. No, a really mad dog should not be approached because it is like a suicide bomber. It is not only doomed itself, but it may destroy others in its date with death. A really mad dog has rabies. In fact, the term 'rabies' comes from the Latin word for madness.

Fortunately, by enforcing strict quarantine regulations and pursuing eradication programmes, islands like Britain, New Zealand, Japan and Singapore are rabies-free, but the disease is present in many other similar countries and on all continents except Australia. It is infrequent in most of the developed world, but not uncommon in many third-world countries. Rabies is usually contracted through a bite wound and it can infect a variety of mammals, including foxes and bats, but humans usually catch rabies from man's best friend.

'A patient has been admitted to the Batten Unit with probable rabies,' a fellow registrar informed me one morning. 'I thought you would like to know. He's called Douglas Smyth and I think he's a Kiwi. He's been working in Africa and was nipped on the lip by a puppy a couple of months back. He has just been flown here for treatment, but his prospects don't look too good.'

The Batten Unit was the National Hospital's intensive-care unit and was used particularly for patients with potential or established respiratory difficulty.

'Thanks,' I replied. 'I'll follow his progress with great interest.' If he wasn't immunised before or straight after the nip, then it wouldn't be too promising, no matter how small or playful the pup might have been.

Most people have a reasonable knowledge of meningitis, which is an inflammation of the cerebrospinal fluid and the meninges, the membranes that cover the brain and spinal cord. Meningitis can be due to infection by a virus or bacteria, with the latter generally being much more serious. Less well known are the entities of encephalitis (inflammation of the brain) and myelitis (inflammation of the spinal cord). They sometimes occur together, in which case they are referred to as encephalomyelitis. They are usually the result of a viral infection. Occasionally a common virus may cause an allergic reaction in the white (leuco-) matter of the brain and/or spinal cord of a particular individual, whereas it might produce only a mild respiratory infection in most of us. This would be called a leuco-encephalitis and it damages principally the electrically insulating sheaths around nerve fibres. These sheaths are composed of myelin, a white fatty material. Certain sorts of viruses, however, can directly infect and damage or kill the nerve cell bodies that form the grey (polio-) matter. This would be called a polioencephalitis. Poliomyelitis is a virus that principally infects the motor nerve cells (grey matter) of the spinal cord and the brain stem, which connects the spinal cord with the cerebral hemispheres. Rabies is a particularly nasty virus that enters the nerve fibres in the area of the bite and then spreads up the fibres into the nerve cells of both the brain and the spinal cord causing a polio-encephalo-myelitis.

Prevention is better than cure, and nowhere is this adage more applicable than with rabies. Because it is due to a virus, antibiotics are completely ineffective against it. As with many viral diseases, prophylactic immunisation before the virus attack is best. Second best is to start immunisation immediately after the bite and before symptoms have developed. It was seven weeks before Douglas developed his first symptoms, a period during which he was blissfully unaware of the gravity of his situation, which had arisen from such an apparently trivial event. It was a further three days before he could be immunised in Africa.

The first symptoms of rabies tend to be non-specific, with a temperature, chills, headache, tiredness and a sore throat. Most patients then develop 'furious rabies' in which they become agitated, aggressive and delusional with hallucinations. They may lash out at and, like a mad dog, try to bite others. A striking feature can be hydrophobia or fear of water. A sight, a sound or even a mention of fluid can precipitate panic and produce painful spasms in the throat. A minority have 'dumb' or 'paralytic' rabies in which they develop severe muscular weakness from the onset rather than being overexcited, but even those with furious rabies eventually become paralysed. Douglas had 'furious rabies' with hydrophobia. Most deaths from rabies are due to failure of the respiratory muscles or the heart. There had been virtually no recorded cases of survival of patients in whom treatment had been delayed until after the onset of symptoms, as in Douglas's case.

At that time, however, it was considered that some of the damage to the nervous system resulted from swelling and inflammation, particularly of the brain, rather than direct destruction of the nerve cells by the virus. It was hypothesised that if the swelling and inflamation could be controlled and the victim was kept on life support for long enough, then possibly his body could eventually overcome the infection and he might make a reasonable recovery.

Some months earlier I had been in a busy outpatient clinic when I received a frantic telephone call from a newly qualified American neurologist who was expanding his horizons by doing some additional training at Queen Square. Sam was a serious but instantly likeable, freckly-faced young man with closely cropped straight red hair that not unsurprisingly defied his every attempt to plaster it to his scalp with liberal quantities of hair oil. Just that morning he had been attached to my firm to act as an additional house officer and general rouseabout. Sam had received a thorough training in New York and he had a good theoretical knowledge, but he lacked clinical experience, hence his attachment at the National.

'Ivan, I thought I should tell you that Mr Robertson is having trouble breathing so I have intubated him and alerted the intensive-care unit. They have a respirator available so I'll bag him until we get there.'

'Mr Robertson!'

'Yes, you know — the old man with the ALS,' Sam replied, mistaking my exclamation for a question.

I knew Geoffrey Robertson very well. Tragically, at 55 years of age he was terminally ill with motor neurone disease, or MND as we were used to calling it; the British reserved the name amyotrophic lateral sclerosis, or ALS, for one particular type of MND, contrary to the practice in the US. The cause of MND was, and still is, unknown. The motor neurones throughout the nervous system gradually die and disappear, which results in progressive weakness and eventual paralysis of all muscles, including those that are responsible for talking, breathing and swallowing. There is no effective treatment that can alter the course of the disease, which from first symptoms to death typically takes two to three years.

Geoffrey's course had been entirely typical, and it had progressed to the stage where he could no longer breathe effectively for himself. He had been due to be transferred to a hospice where he could end his days in peace and quiet surrounded by his family. Sam, however, had now skilfully placed a tube into Geoffrey's windpipe and was rhythmically squeezing a self-reinflating rubber bag to ventilate his lungs. Like many of Sam's compatriots he had come up through a system in which no expense was spared and he had been taught that preservation of life was paramount, seemingly without regard for quality.

Placed on a respirator, such unfortunates may eventually live long enough to lose all ability to communicate, even by moving the eyes or opening and closing them, although they may still be conscious, surely a fate far worse than death.

'Sam,' I said, 'the approach to the management of terminal motor neurone disease is rather different here from that which sometimes occurs in the United States. We know that the motor neurones have been largely destroyed and our main concern is to minimise suffering rather than just prolong life. The situation has been fully discussed with the patient and his next-of-kin. They do not want us to do anything to unnecessarily prolong Geoffrey's life. I'm afraid I'll have to get you to remove the intubation tube and tell the intensive-care unit that the patient won't be coming.'

Unlike Geoffrey, Douglas Smyth had a possibility of recovery. So began his intensive care with all the skill, meticulous attention to detail and dedicated medical, nursing and paramedical teamwork that a long period of total life support demands. For 24 hours a day, seven days a week, breathing was done by machine, food and fluids administered artificially, bladder drained, blood tests monitored, body regularly repositioned to prevent bedsores, skin, mouth and eye care given and intercurrent bacterial infections, which are the inevitable bugbear of the immobile, were treated. In short, he had all of the things done that were necessary to support his body, and all that was possible to treat his infection and inflamed brain.

But what about his brain? How was that getting on? When a brain-damaged patient is put onto life support, sedation is often necessary to control agitation and help reduce intracranial pressure. As time progresses the need for this lessens. When sedation is eventually withdrawn, the reappearance of restlessness is an encouraging sign, signalling ongoing function in the nervous system. Douglas, however, remained ominously immobile and his electroencephalogram or brainwave test showed no evidence of cerebral activity, much to the distress of all. Eventually, it was concluded that he was not only brain-dead but that there was absolutely no evidence of neurological function, even in his spinal cord or peripheral nerves. When, a month after he had started intensive care, he was disconnected from his respirator, he was unable to breathe for himself and death was inevitable.

An autopsy revealed the dreadful truth. Not only had the motor neurones disappeared, as will occur in MND, but nowhere in his body was there a surviving nerve cell to be found. The dreaded rabies virus, which even today kills over 50,000 people annually throughout the world, had claimed yet another victim, and because of the skilful care and attention that Douglas had been given the virus had been free to destroy his entire nervous system! What a bitter disappointment.

**'WHAT ON EARTH DO YOU THINK** you are doing dressed up like that, Dr Haas?' the consultant asked sternly. 'Have you absolutely no sense of standards of dress? Are you wearing any pants under your white coat?'

Lindsay's white clinical coat finished a little above his knees, while a pair of long fawn-coloured socks ended at mid-calf, exposing a stretch of pale hairy flesh in between. While admittedly perhaps not the most attractive of sights, it was not an uncommon one in hospitals around Australia and New Zealand during summer, where the dress code was somewhat more relaxed than at the National.

'It's such a hot day, sir,' Lindsay stammered, 'that I thought I would be all right in this.'

It was indeed hot, to the point of being sweltering. The mercury had been hovering at a little over 30°C for several days and, combined with high humidity, had made the un-air-conditioned hospital stifling.

'Well you are not! Go and change into something respectable and don't show your face again until you are decently dressed.'

'But I have got shorts on under my white coat, sir.'

'Dr Haas, I don't care even if you are wearing a grass skirt and you are prepared to give us an animated performance of your national anthem, the haka. You are not at the beach. This is a prestigious hospital in London and there is a standard below which we will not allow ourselves to be dragged. Come back when you're properly attired, and don't be too long about it!'

'I'm dreadfully sorry, sir,' said a remorseful Lindsay as he began to make a hasty exit.

As he reached the door he was pursued by an irate voice that continued to thunder: 'The next thing you know he will be coming in here with cow manure on his boots!'

It was one of the things that I liked about Lindsay; he was always prepared to tell a story against himself and to laugh it off. We agreed that it was difficult for us 'colonials' from down under to know what was acceptable and what was not. It was best to tread cautiously. When I first arrived in London I found the medical hierarchy's 'uniform' rather formal. The days of black frock-coats and top hats had disappeared to be replaced by the dark-coloured three-piece pinstripe suit. Some of the accessories, however, appeared to me to be rather flashy and cheap. The patent leather shoes with shining gold buckles, the brightly coloured matching tie and pocket handkerchief, and the tightly rolled black umbrella all appeared old worldly and overdone. But after just a few months of living in London they seemed perfectly normal. In fact, they became the preferred items of attire and a style to be mimicked. The disadvantage of this uniform, however, was that it was decidedly uncomfortable in hot weather; fortunately, this was not something that proved to be a bother very often.

One of the consultants for whom I worked was a very dapper little man in his sixties, with white hair and fashionable dark-rimmed spectacles. He always wore the three-piece black pinstripe, the highly polished black shoes, and the matching accessories. On one of the all too infrequent hot summer days he greeted me cheerily as I arrived to accompany him on a ward round of his patients. He had been sitting at the ward office desk, writing. I had a feeling that there was something unusual about him, and as he rose to join me I realised what it was. He was sporting Roman sandals and bright yellow socks. Naturally the socks matched his tie and handkerchief.

The picture of this charmingly eccentric Englishman's concession to summer could only have been improved by a knotted yellow handkerchief on his head. The other consultant neurologists whom we met in the hospital showed no sign that anything was amiss and made no mention of this little break with tradition, but I noticed that one or two of them gazed after us when we continued on our merry way. Perhaps they were wishing they had the courage to do something similar.

**NEUROLOGY IS UNUSUAL AMONG** medical specialties in that rare things occur commonly. That is to say, a considerable proportion of a neurologist's work consists of helping patients with disorders that are individually rare but together make up a significant proportion of the working week. Because the National Hospital at Queen Square was a tertiary referral hospital, patients with difficult neurological problems were referred there from regional and other London teaching hospitals. Hence, by working there it was possible to gain experience of a wide range of rare conditions in a relatively short time, something that would have taken a lifetime working in a general medical hospital. The training was thus excellent. Most of the consultant neurologists were astute clinicians, pleasant, helpful, good teachers and fine role models. Neurologists, however, by the very analytical nature of their specialty, tend to be rather obsessive and like things well done, a trait that Chris delights in pointing out to me. A good example of a man with such an affliction was Shaun McArdle.

Dr McArdle was, reluctantly, nearing retiring age when I worked for him.

He was a plump little man with thinning sandy grey hair, a twinkle in his eye and a ready smile. Like most consultant neurologists at The Square he had an additional appointment at another hospital, so that he only worked at the National part-time. On the days that he was there he spent the morning working in the outpatient clinic. At 2 p.m. he would start teaching the postgraduate students who had enrolled for neurology courses at the hospital. I would have to arrange for three patients, with conditions that were interesting or difficult to diagnose, for him to teach on. His manner with these people and the students was open and friendly, just as he dealt with his own patients. He would talk with them, joke with them, lay a friendly hand on their shoulders, or perhaps pat their hands in empathy. Physical contact was important to help him develop a rapport and express concern, sincerity and sympathy. Unfortunately, today such behaviour has become liable to misinterpretation and is perhaps no longer 'politically correct'. Medicine has become the worse for this loss of friendly contact.

At 4 p.m. Dr McArdle would return to the outpatient department to dictate letters to the referring doctors of the patients he had seen in the morning. There was a highly secret, unwritten instruction in the hospital that was handed down from one generation of registrars to the next. Thus, at 6 p.m. precisely, I would pick up the telephone and dial the number of Dr McArdle's outpatient room. I would let the phone ring twice then hang up. A few minutes later the gentleman himself, often yawning and looking as though he had just woken up, would appear to start his ward round.

Now, being of an obsessive bent, Dr McArdle's ward rounds were never short, because every single fact that the house officer and registrar had recorded in the hospital case notes had to be verified. The round would not usually finish until 8 or even 9 p.m. But no, the day was not then over, for at that stage the dear doctor would, as like as not, do an injection for trigeminal neuralgia, also known as tic doloureux. This condition, which causes excruciatingly severe stabbing pains on one side of the face, could usually be controlled by tablets although it sometimes required surgery. But in a small number of patients it was best treated by an injection that permanently numbed part or the whole of one side of the face. The hypodermic needle had to be slipped into the cheek and advanced into a small canal at the base of the skull, where the nerve and ganglion that supply sensation to the face emerge from the brain. It is tricky to get the needle into the right place, even with x-ray guidance, but Dr McArdle did not use x-rays. He was the recognised expert in this procedure and he had referrals from all over Britain. I would have to assist him with the procedure.

Now, unfortunately, Shaun McArdle had a neurological condition himself, one called essential tremor. This meant his hands shook uncontrollably when he tried to do anything fine or delicate, or even when he just held them out in front of him. This little affliction did not inspire great confidence in the patients who were having these injections, especially as the very long and generously wide hypodermic needle approached their cheek, a little below the eye. A sudden shriek from some terrified little lady was absolutely the worst thing that could happen, as Dr McArdle was prone to jump or jerk in fright. Hence he warned the unfortunate victims that they were not to make a sound, which had the effect of winding up their overactive nervous systems by several more notches.

These were always tense times and part of my job was to wipe my boss's sweating forehead, and possibly that of the patient. The amazing thing, however, is that just as the wildly gyrating razor-sharp needle was about to inadvertently slice into the face or eye it would freeze in mid-air and he would gently slide it into the cheek, advancing it steadily until it found that little canal buried deep below the base of the skull. In the many such procedures that I saw him perform he never missed once.

But no, it was not just a matter of giving an injection then going home. Dr McArdle next administered a tiny dose of local anaesthetic and then, using a pin, he mapped out on the patient's face the area of numbness that this injection had produced. He then gradually moved the needle, injecting further tiny amounts of local anaesthetic until he found and injected the exact part of the nerve that corresponded to the focal area of the face where the severe pain started. The troublesome region of the patient's face would then be numb. But this local anaesthesia would only be transient so we then had to wait for another half or three-quarters of an hour for this numbness to wear off and for the sensation on the patient's face to return to normal. All this time the hypodermic needle was resting in the same place in the nerve and the fully conscious patient had indeed to be patient. At this stage the final injection, which would kill that part of the nerve, would be given and the corresponding area of the face would become permanently numb. Only when that was done could we pack up and go home. Usually it was quite late at night, and there were times I was anxious that I might miss the last train home. And what was injected into the nerve? It was pure alcohol!

Dear Dr Shaun, however, must have been tiring and winding down by the time I worked for him. A younger consultant neurologist, for whom I had also been a registrar, assured me that in Dr McArdle's heyday he regularly did not finish his ward rounds until close to midnight, so that patients were often awakened from sleep in order to be examined. On one occasion this neurologist, who had also been Dr McArdle's registrar, had seen him sitting on one of the ward lavatories testing a patient's vision at 2 a.m., because it was the only place where there was sufficient illumination without putting on the ward lights and awakening the 20 or so other patients! It seems unlikely that such idiosyncratic behaviour would be tolerated these days.

**'GOSH! JUST LOOK AT THAT!** You can see the gyri and sulci of the cerebral hemispheres, and there are the lateral ventricles; they look normal in size and in the right position. You can even see the third ventricle in this lower slice. The pineal gland stands out like a sore thumb due to the calcium in it. The cerebellum is clearly visible, and the brain stem. There's no sign of blood, a mass, or displacement of any part of the brain.'

We were looking at one of the very first computerised axial tomographic (CAT or CT) brain scans to be taken at the National, which was the third hospital in the world to have a CT machine installed. The middle-aged woman whose scan we were looking at had been admitted that morning, having suffered excruciating headaches for several days, something that was completely out of character for her. She had suffered a nasty bang on the head several weeks earlier and it had been suggested by the referring doctor from the nearby teaching hospital that she might be suffering from a subdural blood clot that would need surgery. However, we could see immediately that there was no sign of a clot or any other sort of lump inside the patient's skull and that her brain did not seem swollen or in any way deformed.

'We will need to do a lumbar puncture on Mrs Savage to make sure she does not have meningitis, as she does have a low-grade fever. When you do this be careful to straighten her legs out and make sure she is breathing normally so that you can measure the cerebral spinal fluid pressure accurately,' I told the house officer. 'We still need to make a diagnosis so that we know how to treat her.'

The CT scan we had been looking at was grainy, blurred and showed little of the internal anatomy of the brain compared with those produced by the more sophisticated machines that were to follow. Yet it was strikingly clear to all of us that we were witnessing an amazing revolution in neurology and neurosurgery. For the first time it was possible to view the form of the brain in a living person without subjecting them to unpleasant and potentially hazardous procedures. At last you could go to bed feeling confident that during the night your patient was not liable to succumb to the brain being squeezed from one compartment to another inside the skull or from the skull into the spinal canal, like toothpaste being forced out of a tube.

The CT scan had been developed to solve the type of problem that Mrs Savage presented. Its ingenious inventors had created it to show the inside of the head. It was only later that this technology was applied to other parts of the body. The same was true of magnetic resonance imaging (MRI), which subsequently took scanning of the nervous system to a level that was previously unimaginable to a simple clinical neurologist like me. Looking back, I feel privileged to have been there during these early stages of the technology.

So what tools were available to neurologists in the pre-CT days? First and foremost, we had the clinical skills to take a reliable history and perform a detailed physical examination that allowed us to localise the site and determine the nature of the patient's problem. In fact, at the beginning of the twentieth century this was all that neurologists and neurosurgeons had at their disposal. Thus, a poor unfortunate's skull might be opened at a particular spot that had been determined by the neurologist or neurosurgeon, only to find that it was not the correct place. The location of pathology would have to be judged by a detailed analysis of symptoms and physical signs, the latter being largely obtained by neurological examination of the patient's face, body and limbs. Seldom was a patient able to give any direct indication as to where the pathology was located, as the site of head pains and the like was notoriously unreliable. It was rare to find any sort of external skull deformity or swelling to hint that there was something sinister lurking underneath the surface.

The homunculi or cute little pictures of ourselves that are painted on each of our cerebral hemispheres are so hideously deformed that they look like gargoyles. Our faces are huge, with bloated lips and tongue, while our semi-outstretched arms are also overemphasised, with massive paddle-like hands. Our legs and feet are somewhat more normal in proportion but our bodies are wizened up, like those of dwarfs. These homunculi are the maps of the cortical nerve cells or neurones that correspond to parts on the opposite sides of our bodies. Thus, the nerve cells in the thumb areas of our motor homunculi on the left side of the brain control the movement of our actual right thumbs, while pinpricks in those same thumbs will be felt in the thumb areas of our left sensory homunculi.

What these homunculi tell us is that in neurological terms our bodies, from our necks to our thighs, are relatively unimportant. This is particularly convenient for neurologists and their minions, i.e. trainee neurologists, such as we registrars at the National. It means that neurology can largely be practised with the clothes on — the patient's clothes, I mean, not the neurologist's, for that is generally taken as a given. Yes, there are circumstances when neurological examination of the trunk is vital, such as when you are trying to establish the level of some mischief in the spinal canal. Then you might find the patient is numb below a certain level on the trunk or that the abdominal reflexes are abnormal.

These are cute little reflexes elicited by briskly and obliquely scratching the skin of the tummy from the midline to the flank and watching the belly button flick towards the stimulus. We must also not forget the cremasteric reflex, in which the scrotum and testicle on one side elevate in response to a brisk scratch on the upper inner thigh on the same side. In reality, these little neurological delights are really only necessary or appropriate to perform every so often, in very specific situations. Generally speaking, this does not include student parties!

Thus, 90 per cent of the neurological examination can be done without undressing the patient. You do have to roll up the sleeves and the trouser legs and, unfortunately, slip off the shoes and socks to test the plantar reflexes, but if the patient has conveniently worn rubber beach sandals even this little trial may be unnecessary. Colleagues in other medical specialties are not nearly so fortunate.

An appreciation of this neurological secret was essential to survival in the busy, cramped, stuffy little outpatient examination rooms at The Square, especially in the winter when the central heating was going full bore. When I was a boy my mother had told me that Russian peasants never changed their clothes; as one set wore out, they merely put on another over the top. I am uncertain how she knew this little gem of information as she had never travelled overseas and had no Russian friends. Nonetheless, I did find myself subconsciously trying to avoid choosing the notes of waiting outpatients who had Russian-sounding names, which I told myself was a little rich, given my first name. The situation at The Square was not all that bad, but in those days many flats had no showers, which to some Londoners seemed to be strange newfangled American contraptions, and bathing was clearly not a favourite sport, especially among the elderly. A general medical examination of some sort was usually tacked onto the neurological assessment, but how far one took this had to be assessed on a case-by-case basis.

In the pre-CT days the first imaging investigation to be undertaken was generally a plain x-ray of the skull. These, however, only showed the bones or anything else that was calcified. Apart from the pineal gland in the centre of the head, which frequently calcifies from about middle age onwards, few other things ever showed up. Occasionally, displacement of the pineal gland towards one side of the head might indicate the presence of some sort of mass on the opposite side. Sometimes similar displacement could also be inferred from an echo-encephalogram, in which ultrasound was bounced off a thin sheet of brain tissue that is normally midline. Injection of a radioactive substance into the blood followed by scanning the head with a glorified Geiger counter could reveal a hotspot, indicating a tumour or accumulation of blood. All of these tests, however, were often frustratingly negative even in the presence of gross pathology. Thus, other tests were generally required, and these were all invasive, unpleasant and carried an element of risk for the patient.

By doing a lumbar puncture or spinal tap, with the patient lying on one side, the pressure inside the head and spinal canal could be measured and cerebrospinal fluid obtained for analysis. Lumbar puncture was vital in diagnosing subarachnoid haemorrhage, inflammation and infection. The procedure was highly dangerous, however, if there was increased pressure in the head due to a mass of some sort. In this situation, lowering the pressure in the spinal canal by performing a lumbar puncture could result in the brain being squeezed further out of shape by the high pressure in the skull, bringing on the 'toothpaste' effect mentioned above and causing death. For that reason, cerebral angiography (as described in Chapter 1) was used to diagnose sites of bleeding and the presence of abnormal masses in the brain. Some brain tumours contain myriad small blood vessels and these might show up on the x-rays. The presence of other less vascular tumours might be inferred from disturbance of the normal anatomy of the brain's very complex network of arteries and veins.

As if this little Pandora's box of nasty tests was not enough, there was yet another that was frequently called for. This was the air-encephalogram or pneumo-encephalogram. The patient would be strapped into a seat attached to an x-ray machine and a lumbar puncture performed. Air would be injected into the cerebrospinal fluid and bubbled up into the head, where it would float up over the surface of the brain and find its way into the ventricular spaces, that system of symmetrical cavities within the brain. Because air and the cerebrospinal fluid look different on an ordinary x-ray it was possible to delineate the outer and inner surfaces of the brain, but nothing of its structure in between. Since air always rises to the top it was necessary to rotate the patient in order to see the whole brain — which meant making the patient do a somersault while strapped in the chair. As you might imagine, it was not particularly comfortable to be suspended upside down with air inside your brain while having x-rays taken, and many who were so assaulted would become nauseated and vomit. I personally hate vomiting, and think that doing this upside down must be especially revolting. A general anaesthetic solved this little aspect of the problem but not all x-ray departments used it. I never sent a patient for an air-encephalogram if it could be avoided.

The CT brain scan I was now looking at had just kicked the air-encephalogram into the rubbish bin, and made many of the other tests mentioned above redundant or less frequently required. This was a turning point in neurology and, apart from the lumbar puncture, Mrs Savage did not have to undergo any of the other tests. Her cerebrospinal fluid pressure was substantially elevated but the analysis of its contents was normal. She had a mysterious but not rare disorder called benign intracranial hypertension. This caused miserable headaches but was, as its name suggests, generally benign, in the sense that it would not kill her, although if left untreated it might damage her vision. Fortunately she responded readily to treatment and the headaches disappeared. She needed to be seen in outpatients for several months but she made a complete recovery.

**HIDDEN INSIDE THE BROWN STONE** Victorian façade of the sleepy-looking National Hospital was a bustling institution. Nowhere was it busier than in the outpatient department, which was generally swarming with a combination of new patients referred by other doctors and follow-up patients. The situation would have descended into chaos had it not been for the work of the very able senior registrars. Generally, they had finished their time as registrars on The House and were in a holding pattern while trying to gain appointments as consultant neurologists somewhere in the UK. In the outpatient department it was their job to rapidly evaluate all new patients, sorting them into those who were likely to prove fascinating, instructive, interesting, commonplace, ordinary, boring, non-neurological, non-organic, hypochondriacal and so forth.

Where these patients went depended on these rapid-fire assessments. A few of the selected neurological gems were sent to a lecture theatre where they would be seen by the teaching consultant of the day and the postgraduate medical students. The remaining patients would be sprayed out into an alphabetically arranged array of modestly sized consulting rooms, with the bona fide neurologists in the largest suites being more likely to see those at the start of the above list and the junior staff in cubbyholes picking over those at the end. I never ceased to marvel at how often the senior registrars got it right, given that they could only devote a few minutes to each preliminary assessment.

If it was a registrar's misfortune to descend to consulting Room D or below then he or she was probably going to have a fairly dull day, at least so far as new patients were concerned. The unfortunate follow-ups were usually there for genuine reasons, sometimes serious. There were, however, exceptions to this general rule, as I was to find out one day.

'I say, Ivan, Dr Golden has telephoned to say he is sick. Would you be kind enough to do his clinic?' Kim said to me one morning as I rushed into the outpatients late, following a delay on the underground. 'It will be in consulting Room A. As usual he seems to have a lot of follow-ups. Your first patient is a follow-up; I have already put him in the consulting room as the waiting space is very crowded.'

'Good morning, Mr Finkelstein,' I said cheerily as I installed myself in the comfortable, padded leather chair behind the desk and prepared to carry out my boss's clinic.

The dowdy, grey-headed old gent, who had smiled at me as I entered, now looked bewildered.

'I am Dr Donaldson. Dr Golden asked me to apologise to you because he is unable to be here today, and he has specially asked me to fill in for him,' I continued, taking the liberty of mildly misrepresenting the real events behind my elevation to Room A.

The old gent's visage seemed to harden and it appeared to me that Mr Finkelstein had made some sort of decision. He rose in front of me, pulling himself to the full extent of his unimpressive height, and stretched his right arm towards me. I also stood up and went to shake his hand, mistaking his intention, but he ignored my gesture. His wrinkled fingers clutched the neck of a bottle that was sitting on the corner of the desk closest to him, and he resolutely thrust it into the depths of an old shopping bag. The bottle had been largely concealed in a crinkled paper bag, but I had been quick enough to see the Glenfiddich insignia. Mr Finkelstein might look downtrodden but it was clear he could afford a good bottle of single malt whisky. He flopped back into his chair as though exhausted after expending a great effort.

After thumbing through his hospital records and talking to him I came to the conclusion that Mr Finkelstein had suffered from epilepsy as a young man but that over the past 30 years, while on his current medication, he had been free of all seizures. Was it that he wanted to try and gradually come off his antiepileptic therapy? I enquired.

'No, definitely not,' was his response.

I was uncertain why he was still being regularly followed up in a specialist clinic after all these years. Why was his family doctor not managing this case? Mr Finkelstein looked decidedly unhappy when I gave him the good news that he no longer needed to come to the National Hospital, and that I would write to his GP and advise him that Dr Golden would always be happy to review the situation should there be any future difficulty. He gave me an evil look as he picked up his shopping bag and stalked out of the room.

Mrs Beagle, a chubby middle-aged shop assistant, suffered from migraine, or rather, had suffered from migraine. As a young woman it had plagued her life but, as is common, it had settled when she 'lost her monthlies' some years earlier. She still got rare attacks but could control them with ergotamine tartrate tablets, which constrict dilated blood vessels, and aspirin. Again, I could see no reason why she was still coming to see Dr Golden. She seemed genuinely relieved when I told her that I would hand her management back to her own family doctor. She seemed to have a moment's indecision after she had picked up her shopping bag but, after a fleeting look of embarrassment, she then turned and left the room.

Mr Paget had been a hypertensive smoker and overweight when he had suffered from a series of small strokes a decade earlier. He was found to have severe narrowing of the right carotid artery in the neck, which is the artery that supplies blood to most of the cerebral hemisphere on that side. A vascular surgeon had performed an endarterectomy to remove the inner lining of the artery with its constricting mass of atheroma or hardening. He was now a slim non-smoker who had turned into a fitness fanatic and whose blood pressure was well controlled by medication.

'Congratulations. Your blood pressure is 125/75, Mr Paget, and you seem fighting fit. You have made an excellent recovery and there is no sign of those small strokes that you had many years ago,' I enthused after examining him.

He smiled widely and looked proud. Perhaps it was my imagination, but I thought I saw him lean forward and reach towards a bag that was resting beside his chair. As I continued, however, he straightened up and looked as shocked as if I had hit him in the face with a brick.

'You are so healthy that I think your own GP can now carry on your treatment without our help. You are only taking the blood pressure medication and it's doing a great job.'

'You can't do that, Dr Macdonald … or whatever your name is. Dr Golden saved my life and he needs to keep an eye on me. I am not going to let you just throw me onto the street like that,' he protested loudly.

'I'm sure that you're in no danger, Mr Paget,' I countered. 'I'll write a full report to your own doctor and say that if your condition changes we would be happy to re-see you at any time. I will send a copy of the letter to Dr Golden so that he can make another appointment if he disagrees with me.'

Mr Paget eventually acquiesced and reluctantly left the consulting room.

'How did your morning go?' Kim asked as I finally staggered out of consulting Room A, carrying a stack of case notes that I was taking away to dictate letters on.

'Fine. There were some interesting patients, but quite a lot of follow-ups that seemed to have no active problems. There didn't seem any point in them coming back so I discharged probably a third of them.'

'You might have been a bit rash,' Kim said, raising an eyebrow. 'I'm not sure that your boss would like that.'

'What do you mean? He surely wouldn't want to keep seeing these people just for the sake of it,' I replied, feeling perplexed.

'A few of the older consultants, like Dr Golden, have developed a special rapport with certain patients over the years. There's a sort of mutual bond, almost amounting to dependence on the part of the patient. They're extremely grateful for his ongoing interest and concern. It makes them feel as though someone important cares for them, even though Queen Square is just another part of the big impersonal National Health Service. As they don't have to pay they like to express their appreciation in other ways.'

Three weeks later, as I was leaving the outpatient department after my last clinic of the year, I thought I spied Mr Paget heading towards the exit. I rounded the Christmas tree at speed, hoping to see if I had been correct, and ran straight into Dr Golden.

'Oh, gosh … I am so sorry, sir,' I spluttered, not really knowing what to say and feeling rather stupid.

'Ah, there you are, Dr Donaldson,' beamed my amiable boss. 'Think nothing of it. You young doctors are always in a great hurry these days. No doubt rushing off to save a life,' he added with a wink. 'I seem to have collected a few packages and things and I wondered if you would be kind enough to give me a hand to carry them to my car? They are in consulting Room A.'

One of the parcels had had the wrapping paper pried open and I could not help noting that the six-pack of champagne bottles that I was carrying sported the Moët & Chandon label.

I have long regretted that a certain admirable custom, which reflected the public's fondness of the UK's National Health System, never found its way to what was once the most far-flung colony of the British Empire.

**'WHAT PARTICULAR SUBJECT** interests you?' asked Roger Gilliatt.

'I would really like to do a research project in neuropharmacology, Professor Gilliatt,' I responded.

My time on The House at the National was coming to an end and I had decided that I would like to follow my clinical training by doing a period of research, one that would enable me to obtain a doctor of medicine degree (MD). New Zealand universities followed the British model and at the end of a six-year medical course I had graduated with two bachelor degrees, bachelor of medicine and bachelor of surgery. The MD was a research degree, somewhat like a PhD, but rather more restrictive in that the thesis could only be submitted a minimum of five years after the double bachelor qualification had been obtained. It was thus unlike the general European or American MD, which is the basic qualification necessary to be a medical practitioner. I had spoken to Ian McDonald, earlier my mentor and now a close friend, regarding my aspirations. He had suggested I discuss them with Roger Gilliatt.

Only a few years earlier L-dopa had been found to be a remarkable treatment for Parkinson's disease, a result that had been accurately predicted from neurochemical studies of the brains of dead sufferers. The stunning transformation in the lives of patients who had been confined to wheelchairs, immobile, rigid and trembling, and who, with treatment, could get up and walk normally, had made a deep impression on me. It had inspired the neurologist Oliver Sacks to write the book *Awakenings*, which was subsequently made into a film of the same name. I had decided I wanted to be part of this exciting new world.

Professor Gilliatt now continued: 'I have been approached by a German drug company regarding a new medication that they want to try on patients with severe postural hypotension, the sort of thing that you get in Shy-Drager syndrome. We could set up a trial and you could run it for me. I'm not sure whether there would be enough original work for you to get an MD out of it, but it would be good experience for you.'

My heart sank. This was not exactly the sort of thing I had in mind. Patients with Shy-Drager syndrome were rare. In those days the condition — whose rather odd name comes from two authors who had described it in the 1960s — was regarded as a form of primary autonomic failure, although it is now known to be just one type of clinical presentation of a more common disorder called multiple system atrophy. The autonomic nervous system consists of the nerves that control all those bodily functions that occur automatically and over which we have little if any voluntary control, such as blood pressure, digestion, sweating and the like. Patients with Shy-Drager could become very faint and even lose consciousness when they stood up because their autonomic nervous systems could not adjust their blood pressures to cope with the upright position. Their brains would thus become starved of blood, which would accumulate in the lower parts of their bodies.

Reluctant as I was, I decided that it would be politic to go along with Roger

Gilliatt's suggestion. In addition, there was nothing better on offer at that moment.

'That sounds interesting,' I ventured.

'Yes. Preliminary tests show it will increase the heart rate and cause narrowing of the small arteries, thus raising the blood pressure. The company hopes that it will lessen the amount of postural hypotension, or even abolish it.'

'Would it make the patients hypertensive lying down?' I enquired.

'It might. We would have to monitor carefully for that in case the supine blood pressure became dangerously high. The main difficulty at present is that I don't have any patients with Shy-Drager syndrome. I know that Roger Bannister has been working in this field and must have some cases. Why don't you make an appointment to see him and ask if he would be prepared to let us include them in a trial? Hopefully he'll give you their contact details. I'll give you all of the data I have on this new medication so you can swot it up before you see him.'

I was known to Roger Bannister as I had earlier been his registrar for several months. In some respects he resembled Roger Gilliatt, being rather formal and distinguished-looking. He was, however, the more celebrated of the two and his name was virtually a household word. His particular claim to fame was that as a medical student he had broken the four-minute mile, something that a number of other runners had tried to do without success. Roger's triumph had been achieved in 1953, the same year that an equally tall, lean, muscular Kiwi, Edmund Hillary, had also done the seemingly impossible and Mt Everest. It was the year of Queen Elizabeth's coronation and the press of the day hinted that these great endeavours showed the superiority of the British sporting spirit.

Both men were subsequently knighted, but when I made my appointment to see Roger he was simply Dr Bannister. As a neurologist, he was in the process of carving out a niche for himself as an expert in the field of the autonomic nervous system, which was a Cinderella of neurological subspecialties. He was also the only consultant neurologist who kept up the bygone tradition of having his junior medical staff meet him at the door of the National when he entered. It was with some trepidation that I made my appointment to see him.

Dr Bannister was welcoming but rightly somewhat cautious when I explained the purpose of my visit. Naturally he did not wish to expose his patients to any unreasonable risk, and he wanted to know all about the medication and the tests that we proposed to undertake in order to assess its effects. I provided him with the relevant material that I had, but I felt less confident about which were the best measurements to assess the medication's effects. After all, he was the expert. He was, as I expected, noncommittal, but he agreed to consider the matter and suggested that if I liked to make a further appointment we could discuss the project in more detail. In the meantime, it would be helpful if I could obtain more information about the intended tests from Professor Gilliatt.

I spent the next few weeks running about like a headless chicken, and I felt like one. It is well known that if a hen's head is cut off it can still run about for a short while. The reason is that the neurological machinery that allows it to run lies in the spinal cord, nerves and muscles. The head directs where it is to run. I had attended a meeting of the Association of British Neurologists at which evidence was presented that some mammals react similarly. Roger Bannister left the session just before it finished. My ex-boss, the mischievous Dennis Williams, was the chairman.

'What a pity Dr Bannister has just left,' he announced before asking for questions. 'I was going to ask him to comment on how it is possible to run so well without a brain.'

The whole hall erupted into laughter.

Meanwhile I acted as a human tennis ball, bouncing back and forwards between the two Rogers. At each meeting I felt as though I was boxing with one hand tied behind my back; I was able to give an occasional good jab but my thrusts were largely ineffective. In return, I had to take the expected punches on the chin without complaint; punches that appeared to be directed between my two superiors while I was the punchbag in the middle. There seemed to be coded messages hidden behind the cordial words that I took from one side of the abyss to the other. Deciphered in one direction they read 'Give me access to your patients', while in the other they read 'Let me have the medication'. The two gentlemen never met face to face. In the end I felt completely rogered, and I decided it was time to pull out.

'I don't think we are likely to get any patients for a trial,' I told Professor Gilliatt at our last meeting. 'Dr Bannister says he doesn't think he can find the details of any who would be suitable. Is there a project related to Parkinson's disease and brain neurotransmitters that I could get involved in?'

'I see. Yes, I think that you are probably correct and we are not going to get any further with this Shy-Drager project. Professor Marsden at the Institute of Psychiatry would be the best man to see in relation to research into Parkinson's disease. Telephone him at the end of the week, and in the meantime I'll talk to him about you.'

My heart gave a little leap of joy. I had heard of David Marsden but knew little about him, apart from that he was rumoured to be brilliant and he was the youngest medical person ever to be appointed to a professorship by the University of London.

'This could prove to be very, very interesting,' I thought to myself as I put through that fateful telephone call later in the week. Nevertheless, I had no inkling of the far-reaching consequences it would have for my life.

**IT WAS A COLD, DULL GREY DAY** when I boarded the number 68 double-decker bus at Russell Square, which is just adjacent to Queen Square. As it crossed the Thames and headed south of the great river towards Denmark Hill and the Institute of Psychiatry, the sky was filling from the northwest with threatening black clouds. Rain had started to fall by the time I reached the Department of Neurology. The department was housed in a somewhat sinister-looking, dark brown-black, three-storey laboratory block set at one corner of the campus, apart from all the other buildings. It looked as though the psychiatrists had only accepted its presence very reluctantly. The department was shared with King's College Hospital, a large general hospital across the street, and it was there that the neurological patients were seen. Although it was only 3.30 p.m. the daylight was already starting to fade, but inside the neurology laboratory block it was bright, warm and buzzing with activity.

'Professor Gilliatt has told me you are interested in doing a research project in neuropharmacology,' Professor Marsden began. 'Would you prefer to do something that was clinically or laboratory-based?'

'As all of my postgraduate experience to date has been clinical,' I responded, 'I thought I would like to have a change and work in a laboratory situation.'

Professor Marsden was an instantly likeable, charming, almost debonair man with a handsome, boyish-looking face and dark wavy hair. He was slight of stature, although not conspicuously short, and at that moment he was slumped back in his office chair looking completely relaxed. Judging by the bottle of sherry on the shelf, the ashtray and the smoke fumes in the room, it was clear that, in spite of his innocent appearance and his reputation as a clinician and scientist, David Marsden was a man of the wider world.

'Well, there is a project that I have been thinking about which may suit you,' he now said. 'We know that dopamine, which is so vital for normal movement, is severely diminished in the brains of patients with Parkinson's disease. However, the number of brain receptors on which dopamine acts is not similarly decreased. That, of course, is why giving dopamine's precursor, L-dopa, results in such dramatic improvement. In spite of this, however, patients' movement may not return completely to normal, and L-dopa has a number of troublesome side-effects. As well as the network of dopamine-containing neurones in the brain there is a highly developed system containing noradrenaline or epinephrine, as the Americans call it, and this is also badly damaged in Parkinson's. The project will investigate the possible role of this noradrenaline system in locomotion and motor activity in rats and mice. It is vital that we find out if it is concerned with movement. If it is, then perhaps we should be searching for new medications to modulate the brain's noradrenaline receptors in Parkinson's disease.'

I was completely seduced by Professor Marsden's unassuming but authoritative manner and the clear logic of his argument.

Later, as I stood crouching under my umbrella waiting for my return number 68, I mused over what we had agreed. I would read up the literature in detail and come to the laboratory one day a week over the next few months to do a pilot study. The results of this, if successful, would allow Professor Marsden to apply to the Medical Research Council for funding to cover the costs of my doing a full-scale investigation. He would then become my supervisor in this MD project.

And that is how I became a research fellow employed by the University of London, working in a neurological laboratory at the Institute of Psychiatry. I think it helped that it was summer when I started there full-time, but even so I found that adjusting to laboratory work was not as simple as I had imagined. I had previously worked as part of a team and now I was solo, paddling my own canoe upstream as a flow of obstacles came down to meet me. They often rocked my little craft as they passed by, but never caused serious damage or hindrance. It felt lonely, although I was surrounded by other friendly, helpful laboratory staff who were working in teams on a range of different studies. It seemed to take a very long time and a lot of effort to get apparently small results. Where was the excitement, the *frisson*, and the sense of purpose that I had found in the wards and clinics? In spite of having been brought up on Beatrix Potter, talking to rats and mice did not give the same sense of satisfaction as interacting with real people and their problems. It made me realise that I truly loved clinical medicine.

Although I found laboratory work somewhat dull, it was busy, and all the more so because I was determined to finish with it as soon as possible. Not only did I want to get back to real doctoring again, but the troops were also getting restless. Chris had soldiered along bravely throughout yet another winter in our little flat with our two boys, but now a third child was on the way. Although I had been tempted by the offer of a good clinical job at a London teaching hospital I had never seriously entertained it. Like a flock of swallows we felt that our season was coming to a close, and with other friends from down under we were chirping and twittering excitedly about flying to the other side of the world. It wasn't a matter of *if* but *when*, and the *when* had a distinct sense of urgency about it; all the more so because it was imperative to leave in autumn so that the children could have two summers. It was never mentioned that, should we mistime our departure, the ensuing two winters indoors with the youngsters would be hell. Surely, it would severely test the strongest of marital unions. Work in the laboratory was augmented to fever pitch, with early arrivals and late departures becoming the norm, even during weekends.

I had lost summers before, studying for exams that were habitually held in the autumn so as to inflict maximum pain, suffering and loss on the candidates. I was also to miss a good number of summers in the future, pursuing mad dreams. I am certain, however, that the last year I spent in that laboratory contained no summer. I did not see it, smell it, taste it, hear it or in any other way sense it. I have raised the subject several times with my closest friends and they all look at me in the same peculiar way. It makes me highly suspicious that there was an international conspiracy that resulted in a stolen summer, a crime so cunningly executed that only a few of us astute people are aware that it was perpetrated. After spring there came autumn, and as the final days of that season flowed through the hourglass I prepared to leave the laboratory. It was well after midnight and the rain had set in when I heard the self-locking door click behind me for the last time and I walked the block or so to the nearest bus stop. Following a long, cold wait I boarded a London Transport night bus, and after an interminable journey I at last let myself into our little flat.

Before me lay a scene of devastation. The room was strewn with wooden crates. From some of these, objects thrust upwards at jaunty angles, as if to defy a smothering lid, while others were quite empty. Jumbled between them were piles of crockery, saucepans, ornaments, clothing, mats, books, pictures and all manner of other household and personal items. I couldn't believe that so much paraphernalia could fit into such a tiny flat. In the centre of all this sat a determined Chris, who was methodically packing the bulging crates with all the skill and speed that her flagging strength could muster. We stared at each other in silence. Thank goodness — silence. Our three boys were asleep.

'What on earth …' I began, and then stopped abruptly. Chris's look was menacing.

'Where have you been?' she challenged.

'Finishing off in the lab,' I said weakly. 'I didn't realise that it had got so late. I'm dreadfully sorry.'

'So you should be. Get your coat off and start helping me. You sort stuff out and pass it to me while I pack it into these boxes. In between times start securing the lids. I'll come and sit on them if you can't get them down.'

I don't know why, but I had blithely imagined that everything would be packed and that Chris would be asleep in bed. As usual, I had left her to organise everything and to do the hard work while I continued on my own self-centred little way.

'When do the transport company's men arrive for all this?'

'In about three hours, but the boys will start waking and demanding breakfast before then so we do not have a lot of time,' Chris said. 'By the time we deal with the transport men it will only leave us two hours to get out to Heathrow.'

I had expected to flop into bed and get a few hours' sleep before our departure for New Zealand, but it was clear that neither Chris nor I would lay a head on a pillow that night, or rather that morning. Silently we set to work, packing as quickly as we could. I was just securing the lid on the last crate and Chris was washing the breakfast dishes when the doorbell announced the arrival of the transport men.

'Did my thesis come back from the binders?' I asked belatedly.

'Yes. I've wrapped up the required number of copies and addressed the parcel but I didn't have time to take it to the post office to get the stamps. We'll have to do that on the way to the airport.'

There was a frustratingly long queue, but eventually the precious parcel was weighed and adorned with the sovereign's head, which was duly kissed, wished good luck and entrusted to her own Royal Mail. Even before starting at the laboratory I had been determined that I would submit my thesis before leaving London. I had seen colleagues who thought they would finish their magnum opus back home, only to find themselves swamped in their new jobs. Meanwhile their red-hot and very publishable results cooled before eventually rusting, never to be forged into a meaningful shape. Being of an obsessive bent I was determined that my undoubtedly Nobel Prize-winning piece of work would not be cast on the same slag heap.

So what did I discover in the dim, dark recesses of that laboratory, where I learnt to become a neurosurgeon, performing, under general anaesthesia, tiny stereotactic injections of a substance called 6-hydroxy-dopamine into very precise and localised predetermined regions of the brain? The damage inflicted by this chemical was specifically restricted to the noradrenaline-containing pathways. Firstly, I found out that damage to these pathways does affect locomotion, but that the brain's wonderful capacity to adapt, sometimes referred to as plasticity, means that the outward signs of this disappear after a week or two and to all intents and purposes function returns to normal. Given an appropriate stimulation or injection of medication, however, locomotion again becomes abnormal. It is just so with people who have suffered brain damage. They may be able to function quite normally in most circumstances and any external evidence of the problem may be lacking, even with sophisticated testing, but in some situations or under stress they may not be able to perform as well as before the injury.

None of these findings was novel, except in so much as they applied to the noradrenaline-containing pathways in the brain. In essence, noradrenaline does have a role in motor activity, but it seems relatively minor compared with other influences. Secondly, and more importantly, I found out that rats, contrary to general opinion, are much nicer than mice. I am sure their large, scaly tails have much to do with their infamous reputation. Never judge a book by its cover or a person by his or her appearance. This was a more valuable lesson than anything I learned about the brain's noradrenaline-containing neurones and motor activity, which has been largely consigned to science's box of curiosities, if not its slag heap.

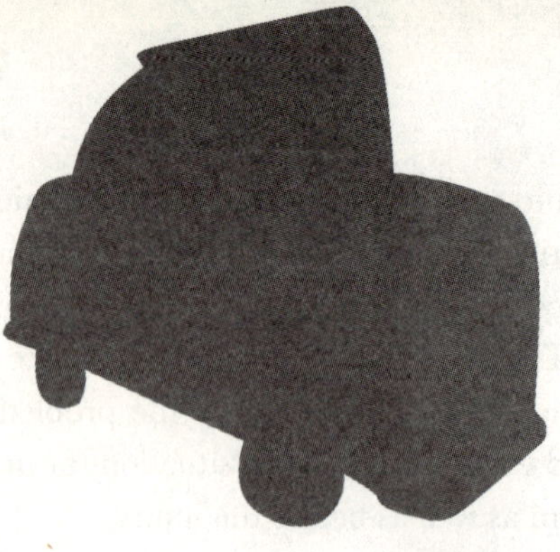

## CHAPTER 4

# Wine *and* Wine Country

### 1973 and well beyond

**WHEN WE LIVED IN LONDON DURING THE 1970S,** did that great city, which has been called the world's wine centre, introduce us to fine wine? Unfortunately, the answer is most definitely no. We simply could not afford it. London, however, gave us something that was much more valuable. It expanded our vinous horizons. Because economics forced us to buy from the lower shelves we became particularly adept at finding value for money. To do this we had to read up about and experiment with the wines from many of Europe's lesser-known wine regions. We became familiar with the tastes of Gaillac, Madiran, Ribera Baja, Bairrada, Puglia and the like. We also had our share of the bottom-end, and hence cheaper, wines that were on offer from the better-known viticultural areas, such as Bordeaux, Rheinpfalz and Tuscany, but we generally found it more exciting and satisfying to fossick in the obscure dark hills and valleys that lay well beyond the price-hiking spotlights of the world's wine stage. We thus built up a fairly complete palatal picture of Europe's wine map, one that extended considerably further than just the classical regions. This was to stand us in good stead during our travels.

We also continued to make wine, although our London lifestyle did not exactly lend itself to such hobbies. A cramped flat packed with small, curious children and surrounded by similar apartments is not the best milieu in which to situate a winery, with its all-pervading fermentation aromas and magnetic attraction for fruit flies. Nonetheless, the fruit barrows in the local market often held large quantities of super-ripe, oozing bargains, which Chris could not resist and even our growing family could not possibly eat. Circumstances forced us once more to become oenologists, like the time she brought home 30 pineapples. We would spend the evening cutting out any suspicious brown patches and juicing the remainder. Occasionally we would buy cans of concentrated grape extract from a home-brew shop, add water and ferment it. The result was inevitably unexciting.

One evening I had an experience that I found so startling that the memory of it remains vivid, even though 40 years have passed. I was at a mess dinner at The Square, for which we were given the privilege of being allowed to use the boardroom. The only other times I had been admitted to this sacred chamber were for job interviews. These dinners were formal affairs, held once every year or so by the registrars to farewell those of their peers who had finished their stints on The House and were departing for new jobs. Although there were a fair number of speeches, they tended to be light-hearted and everyone had a lot of fun. On this evening the speaker was making a joke at the expense of one of the 'dear departed' when I first sniffed the wine that was to be matched with the fish course.

'What a stunning bouquet! It smells like passionfruit, lychee, honeysuckle, peach and I don't know what else. Yet it has a twist of dried herbs and perhaps tobacco. I have never smelt anything like it. It's racy and exciting but at the same time very refined,' I mused pompously, as though trying to impress myself with my newly acquired wine-speak.

I turned to my neighbour as I desperately needed to talk to somebody about this sensational wine, even though I guessed he would not be faintly interested.

'This is the most fantastic wine, but why are they serving a sweet wine with the fish? I know they do it in Sauternes as they claim their wine can match any dish, but here?'

I took a sip of the wine and sat bolt upright with shock. The wine was totally dry and as crisp and fresh as the frost had been that morning. It felt like sucking on a smooth riverstone — firm, cool and minerally. I had never experienced a wine like it. It smelt deliciously sweet but was so steely and dry. The contrast between the nose and the palate was extreme, and made it very appealing. I kept sipping, savouring and luxuriating in its clashing but complementary characters. It was undoubtedly the most schizophrenic wine I had tasted, but its madness was that of an artistic genius. I managed to catch the eye of one of the usual kitchen staff, who was filling in as a waitress that night.

'Could I please have another glass of this wine,' I asked her, 'and I would like to see the bottle. I am really enjoying it.'

'There you are, sir. I will leave the bottle with you.'

It was quite dim in the boardroom so I held the bottle up to the candle. Sancerre, the label stated. I had read about this wine from the Loire Valley but had never before had the opportunity to sample it. It was the first sauvignon blanc I had tasted and, of course, I had no inkling this would one day become New Zealand's most celebrated white wine.

'Don't you want your fish, sir?' enquired the waitress.

They were serving beef Wellington with a medley of vegetables while I was still turning the bottle over in my hand and sipping the last few precious drops. Unfortunately, I had forgotten the now half-cold dish in front of me, but I didn't feel aggrieved to have missed the accompanying speeches.

'How could we get some decent wines to drink at a reasonable price?' I asked Chris on returning home that night; spouses, of course, being *interdit* at mess dinners.

'Let's have a really good look in some of the bargain bins,' she suggested. 'I know we have searched before, but our attempts have been rather desultory and sporadic.'

So over the next few weeks we made a concerted effort to visit quite a range of wine merchants, without experiencing that quasi-orgasmic feeling of believing you have found a really great bargain. Yes, there were the usual cheap Bordeaux from imaginary châteaux, and even those of reputable Bordeaux producers from off-years, rosés, wines made from grapes that would have been better served by being distilled into industrial alcohol and all other sorts of exotica, but nothing that really tickled our combined fancies. While we did have a flirt on the odd bottle, the result was inevitably disappointing. We got what we paid for.

I discussed the problem with another registrar at the National who was afflicted by the same vinous bent from which Chris and I suffered.

'Is there any way you can buy decent wine more cheaply than what's on offer in the merchants, without going to Europe?' I asked.

'You can get some quite good bargains by going to a wine auction. You have to know what you're doing, of course. You need to get a catalogue in advance and read up about the wines on offer, including checking out the vintages, but otherwise it's quite simple.'

'Where do you go?'

'There are several options but I usually go to Sotheby's.'

'It sounds very high-class and posh. I thought Sotheby's just sold expensive wines.'

'That's what they are best known for, but they also sell quite a lot of ordinary wine. It just depends on the exact auction. If there aren't many people there and competition is not strong you can pick up some really good bargains.'

And that is how I found myself sitting at the back of a small crowd as the auctioneer worked his way through a part of the list that abounded in indifferent wines. It was sprinkled with a few more distinguished offerings that were meant to quicken the pulse and arouse the somnolent. I had conscientiously done as my colleague had advised and I had marked in my catalogue the wines in which I was interested and the maximum price that I was prepared to pay. I had arrived late as a result of an outpatient clinic that had been drawn out interminably by a charming but garrulous *migraineuse*, whose headaches were inconveniently triggered by alcohol, which she found 'frightfully limiting socially'. On arriving at the auction room I had given my personal details and in return had received a card with my bidding number boldly printed on it. My friend had told me that I would have to display this proudly each time I made a successful bid. I looked at the bottles being held up by the auctioneer's assistant and eventually worked out how far the auction had progressed. I had missed a couple of lots that had tweaked my interest but there were still plenty more to come. The wines that I was bent on acquiring were listed in dozens, whereas those in the more rarefied atmosphere of vinous fame, i.e. likely to be excessively expensive, were listed singly.

As we approached the first offering that I had marked as being worth pursuing I felt my heart beating more forcefully, my body tense and my throat becoming dry. I may have been an auction virgin but I fancied myself as something of a hunter, and in the art of the pursuit I was as experienced as a hardened prostitute. I was determined to get my prey, and as I lay in wait it was slowly and unsuspectingly ambling towards me. The bidding was a bit lacklustre to start with, and it annoyed me that I could not see my rivals and how the bids were being placed. As I was at the back of the room I felt that I had to hold up my arm and wave it about in order to be certain that my cunningly timed and strategic moves were not overlooked. For some strange reason I felt that this placed me at a disadvantage to my unseen opponents. How were they doing it? Winking, raising an eyebrow, scratching a nose or something similar? No doubt they thought they were more experienced and sophisticated, but I would not let them beat me. When the hammer fell I had prevailed, and what a bargain. It was only a fraction of the price that I had been prepared to pay. I held up my bidding number victoriously and noticed one or two of my enemies look around to see who had outsmarted them.

'Eat your hearts out, suckers; you are up against a real professional here!'

The auction progressed in a similar vein and all the lots I had marked in my catalogue came my way. My friend had been correct. This was definitely the way to buy wine. It was so cheap and accessible. I decided to branch out and go after a few parcels that I had not researched but that my background knowledge told me must be good bargains, especially given the crowd of dumb wimps who were at the auction. I might never be lucky enough to get the same chance again. When the hammer fell for the last time I looked at my catalogue with satisfaction. Yes, I had exceeded the budget that I had set myself, but I had enough decent, if not really fine, wine to start a small cellar. Chris might be annoyed at my extravagance but she would soon get over that, especially after we had savoured a few bottles.

The auctioneer informed the lucky buyers that we should collect our invoices from the office as we left and that the wine would have to be collected and paid for within the next week. After that we could be liable for storage charges. I proudly presented my bidding card and collected my invoice. I checked down the left-hand side to make certain they had included all of the valuable lots. You could never be too careful, and I did not want one of my competitors to make off with something that really belonged to me. Yes, according to the scrawls in my catalogue all were present and correct. Then my eye caught something at the bottom right-hand corner of my precious invoice that suspended my respiration, made my legs feel like jelly and caused me to feel faint. The total was well over 1000 per cent more than I had expected!

'I think there must be a mistake,' I stammered.

'Why is that, sir?' replied the clerk in a distinctly disbelieving and supercilious voice.

'Well, for example, I only bid £4 for Lot 53 and it says here £48.'

'£4 is the price per bottle, and you have been lucky enough to have got a dozen. The auctioneer explained it very clearly at the start and it is written right there in your catalogue.'

He pointed to some fairly obvious print that I had carelessly overlooked. No wonder I had outbid all my competitors, and it was all my own stupid fault.

'How did the auction go?' Chris asked enthusiastically as I walked through the door of the flat.

'Not so well.'

'What was the matter? Didn't you manage to get anything?'

'It's not exactly that. I got quite a lot. In fact, I got too much.'

'That shouldn't be a problem. If we ask friends around for dinner on a few occasions we'll soon make a dent in the supply.'

'It won't be fixed quite that easily. Here, let me show you this invoice and you'll see what I mean, but you had better sit down first.'

Chris stared long and hard at the piece of paper. She had turned quite pale, and the only time I had seen her look so pained and unhappy was during labour. I gave a hesitant and apologetic version of the thrashing that I had given my opponents in the auction ring, then told of how victory had been snatched from me by a miserable little clerk, well after the bell had been rung by the final fall of the hammer.

'There is only one thing you can do,' she said decisively. 'You have to go back tomorrow and say that we cannot possibly pay. If you offer them some compensation they might agree to let you off the hook. After all, they still have the wine and they can no doubt auction it again.'

And that is what I did. I returned with my tail between my legs and explained the whole situation. Fortunately, the Pickwickian-looking gent before whom I had to plead my case turned out to be understanding and even sympathetic. No doubt he had previously come across the situation of young bucks getting carried away, overextending their means and making fools of themselves, or possibly even worse. Using the retrospectoscope, which I have found to be a very powerful instrument, I have come to the conclusion that he thought I was just going to walk away from the situation. His eyes lit up like burning coals and a broad grin looked as though it would shatter his generous jowls when I naïvely offered the compensation, which he accepted with alacrity.

'It would be particularly convenient, sir, if you could make the cheque out to "Cash", and there is no need to cross it.'

To punish myself even further I walked the not inconsiderable distance back home, but as my pockets and my spirit were now much lighter my steps seemed to fairly spring along. For the next few months we were reduced to drinking what the French call *vinasse*, which is not some mysterious or new appellation, but simply *plonk*. Never again did I venture into a London auction room, so while I cannot say that I am completely unsullied, I remain to this day a wine auction semi-virgin.

**AFTER MY LITTLE AUCTION FIASCO**, our London wine experiences became rather restricted for a period. Fortunately, it was not too long before I was due for a holiday. Chris and I had selfishly decided that we would spend all of our holidays touring around Western Europe's vineyards and that the kids would just have to tag along. They were so young that they could be happy almost anywhere, so long as there was sunshine, plenty of fresh air and space, new worlds to explore and exciting adventures around every corner. The odd stream or occasional beach would be a bonus. We would take just a few books and basic toys to keep them amused should it dare to rain.

For transport and accommodation we were reliant on our beaten-up old campervan, which had a pop-up roof that contained extra bunks for the children. We had bought it with continental holidays in mind. Our first summer vacation was in 1973, but we had a number of similar ones over the ensuing years. Each time we were away four to six weeks, and we visited just about all of the viticultural regions we had read about or whose wines we had tasted. It was travelling at its most basic, with every expense spared, except that of buying and tasting the wines of the regions through which we passed.

We always tried the local foods and cooked up each area's special recipes, but eating out with the boys and our thin wallet was a no-no. Sometimes Chris and I felt guilty and wondered if we were just a couple of old soaks, indulging ourselves while our children suffered. The long distances we travelled were lengthened by the slow lumbering of our growling beast of burden, and in order to quell restlessness and occasional rebellion amongst the troops we had to limit our times on the road and intersperse them with plenty of outdoor action.

The wind was buffeting the side of the campervan and dark clouds were boiling overhead as we drove onto the quayside in Dover at the start of our first Continental excursion. We were glad to park our ageing accommodation — in first gear and with brakes on, as instructed — and to scuttle out of the dark, claustrophobic and fumy hold of the ferry. We made our way up the internal stairway towards the inviting light and fresh air, our spirits buoyed by excitement. We felt rather like insects coming up from wintering over in the depths of the earth to emerge into a bright and entirely new world; we were on our way to meet Europe head on, with all her vinous delights.

The lounge was brightly lit and furnished in cheerful, vibrant colours and we felt utterly contented as we relaxed back into the comfortable chairs. It had been hectic leaving London as I had been on duty at the National the night before and I was late getting back to the flat. Chris had packed the campervan by herself and was ready for immediate departure. We had had to rush to avoid missing the boat. Now at last we were on the high seas, or rather on the little ditch that separates England and France.

'Look, boys!' Chris said. 'There's a little house that's full of toys. Why don't you go and play in there?' She turned to me with a knowing wink. 'It will amuse them perfectly while we read our books.'

In the centre of the room was a clear plastic cube, like a big playhouse, which was half-filled with brightly coloured plastic balls. Entrance was by way of a door halfway up the wall, with a ladder leading up to it. The kids did not need any encouragement, and soon they were romping around on top of the balls and biffing them at the other children who were similarly ensconced in this gaudy piece of plastic paradise.

I had never admitted to being a rotten sailor, but then again, I had never claimed to be a good one. All was well while we were firmly tied to the wharf, and to this day I pretend that it may have remained so if I had not continued reading with my head down. Whatever the truth of the matter, I cannot dispute that not long after we cleared the white cliffs I became decidedly queasy and began to look around me for a handy receptacle.

'I'm feeling a little the worse for wear,' I confided to Chris. 'I think it must have been the late night.'

'Go out onto the deck and get some fresh air,' she said. 'You'll feel much better in no time.'

'What about you and the boys? You may need a hand with them.'

'You know me, I'm a good sailor, and the boys are fine.'

I rose tentatively, and slowly and unsteadily made my way towards the exit. The ferry was certainly swaying, although not too badly at that stage. Suddenly I had that rising feeling and I made a mad dash for the door. A blast of raw wind hit me full face and I swallowed hard. I had succeeded in escaping and I knew that if I stayed facing the elements I would probably survive with my dignity intact. I clung miserably to the rail, breathing and tasting the salt spray throughout the entire trip. The 'ditch' had certainly become very rough, but somehow I had managed to keep my gastric contents in their place. However, the trip had given me a new respect for this short stretch of water.

It was not until the good Lord had poured oil on the troubled waters of the English Channel, more properly at that point called La Manche as we were entering the harbour at Calais, that I felt secure enough to venture towards the cabin door again. But where were Chris and the boys? All about me was a scene of devastation, and they were nowhere to be seen. The lounge was full of pale, green-looking people, sprawled over or slumped in chairs. Some were clutching bulging paper bags. There was the thick, fatty, unmistakable stench of partially digested fish and chips hanging in the warm, putrid air.

I became alarmed and a melodramatic vision suddenly forced its way into my mind. In it Chris and the boys were following me onto the deck, where they were washed overboard by a huge wave.

'Do you know what happened to the blonde woman who was sitting there?' I asked a passing crew member, pointing to the spot where I had left Chris. 'She's my wife and she would have had our sons with her.'

'They were so miserable that the captain put them in his cabin,' the man responded. 'Follow me.'

And that was where I found them, lying together on the captain's bed looking quite a bit the worse for wear.

'What happened to you?' Chris demanded somewhat abruptly.

'I was on the deck, trying not to vomit.'

'Lucky you!' she replied, with more than a tinge of bitterness.

'But I thought you must all be all right as you didn't come out on the deck after me,' I said weakly, suddenly feeling very self-centred and selfish. 'What happened?'

'Not long after you left it began to get very rough. Some of the children in the little house became ill and started to be sick. You could see all the vomit running down between the coloured balls! Then I realised that this must have happened before in that cube. It's obviously not the first bad crossing this boat has ever experienced, and there is no way the staff could get out all those balls and wash them after every bit of rough weather. They must be filthy.

'I rushed and rescued the boys before they fell onto or were pelted with fresh vomit. I only just managed to get them out before they became sick as well. Then I became nauseated. We were totally miserable, so I waylaid one of the crew and pleaded for somewhere where we could all lie down. Fortunately, he took pity on us, and that's how we ended up in here. We all felt much better when we were lying flat.'

I described the scene of desolation in the lounge.

'It's too bad about all the others, but they didn't have the gumption to ask,' Chris said with a flicker of a smile.

It wouldn't be the last time on this trip that I would admire my wife's ingenuity and resourcefulness.

**'LOOK OUT!' I SCREAMED** as the large, heavily laden truck flung itself out of nowhere and came hurtling towards us.

'The bastard is going completely the wrong way around!' Chris exclaimed as we narrowly missed being pulverised.

We had just driven away from the docks, and had been saved by Chris adeptly pulling the campervan onto the centre of the roundabout or, as the French quite irrationally insist on calling it, *le rond-point*. There it rested immobile while she honked loudly and persistently with indignation.

'I've heard the French are lousy drivers,' she complained.

'No. No. No! It is us who must be going the wrong way around,' I stammered as it dawned on me.

We both knew that we had to drive on the right side, or rather, the wrong side of the road in Europe, but we had no idea the continentals would be mad enough to turn to the right side, or rather the right-hand side, when entering a roundabout. We just had not thought it through to its logical conclusion, this driving on the opposite side of the road.

'For that matter, to which side do we give way when we come to an intersection?'

We stared dumbly at each other as a number of other vehicles circled around us, each entering and leaving the roundabout correctly before going on its merry way. The occupants no doubt thought that we were quite mad. Rather than admitting we had been stupid enough to get it so wrong, we were briefly tempted to have a picnic in the middle of the roundabout and pretend we were merely eccentric English. There was plenty of room on the slightly raised dais, and not a single 'No Parking' notice in sight. Sanity ruled, however, and when the coast was completely clear we gingerly eased ourselves off our perch and slowly followed the locals' example of anticlockwise rotation.

To our credit, we never, or hardly ever, made that mistake again. On a certain hot, sultry afternoon in central Spain, when only mad dogs and Kiwis were about, we circled in a clockwise direction around a fat, sleepy policeman. He was standing in a little pillbox, no doubt to provide him with protection from the crazy local drivers, and under a makeshift parasol to give him a little shade. He was evidently supposed to be directing the non-existent traffic and our tricky little manoeuvre took him completely by surprise. As he started to shout and point at us menacingly, we noticed the nasty-looking pistol on his hip. Then he seemed to notice our number plates, shrugged his shoulders, raised his hands, shook his head and smiled.

We could almost hear him saying 'Crazy English woman!'

After extricating ourselves from Calais we headed towards the Loire Valley, home to the pretty little village of Sancerre, whose sauvignon blanc wine had earlier made such a startling impression on me. Sadly, in spite of our buying quite a number of bottles from different producers, the wines all seemed but pale, lacklustre imitations of the one that had so fired my imagination at the mess dinner. We then went with the flow, passing downstream along the banks of that mighty waterway into lands where the chenin blanc grape reigned supreme, producing a spectrum of citrusy wines, ranging from the steely dry to the voluptuously sweet.

We passed picturesque old châteaux and quaint troglodyte houses and wineries carved into the limestone hills, only their doors and windows poking out of the earth. Old women all dressed in black, with high lacy headdresses, sat in the doorways, gossiping and crocheting in the last rays of the setting sun. Of all of the images, however, the most powerful was that of the morning fog, which lay like a fluffy blanket over the river and its surrounds. It insinuated its way into every bush and tree, between every leaf and every blade of grass, leaving on every surface a fairytale gossamer film of droplets that sparkled like a million diamonds in the early sunlight. The hazy shapes of flat-bottomed rowing boats could be seen moored out in the lazy current, while their owners patiently tried to lure lunch onto their hooks. After we had drunk deeply of the Loire Valley and all it had to offer, our little campervan turned its nose towards the south.

It was sultry when we arrived on the outskirts of Bordeaux. The day had been hot, but now a swelling bank of thunderous-looking cumulus clouds was obscuring the sun, its golden-white rays streaming outwards around the dark sides of the cloud. In front of us stood the silhouette of an old iron wayside crucifix carrying its heavy and equally rusty burden, such a common, but never ordinary, sight throughout rural France. Immediately behind our Lord was a gloriously verdant vineyard, and in the middle distance there was an idyllic-looking village, complete with church spire.

'That would make a superb photograph,' I enthused as I pulled over to the side of the road and leapt out of the van, camera in hand. I crouched down to make the foreground crucifix more imposing and took a couple of shots.

'I'm going to take one without the cross ... from within the vineyard itself ... and I'll choose a vine to be the centrepiece against the cloud.'

So saying, I jumped down from the side of the road into the vineyard, a drop of about a metre. Suddenly I felt a sharp pain on the inner side of my right ankle and I stumbled forward, letting out a semi-religious expletive. I looked down and saw that a sharp stick had been thrust through my skin and had travelled upwards underneath it, breaking off to leave a rather prominent swelling quite some distance from the puncture hole. Blood was starting to trickle from the little wound and into my sandal. If I had been wearing long trousers, shoes and socks I possibly might have avoided the injury, but I was supposed to be enjoying myself on holiday rather than being dressed for work back at the National. I looked around the vineyard and noticed that it had recently been ploughed. Ominously, there was a large piece of horse dung lurking amongst the furrows, clear evidence the ground had been tilled by horse. The medical implications of this were not lost on me. I scrambled back up the small bank, forgetting all about the lost photographic masterpiece.

'Time is getting on,' I said to Chris; 'the boys will soon be getting desperate for their dinner. We had better find a place to camp.'

We found a sheltered spot beneath some willows, not far from a stream, and let the children play before getting them a meal and then settling them down for the night. During the small hours my ankle started to feel quite painful and to throb. In the morning light I could see reddish inflammation developing around the swelling. The previous night I had searched for our first-aid kit and had been dismayed to find that in our rush to get away we had left it behind.

'I had better get something done about my ankle. I'm sure there is a piece of stick embedded under the skin and it's so far from the wound that I couldn't pull it out with your small cosmetic tweezers.'

'We passed quite a big hospital about 15 minutes before you jumped into that vineyard. Perhaps you should try there,' suggested Chris.

It was later that morning that I presented myself at the reception and tried to explain my mini-plight. The receptionist called the medical staff, who appeared quite perplexed. Admittedly my schoolboy French was rather rusty, and none of them seemed to speak a single word of English. This surprised me, as most of my colleagues in London had a workable knowledge of French. Explaining about the horse dung brought looks of horror and dismay. Yes, they explained, horses were still used to cultivate the soil in some vineyards, and I was at severe risk of contracting tetanus. As I was also a doctor I must be aware that my life was in mortal danger. I explained that I was up to date with my tetanus immunisation, but this did not seem to appease them. After a brief discussion among themselves in machine-gun French I saw, out of the corner of my eye, a nurse setting up a drip-stand.

'Quel est cela?' I asked suspiciously. 'What is that?'

The young doctor who seemed to be in charge explained that I was to have an infusion of anti-tetanus serum to give me extra protection. I felt a tightening in my throat and a constriction in my chest. Tetanus immunisation enables your body to create your own antibodies to protect you against this potentially fatal disease, but anti-tetanus serum contains another animal's antibodies, usually a horse's or a cow's, which provide more rapid protection and treatment. The problem is that anti-tetanus serum can occasionally induce a fatal allergic reaction. As a medical student I had been taught that it should be avoided like the plague, and it was completely unnecessary for someone who was up to date with their tetanus immunisation.

'Non! Non! Non!' I shouted, much to the amazement and consternation of the small but growing medical group who had assembled around me.

I again indicated the small lump under my reddening skin and said that a piece of stick was lodged there and it needed to be removed. I pointed to a scalpel and made cutting movements over the swelling, but to no avail. No one made a move to touch the knife. I was then asked if I had medical insurance. It was clear that they were reluctant to remove the offending little object. It had taken almost two hours to get to this stage and my patience was running out. More importantly, I was concerned about Chris, who was trying to amuse the children in the hot hospital car park. I reached for the scalpel, my intention clear, but before I could proceed a restraining hand was put on my arm. It was explained through a mixture of sign language and words that I could not perform an operation on myself in the clinic. I would have to go to the operating theatre!

And so it was that I found myself sitting on an operating table under the bright theatre lights, with the foot of my troublesome right leg underneath my left thigh, while I sliced through the skin and removed the pathetically small but very troublesome dirty piece of stick. I swabbed and cleaned the area before applying a bandage, helpfully supplied by my dear French colleagues. After thanking them profusely I sauntered out into the heat of the noonday sun to be reunited with my ever-patient family. I had learnt a hard lesson — *look before you leap* (into a vineyard) — but I would forget its figurative application in years to come.

While we were in Bordeaux we tried to visit a number of producers, thinking that we would be able to buy a few decent bottles of wine. Everywhere the reception was cool and the looks uninterested.

'We are not shopkeepers. We do not have to market our wine. We sell it to the negociants, not to the public,' we were told by one particularly frosty winery owner.

This was true. The winemakers of Bordeaux considered themselves above dealing with the public. The wines of the more prestigious estates would be bottled under their own labels, Château This or Château That. Much of the rest would be sold to negociants, either as grapes or as young wine, often to be blended into the negociant's own brand or into a wine that would be bottled with the generic label of a commune or the region. Such was the demand for the wines of Bordeaux, the powers of the negociants and the dependence of the growers and small producers on the system, that it was simply not seen as necessary or seemly to have cellar-door sales.

The classic wine regions of Europe had no need to market their wine; it was sold to negociants and from them to wine merchants and wine shops. It was an old system that was overripe for a shake-up. With the coming of competition from new world wines and the advent of affordable tourism, attitudes would change. Bordeaux producers now vie with each other for clients as vigorously as streetwalkers in a red-light district, and the same could be said of most famous wine areas.

At that time, in order to slake our thirst, we had to be content with buying our Bordeaux wines impersonally from a shop.

**DURING THE MULTIPLE FAMILY** campervan trips that we made to Europe's vineyard regions we usually camped in the wilds, something that is difficult to do nowadays. We felt it was better and more natural for the children, rather than being stuck in a camping ground with dozens of other families, sharing limited communal facilities and with only playgrounds to amuse them. By staying in the countryside they were closer to all of nature's wonders. They watched butterflies, collected snails, caught lizards and frogs, found 'precious' stones and bathed in streams. They were wet by the morning dew and dried by the noonday sun. They became as brown as little chestnuts during the day and tried to count the twinkling stars at night.

Sometimes the days were impossibly hot, but often, during the late afternoon or early evening, dark cumulus clouds would mushroom overhead. They were heralds of a thunderstorm, with its blinding lightning, deafening thunder, torrential rain and chilling wind. These never lasted long but they were incredibly dramatic, all the more so as we were all alone in a little van in the middle of nowhere. Why was it that such storms always seemed to pass directly overhead? They cleared the air and made everything seem fresher, but over the ensuing days the temperature would gradually rise until it again reached crisis point and the storm cycle would be repeated. We enjoyed these spectacular displays of nature's raw power, whose genesis was fostered by a large land mass. Coming from an island we were unused to such frequent electrical storms.

Snakes were also a novelty, New Zealand being free of these reptiles.

'Look out for that snake!' I yelled to Chris, who swerved automatically, then we both wondered why we had reacted that way. It was a silly and rather dangerous thing to have done on a busy road. We had just caught a glimpse of an elongated, brown-green shape slithering out of the grass and trying to make a sudden dash to the other side of the tarseal. Our spontaneous reactions had no doubt been heightened by the fact that we had never before seen a live snake.

'You ran over it!' I said, looking in the rear-vision mirror.

'Damn! I was trying to avoid it,' Chris replied, pulling over to the side of the road. We all piled out and hurried back to the twitching reptile, whose sleek shape had been somewhat flattened and was firmly embedded in the semi-melted tar. It was going to be another stifling day in the Midi.

'It's so pretty with its different shades of green and those diamond markings running down its body,' Chris said guiltily.

'Can we please keep it? Yes! Please, please?' chorused the boys.

'It will just go rotten and start to smell,' I replied discouragingly.

'You could skin it for us, Dad,' was the hopeful but unwelcome plea.

'Well, I don't think it would work as the skin itself would probably start to rot.'

'Please, please, please! We'll help you.'

Under the excited and expectant gaze of our little tribe, and timing myself to avoid the passing vehicles, I retrieved the unfortunate creature, putting it into a plastic bag and slinging it into the back of the van. It lurked under the back seat and in the back of my mind as we continued on our way. If I was going to do anything about the wretched animal I would have to do it soon, since in this heat it would not take long for putrefaction to set in.

That evening after dinner, I took out a small sharp knife and made a circumferential cut through the skin just below the head, then I nailed the skull onto a tree. Having separated a small amount of skin from the underlying flesh, just below the cut, I grasped these newly formed flaps of skin with pliers and pulled firmly downwards. Lo and behold the skin peeled off as simply as removing a glove. There was a little bit of flesh left clinging to the hide, but after it had been wrapped up with salt for a week this unwanted tissue came away from the skin very easily. And that is how our family came to have a snakeskin proudly displayed on the wall of our lounge. It became a memento of a fight with an enormous and venomous serpent that was guarding a hoard of stolen treasure in a dark forest somewhere in the wilds of the kingdom of the South of France.

**CAMPING IN THE WILD** carries certain responsibilities and risks. We tried to be as responsible as we could, never leaving litter, lighting fires, damaging plants or interfering with people's property. 'Take only photos and leave only footprints' seemed a worthy motto. Chris and I were always mindful of security. We were careful to choose a concealed and sheltered place in the countryside in which to park for the night, one that could not be seen from the road and was not near houses. We preferred being on a riverbank, by a stream, under some trees or the like. We always backed into our camping spot and made sure there was nothing in front of the van that could obstruct our departure should we need to make a hasty exit. Generally, we needed to discover a place to stay by 3 p.m., in order to give the children a chance to explore the area and frisk about before the evening meal. However, not everything in this life is perfect and very occasionally we had to compromise.

One afternoon in the south of France we just could not find anywhere that looked at all suitable. The places we did see were too public, too dirty, too noisy or too dangerous. In other words, we were being too fussy, and there was not a camping ground in sight. Consequently, we kept driving and searching, but to no avail. Eventually the kids became so scratchy that they would neither be appeased by another offering from Chris's never-ending supply of novel stories nor fobbed off by an offered snack. We had to take the next camping possibility, no matter how bad it might be.

It was about 7 p.m. when we pulled into a large tarsealed space beside some public gardens in a medium-sized town. There were about 20 or 30 motley campervans, caravans and the like already parked there, so we assumed that it would be all right. I backed into a suitable-looking place and we immediately let the boys out, popped up our elevating roof and started to cook a meal.

It was only then that we bothered to have a good look at our neighbours. It was clear that they had been there for quite a long time. There was washing flapping in the breeze, TV aerials perched at odd angles, meat cooking on several dilapidated barbecues, and a fair scattering of rubbish littered about. Propped against the van next door was a badly stained mattress that had been left out to dry, complete with a protruding innerspring. We gave a friendly wave to a group of grubby little urchins who had stopped their game to stare at us disbelievingly. There were about half a dozen flea-bitten dogs, of uncertain but undoubtedly aggressive pedigree, that strained at their flimsy leashes while snarling and barking their combined welcomes. The noise had roused a number of bleary-eyed, dishevelled-looking males, who must have been disturbed during a prolonged siesta or *sexesta*, possibly preparing them for a nefarious night on the town or countryside. They now appeared from their makeshift accommodations without displaying any enthusiasm or reciprocation of our cheery 'Bonsoir'. It was clear that we had unwittingly joined a group of gypsies, who looked as though they were there for the duration.

'What shall we do?' I asked Chris. 'Perhaps we should just pack up and try to find somewhere else.'

'No. We'll just stay here. They can't do anything about it. It's not their place and we are too tired to look for anything else. I doubt that they would damage our van, as then we might not be able to leave in the morning.'

'Boys! Come here!' I shouted out, as I could see the children making a beeline towards the other youngsters and their dubiously restrained dogs. 'We've got your dinner!'

Dinner was not really ready, but I did not feel like sorting out juvenile ethnic rivalries or arguments with our new neighbours. Nor did I wish to start practising my limited surgical skills on rabid dog bites.

It was dusk and we had just finished our meal when unexpected company arrived.

'The gendarmes are here,' I said to Chris as she was boiling the kettle for a postprandial cuppa. 'I wonder what they want.'

I didn't have long to wait to find out. They marched straight over to our campervan.

'*C'est interdit rester ici*,' commanded a ruddy-faced brute of a man in a blue uniform. 'You can't stay here.' He was flanked by several equally impressive, serious-faced colleagues who also had pistols dangling casually from their hips.

In spite of the line-up of heavies and their obvious display of firepower, I did not feel like going down without a fight.

'But where will we go? We can't find anywhere else to camp. Couldn't we just stay here for one night? Can you suggest somewhere else that we could go?'

'It is not our job to find people camping places, and no, you cannot stay here tonight' was the brusque reply.

'But what about all these other people here?' Chris chipped in, waving her arm in the direction of the now-assembled multitude who had collected outside their homes. 'We are not doing any more harm than they are. If they are allowed to camp here, then we should be able to stay here for just one night.'

The gendarmes' spokesman looked at the gypsies and then glanced at his colleagues in blue, shrugging his shoulders. 'I guess that we will just have to remove them as well,' he said resignedly, but he appeared somewhat hesitant and uncertain.

'Just fiddle around and pretend that we are packing, getting ready to move,' I whispered to Chris. 'Maybe they will just go away without shifting anybody. If they come back we can pretend we didn't understand him. It's clear that for some reason they have let these others stay here but they want us out. I don't know why.'

After a bit of shilly-shallying and further discussion between themselves, the gendarmes suddenly catapulted into action, shouting and waving their arms at the gypsies, whose looks changed mercurially from uninterested to amazed, to horrified, and finally to sullen. Naturally, theirs was not going to be a fast getaway. After an hour or so the first of them, with much engine revving, oily-smelling black smoke, honking and internationally recognisable finger gestures aimed in our general direction, pulled out and departed into the gloom. Not long afterwards, when it was clear that this activity was not just a bluff, our little campervan slipped out and, unsurprisingly, turned the opposite way to the horde of disappearing nomads. We had no wish to find ourselves again camped *ensemble* in Elysian Fields further down the road.

By chance, about 15 minutes later, just outside the town, we found a perfect camping spot nestled under some willow trees growing on the bank of a small stream. If we had not turned into the gypsy encampment but continued in the direction that we had been heading we would have stumbled across it earlier in the evening. We felt very sad at having been responsible for the gypsies' decampment. It had not been our intention and we had hoped that by protesting we might have been able to stay there. Did the gendarmes receive a backhander to keep strangers off the gypsies' turf? Did they just want an excuse to move the gypsies on? Was our arrival on the scene just a coincidence? It did not make any sense to either of us, but thinking up possible explanations kept us amused for weeks to come.

**ONE SUMMER'S NIGHT, WHEN** a chilly wind howled its way down the Rhône Valley, seeking to disturb every hidden nook and cranny and gently rocking our campervan, we prepared to settle down for the night. We were camped between the edge of a vineyard and a small, gently flowing river. High above, the stars twinkled and a full moon shone down, unhindered by the last shreds of clouds, which had been torn away by the restless *mistral*. At dusk we had walked upstream for some distance, attracted by the little wisps of music that fought their battered way through the annoying gusts. There, on the other side of the river, we had seen the pulsating coloured lights of a *guinguette*, an outdoor café and dance floor. There were plenty of patrons and they seemed to be having a good time. We were camped well away, however, and even though we were downwind, once inside our little cocoon we could hear nothing of the merriment. All was peaceful in the campervan, and the children were sleeping soundly.

It was about 11 p.m. when Chris and I finished cleaning up and were about ready to hit the hay. We had assembled our bed, which occupied most of the space at the back of the van, leaving only a small gap between the bed and the rear doors. One second I was standing in this space, trying to balance while taking off my underpants, and the next I was lying on my back with my legs and arms outstretched. I was outside the van. My head had hit the hard ground and it throbbed badly. I felt dazed and was seeing stars, but almost immediately they disappeared and everything went black. Then, just as suddenly, they reappeared, only to flicker off again. Then I realised that there were two heads immediately above mine and that they were blocking my vision of the night sky. I had landed on the ground between two strange men, who must have been standing immediately outside the back door of the campervan. Presumably they had turned the door handle as I knew that I had shut the doors tightly, intending to lock them from inside. Because the indoor lights were on, Chris, who had been undressing in the space at the other end of the bed, was unable to see that there was anyone else outside in the dark.

'Are you all right?' she called out, sounding concerned. It may not surprise you that I did not feel like having a jolly conversation with her while I was lying in the rather compromising situation in which I had unwillingly found myself.

'*Pardonnez moi, si vous plait?*' I rather incongruously said to the sinister black shapes hovering above me. 'Excuse me, if you don't mind?'

At the same time I sprang to my feet and bounded back into the campervan, closing and locking the doors behind me with a bang.

'Put out the lights!' I shouted to Chris.

Silently we sat there in the dark for about 10 minutes before we cautiously parted the curtains a chink and peeked out. There was nobody to be seen. We kept a wary eye out during the next half-hour or so and then, as the adrenaline subsided, the fatigue from the busy day's activities began to make itself felt. Sleep overpowered us, although it was not very restful, and we tossed and turned fitfully before waking at sparrow's fart. The *mistral* had departed to lands unknown, leaving behind the promise of a beautiful day.

We chewed over the events of the previous night. They may have been quite innocent, but why had the two men crept up and stood there silently, and why had the doors suddenly opened? Perhaps our stealthy nocturnal visitors actually owned the land and were just checking that we were not wreaking havoc. Whatever the explanation, the delightful camping spot of the night before had become somewhat foreboding and we hit the road after an early breakfast. We were off to seek new adventures, but hopefully they would not be so nerve-racking.

**THE HOT DAY HAD SLOWLY FADED** into a warm, lingering evening and there was not the faintest breath of wind to ruffle the placid hills that were perfectly silhouetted in the small dark lake. This was German wine and vine country at its best. We were sitting outside the campervan, sipping a well-earned and delicious local riesling, having bedded the boys down and cleaned up after our evening meal. It was Mum and Dad's special and sacrosanct time of the day, but it was seldom as perfect as this. We exchanged satisfied smiles and raised our glasses once again to salute the gods of the Rhine and wine. We were completely isolated from the rest of the world, without any sign of other human habitation.

'Would you mind if I went for a stroll around the lake, Chris?'

'Not at all. I'll sit here and read my book. If it gets too dark I'll just enjoy this wonderful evening. You go and get some exercise.'

To say that it was very pleasant walking around the lake would be an understatement. It was intoxicating. The wildflowers came almost to the water's edge and the birds high in the trees were chirping a tranquil lullaby. The air possessed a magical, almost silky quality. The world was at peace with itself and all within it. Unfortunately I lingered rather too long and by the time I came round the small point of land and saw our van just ahead of me, dusk was on the cusp of night. Chris was sitting outside, reading by light that was spilling through the open door of the vehicle. For a split second my blood froze, my whole body became rigid, I stopped breathing and my throat clenched into a tight fist. Creeping silently through the long grass towards Chris were five or six menacing black shapes. They were coming from different directions and all moving stealthily towards her. Undoubtedly, they were human. Suddenly I found my voice.

'Quickly, Chris!' I screamed out. 'Jump in the van, lock the doors, put out the lights and get ready to throw me out the axe! We're being attacked!'

Within a flash she sprang inside and swung into action. I had seen the dark shapes flatten themselves on the ground and they were now quite imperceptible, but I knew that they lay fanned out in a semicircle between me and my family. I could only just make out the obscure blob of our immobile mobile home. I would have to either pass through the group of intruders or make a wide and time-consuming detour around them in order to get to the van and the axe. Every second counted because our would-be attackers had been taken off-guard and my advantage of surprise would not last long. Fortunately, I had learnt a little German at night school in London. I sprinted to the spot where I guessed the closest person was lying and grabbed hold of the invisible form.

'Who are you? What are you doing?' I shouted.

'Please don't hurt me!' came the pathetic response. 'We are all Boy Scouts. We are camped over the hill and we were just out walking. We saw your van and thought it would be fun to practise our camouflage skills and creep up on you.'

'All of you stand up!' I ordered. 'Come over towards the campervan.'

The little band of shiny-faced, bright-eyed youths who gathered in the light of the campervan looked very apologetic.

'I think that was not a very sensible thing to do, especially in the dusk,' I gently reprimanded. 'You gave us quite a fright and someone might have got hurt.'

They nodded sheepishly.

'Would any of you like a biscuit?'

They nodded more enthusiastically and smiles began to appear.

'Danke, danke.'

The grateful thanks trailed off as the boys disappeared into the gloom, the way back to their camp being lit by a single torch.

**THE MIGHTY RHINE, THAT** unstoppable river that marches out of Switzerland and through Germany towards the sea, confronts headlong the immovable Taunus Mountains near Mainz. Here it is forced to yield and turn sharply westward for 30 kilometres before skirting around the Rüdesheimer Berg and reforging its northward journey. The vineyards that cover the slopes of that steep-faced hill look down approvingly as the Rhine retreats into the distance.

This almost S-shaped curve of the river cradles some of Germany's most beautiful and fabled countryside. Stately schloss, famous wine estates and picturesque medieval villages provide the perfect backdrop for the heroes, dragons, Rhine maidens, giants and treacherous dwarfs who once peopled this land. Unfortunately, it was not the winged horse of a Valkyrie but our clapped-out campervan that jerked and spluttered to a halt on Rüdesheimer Berg. Nonetheless, the sunlit scene that lay below us was completely breathtaking. It was a warm, windless, peaceful afternoon and it seemed that mankind's attempts to impose his wishes on the world were here in perfect harmony with nature.

'Why don't we treat ourselves to a few days in a camping ground while we visit some vineyards and explore the region?' Chris suggested.

'Yes!' chorused the boys excitedly.

We had been on the road for quite a long time and the idea of hot showers and a playground clearly appealed, even if the thought of visiting more vineyards did not provoke enthusiasm in the lower echelons. In reality, everything in this famous Rheingau wine region of Germany was so obsessively ordered that camping wild was out of the question. There was nothing left that could be called 'wild', and certainly nowhere that it was possible to freedom camp. Even camping grounds seemed thin on the ground, but after a lot of searching and enquiring we were directed to one.

As we pulled in to our intended home-away-from-home for the next few days the boys became very enthusiastic, but Chris and I felt more than a tinge of disappointment. It appeared clean, neat and tidy but entirely soulless. There were one or two trees scattered about to provide a modicum of shade, and a few squares of rapidly balding grass. The latter had been marked out as camping spaces and they looked a little like rows of animal pens without walls. They had evidently been designed to allocate the minimum area and the maximum number of spaces possible. The ablution blocks were no doubt functional but looked as though all expense had been spared on architects' fees. The place was deserted apart from a few desultory-looking campers.

'Do we really want to stay here?' I whispered to Chris.

'Can you think of a better option?'

'No.'

'Well, let's just make the best of it. At least there is a playground that will probably keep the kids happy.'

We drove up to the reception area where the solidly constructed, beetroot-faced welcoming committee of one was standing in a red shirt and blue overalls with his arms folded. His short, spiky, formerly blond hair had greyed somewhat and was now the colour of mouldy straw. I smiled, pointed to our UK number plates and tried to introduce myself in English. I received absolutely no verbal or visual response, so I flicked a cerebral switch and replayed the same track in faltering German. Smiles, nods and 'Ja' were emitted from the automaton. I explained as best I could that we would like to stay for a few days, and received even greater signs of approbation. After signing in and displaying our Kiwi passports, clear evidence that we were not dastardly Albions, I asked him where he would like us to park.

'Anywhere. You can choose your own area,' he said in German, spreading his beefy arms out towards the whole camping ground. It was clear there was not going to be huge competition for space.

We walked around the semi-rural, semi-blissful site and chose the least offensive-looking place, in the furthest corner, well away from the toilet block. At least there was a birch tree to give a little shelter, a few grass remnants underfoot and relative isolation to provide a suggestion of privacy. The kids made a beeline for the swings and slides as I parked the campervan and popped its top, while Chris proceeded to prepare the evening meal.

'Look,' she exclaimed, 'here are some more campers. Isn't it a bit strange that they have chosen to come right over here and park next to us?'

A black Mercedes pulled into the camping space alongside us.

'He's not a camper. It's our old friend, that cheer-germ Frankenstein,' I observed as the multicoloured apparition tried to extract itself from the vehicle. The effort produced wheezing and the visage became a dark shade of puce as at last he emerged.

'You can't stay here! This is reserved,' he pronounced loudly.

'Then where would you like us to go?' I asked in hesitant German.

'Anywhere else is fine,' was my interpretation of his reply, and again he flapped his arms in the general direction of the rest of the camping ground.

This time we chose the next most remote corner, which lacked a tree, had no grass, was a bit closer to the road and hence noisier. Nonetheless, it was okay, but only just. Again we started to prepare for the evening's repast and the coming night, but before Chris could even light the gas stove Boris Frankenstein's black Mercedes showered us in a cloud of dust. An even more agitated, plethoric and sweating host loomed in front of us.

'You cannot stay here! This is also reserved,' he shouted gutturally, as flecks of white slobber started to shower towards us from close range. Chris and I are both naturally cowardly, and instinctively we stepped backwards for reasons of both physical safety and hygiene.

'Where is it that you would like us to camp?' I enquired in a purposely low-volume, calm voice. 'Is there somewhere special that you would prefer that we parked?'

'Nicht. The rest of the camp is fine. Nowhere else is reserved.' This time he merely swept his right arm dramatically in an almost complete circle, which excluded just the spot where we had lowered our anchor.

'We are not going to take the worst place in the camping ground just to please that creep,' Chris said defiantly, 'but we must be careful not to select his best spot.'

And so we looked around carefully for somewhere inconspicuous. We parked at a respectful distance from some other people, more towards the centre of the camp but not too close to the facilities. Again I elevated the roof of the campervan and Chris restarted to cook the meal. By this time the battle between the novelty of the playground and the boys' empty stomachs was swinging strongly in favour of their gastrointestinal tracts and they started to troop back towards our vehicle. We were somewhat surprised that they were able to home in on our moving campsite with unerring accuracy, but perhaps we were underestimating the draw of Mum's cooking aromas. The lads were just settling down to their dinner when the now too familiar black car pulled up unpleasantly close to where they were sitting at our little outdoor folding table. I must have been imagining it but I could have sworn that the piece of lard that emerged had put on weight and had become even more ugly, but there was no doubting that he was sweating more heavily, and the olfactory confirmation of this was overpowering.

'This place is also not suitable to camp,' he started to shout in German.

Now, the French have a colourful little saying that goes, '*La moutarde me monte au nez*', and literally means 'The mustard got up my nose', or more simply, 'I lost my temper'. I have never professed to be a person who can keep my cool under all circumstances, and while I might admire such ability, it seems to me that bucolic people often lack real passion and depth of feeling. At any rate, at that moment I felt anything less than cool and I was experiencing a burning surge of emotion that could not remotely be covered by the term 'mustard'. In *français* it would doubtless qualify for having a red hot chilli stuffed up each nostril and it was driving me insane. In order to get it out of my nose I had to get it off my chest.

'You filthy dirty Nazi!' I screamed in English, as the kids scrambled to get into the van. 'You are a fat, demented bully and an ugly one at that: a psychopath, a sadist and no doubt a sexual deviant. Get out of here and stop molesting us, you despicable piece of horse shit. We will not move again! You don't deserve to have anybody in this rotten camping ground. No wonder it's nearly empty if you treat your guests like dogs that you can chase around.'

Herr Frankenstein looked as though he had been hit by a bolt of lightning. His eyes opened wide, he stood rigidly to attention and I swear his rubicund face blanched a little. After what seemed an age, he said quietly, 'I am very sorry to have disturbed you and your family, sir. Please stay exactly where you are, and if there is anything I can do to make your stay more comfortable and pleasant, do not hesitate to let me know.'

I also stood rigidly immobile, because he had said this in perfect English, with hardly a trace of an accent. He had given no earlier sign of understanding or speaking English and I had let fly with my barrage of insults from behind the protection of what I thought would be an impenetrable wall of incomprehension. He now appeared as comfortable in English as in Deutsche. He turned, got back into his car and drove off slowly, looking deflated.

We spent a very uncomfortable night there, feeling angry, resentful, embarrassed and ashamed in equal measure. Our few days of fantasised rest and recreation within the protective walls of a camping ground had evaporated, like Rhine mist on a sunny morning. We rose early, packed and checked out at the reception. Fortunately, there was a sweet little fräulein behind the desk and no sign of our patron, Boris. Perhaps he was treating himself to a sleep-in before getting ready to terrorise his next customers, or had we got it wrong? Perhaps my German was not as good as I thought and I had misunderstood his instructions and intentions. Whatever the explanation, the experience had a deterrent effect and we did not set foot in another camping ground on that trip.

**IF YOU HAVE BEEN ON HOLIDAY** and treated yourself to locally produced wine with the region's special food, you will no doubt be able to attest to just how magical the combination can be. Perhaps you have dined during a balmy evening on a moonlit terrace overlooking the Mediterranean, or you have savoured a simple country platter while 'discovering' a ridiculously cheap gem of a local wine. Should you have succumbed to temptation and taken a few bottles back home, with the intention of impressing your friends at your next dinner party, it is on the cards that you will have been disappointed, if not embarrassed. Taken out of context your star will have to wing it alone and perform without any props, a hard ask for a talented professional, let alone a rank amateur. Maybe you will shrug it off by saying that the cork must have been faulty or the wine has not travelled well, but the real problem is likely to be the different situation and atmosphere in which your wine finds itself. Many wines, especially cheap ones, are propped up by their picturesque backgrounds. To our surprise we found that Germany proved to be an exception to this general rule.

German winemakers regard riesling as the king of white wines, as do those of neighbouring Alsace, and it was certainly the variety that held most interest for us in those parts of Europe. We were very familiar with German rieslings, as they had been readily available in New Zealand and Britain. We loved their complex spice, floral and fruity characters and their zesty well-balanced structure. We thought they would be just the perfect type of wine to sip and savour against the backdrop of some of the most stunning wine country in the world.

As we travelled through Germany's many wine regions we bought, tasted and drank many of the rieslings on offer, ranging from the cheap to the moderately expensive, at least as judged against our modest budget. Their purported quality was at least equal to those that we were used to drinking, but they never failed to disappoint us. Undoubtedly, they were fruity and reasonably balanced, but they lacked real excitement, seeming simple and one-dimensional. Yes, they had the anticipated apple and citrus attributes, but even these were dumbed-down and the expected mosaic underlay of scintillating flavour nuances had gone AWOL. The wines seemed hollow, lacking in concentration and depth, and their acid was sharp rather than tangy. We purchased rieslings from Rheinpfalz, Rheinhessen, Nahe, Rheingau and the Mosel Valley, but they all underwhelmed us. Were we being miserable cheapskates and not paying enough for our daily tipple? Were the producers trying to palm off their dud vintages? Had the winemakers lost their touch? We simply did not know the answer, but the strangest thing of all was that the wines lacked the true character of riesling.

As we passed south, through Austria into Italy, we were diverted from riesling and explored the delights of Barolo, Chianti and similar robust reds. It was not until a year or two later, when we were back in London, that we found several bottles of the reject rieslings that we had bought while touring Germany and then completely forgotten.

'I can't imagine that they will be much good now, since they were pretty unimpressive before,' I said rather pessimistically. 'Perhaps, Chris, you could use them in cooking.'

'Yes, that's a good idea. I'm doing poached cod for dinner tonight so I'll use some of the riesling in the marinade. I'll prepare it now.'

The cork gave a cheerful pop and out of habit I had a sniff of its wet underside while it was still attached to the corkscrew.

'It's not corked. In fact, it smells quite delicious. Let's try a glass.'

'It's beautiful,' Chris exclaimed, 'and it smells and tastes just like riesling should! How did it manage to change from that wishy-washy wine that we bought back into this one? It's amazing!'

Of course, we were well aware of the changes that occur in wines as they mature, but this appeared to be something quite different. Generally speaking, a wine may take a knock when it is bottled, so that it can appear somewhat muted for two or three months, but then its previous characters reappear. Over the ensuing year or so, its fruity aromas and flavours intensify and its body fills out. Secondary or bottle maturation aromas and tastes progressively develop, making the wine more complex and interesting as it mellows and becomes more harmonious. If left too long, these characters start to fade and the wine goes over the hill, eventually losing its zest and interest. During this process, however, virtually all wines retain the original fruit flavours and aromas that are the unique stamp of the variety or varieties from which they are made. In other words, from day one a gewürztraminer, a muscat, a merlot or a pinot noir will each show its individual flavour profile, which with time will become stronger or weaker and will be overlain by others that result from the maturation process. In spite of this, they retain their identities, just as a cat remains its feline self from kitten to old age and at no stage becomes a dog. Our shock was that our riesling seemed to have completely abandoned this inviolate rule of vinous nature. It was not that it had become a dog of a wine. The reverse had happened and it had metamorphosed from a grub into a beautiful butterfly.

Needless to say, our bottle of riesling from the Mosel Valley did not end up in the fish dish that night but was lovingly savoured with the meal. Even our philistine beer-drinking dinner guests commented how beautiful the wine was. In time we found that this miraculous transformation had occurred in all the rieslings we had brought back with us. What was the explanation? We didn't know it then, but subsequent delving into the natural chemical processes that occur as wine ages shed light on the conundrum. The main and very special flavouring components of riesling are naturally occurring molecules called turpines. These consist of two halves fused together. In this form it does not have a lot of aroma and flavour. As the wine ages these two halves separate, exposing very aromatic parts of the molecule. Hence, the wine takes on a completely new character. Perhaps it should be called a schizophrenic wine, but we prefer to look on it as an ugly duckling. No wonder it is so special!

**ITALY IS A FAVOURITE COUNTRY** of ours and we have been there many times, visiting most regions from the northern Dolomites to southern Sicily. We have trekked through its hills, valleys and villages. Perhaps the most spectacular way to enter the country is through Austria, as we did on the first of our campervan visits. We were fascinated by the primitive but picturesque agriculture on both sides of the border as we watched small terraced fields being hand-scythed for hay, while the dried grass was carefully stacked around poles to form conical tree-shaped haystacks. The customs, people, houses and hamlets all seemed quaint echoes of yesteryear. We were impressed by the raw beauty of the snow-topped mountains and sunny valleys of the Alto Adige, the scenic tranquillity of Italy's northern lakes, the vineyards of Piedmont, the medieval villages of Tuscany and the spectacular architecture of Florence, among many other things.

One thing that struck us as being out of place in this apparently idyllic countryside was the attention paid to domestic security in rural situations. Not only grand country mansions but also quite modest cottages were frequently surrounded by high fences. These were often topped by buttock-menacing metal spikes, scratchy barbed wire or hand-lacerating shards of broken glass that were clearly meant to discourage uninvited guests. The gates were similarly tall, well-fortified and usually locked. Granted, in all communities there are vagabonds, rogues, robbers, psychopaths, cut-throats, and a mishmash of other social misfits, but this emphasis on leading an undisturbed life seemed rather strange.

'I wonder why they have all this security paraphernalia,' I said to Chris one day as we were strolling past a large ugly gate, sporting impressive iron bars, which was guarding a dilapidated and decidedly unimpressive house.

'I suspect that it's a Benedictine monastery and that all the inmates have taken vows of silence,' she replied flippantly. 'They just want to lead tranquil, undisturbed lives of contemplation.'

Suddenly the children simultaneously yelled in terror as a tsunami of adrenaline unleashed the mother of all flight-or-fight reactions in us. Fortunately, our sphincteric guardians were among muscles automatically tensed by the gigantic hormonal release as we swung to face our deadly foe. An enormous, slavering black dog of uncertain but undoubtedly mixed pedigree, which had clearly been bred to dismember gladiators, had sprung from behind one of the bushes in the garden of the house. The brute was snarling and barking savagely only inches from where the boys were standing. It was readily apparent that the dentition of Cerberus was in excellent condition, with every fang sharpened to perfection. With all its might the beast pushed and strained against the gate, which creaked and slowly started to swing towards us.

Only then did I notice that, in spite of being an undoubted testament to the quality of the Italian engineering profession and security business, the gate was not locked. A large rusty chain, with an equally dilapidated padlock, was meant to be securing the gate shut but they had been left un-united. Already the dog's dripping muzzle was appearing around the edge of the gate. Without hesitation I threw my weight at the gate, forcing it back against the gatepost. There was a savage howl of pain as Cerberus's snout was crushed between the two pieces of metal and the offending part was briskly withdrawn back inside. The guardian of the gates of Hell turned tail and fled as Chris reunited the padlock with the offending link.

It is certainly true that the big Italian cities have more than their fair share of low-life and that the tourist needs to keep his or her wits close at hand. Some years later Chris and I were staying in a small Rome hotel, the restaurant of which was several doors away and could only be accessed by walking down the street. We were going to breakfast one morning when Chris turned to see why I was lagging. She was amazed to see me locked in an embrace, with my body pinning a not-unattractive-looking young woman against a shop window and holding her hands above her head. A moment or so earlier she had cheerily called out to me and indicated a photo in a newspaper, which she then thrust towards my face. Naturally, my hands went up to fend it off and at the same time to try to see what it was that had so excited her. Unfortunately for her, I felt a hand slip into my trouser pocket and that is why I grasped both her wrists and pushed her away from me. The back of her head rather unceremoniously collided with the plate glass, making an unpleasant thud. When Chris had relieved her right hand of my wallet I stepped back from my apparently compromising position, released my grip and let the young woman flee into the rapidly assembling, gaping multitude. The second time I did this Eternal City waltz was several years later, with a charming gypsy girl. The newspaper was replaced by a baby that she carried in a sling around her neck but the plot, the dance movements and the ending were identical. Perhaps the production had used the same director.

**BUT THESE BIG-CITY HIJINKS STAND** in stark contrast to our impressions of Italian people in general and country dwellers in particular, whom we have found to be helpful, friendly and honest. One hot Saturday we found ourselves in Tuscany, on one of those tar-melting afternoons on which, with your windows down, you can hear the squelching sound of the road reluctantly parting from your wheels. We were on our way to a prearranged visit to a Chianti producer who, not unreasonably, had seemed somewhat reluctant to spend his valuable family time showing us his estate and wares.

'Would it be possible for you to come sometime during the working week, perhaps on Monday morning?' he had asked when I telephoned earlier in the week.

'Unfortunately, we will be in Umbria by then,' I had replied guiltily, knowing how often his leisure hours must be destroyed by similar visits.

Being a helpful Italian he had graciously acquiesced.

Maps can be deceptive, and we found that we were making very slow progress on the small, winding country road when I happened to glance at the fuel gauge and noticed that it was nudging the red.

'Damn. We're running late but we need fuel. There's a village a couple of kilometres off our route. We'll have to try and get some there.'

Most small-town Italian petrol stations were in the habit of closing for the weekend at midday on Saturday so we were relieved to find one that was open, or so it seemed, as there were a couple of other vehicles having their tanks filled. Frustratingly, my pump would not work so I moved to the next one but the result was the same. A helpful motorist explained that I needed to use a bank card or feed the unfriendly machine banknotes in order to get its cooperation. I had never used an automated self-service pump before, and to find one in a small Italian village seemed remarkable, all the more so because the frustrating beast was intelligent enough not to trust my UK plastic, forcing me to resort to cash.

I only had large-denomination notes but, as I needed a whole tank full of fuel and we were already late for our appointment, I threw caution to the wind and offered the pouting machine one of these, which it greedily ingested. Success! The pump roared into life and a satisfying, erotic gurgling came from the successful union of the Italian nozzle and the British inlet. I watched the litres flow and the price augment with a sense of mastery and achievement. In the silence that followed the cut-out of the pump motor I looked in vain for my change to come submissively tumbling out of the now-conquered beast. It remained defiantly dumb and unobliging. I then noticed that it did not have an appropriate orifice to enable it to render such a service, although a receipt had appeared from a slot, detailing the transaction and confirming that I was owed the equivalent of $20 change. I glanced around and saw that, although the garage and office were closed, there was a small cubicle by the exit, in which sat a bored-looking, acne-challenged youth. With my receipt I would be able to get my change from him. I strode over and thrust my piece of paper through the small slot in the glass that separated us. He looked at it, apparently uncomprehendingly, then passed it back to me.

'Moneta?' I asked.

'No moneta,' he replied. 'Ritorna Lunedi.'

I then tried to explain that I would be in Umbria on Monday and that I could not come back for the change. Did he not have even some of that amount? At that point an Italian voice from behind me explained in English that the teenager did not have any money, and that it was normal procedure to come back at a time when the garage office would be open in order to get change.

'But donta worry. Ia liva nearabuy. Ia giva you change an you giva me receipt. Ia coma back anudda time.'

So saying he opened his wallet and handed me the exact change. I tried to force a small commission onto him as recompense for his generous help but he would not hear a word of it. And this was typical of our experience of rural Italians — welcoming, helpful and generous.

Unfortunately, our Chianti winemaker could not be described by the same adjectives. To cap everything off his vineyard proved to be very difficult to find and we arrived impossibly late. We received a somewhat frosty reception, a brisk and unceremonious tour of the establishment, and were then released to go on our not-so-merry way. For this we did not blame him in the slightest, and we had learnt a valuable lesson. Never underestimate the difficulty of negotiating Italian back-country roads or deciphering that country's unique address system!

**WE WERE, HOWEVER, LEFT WITH** the perplexing enigma of what seemed to be over-the-top security against a largely benign and friendly population. Could it be that there were occasional apples in the barrel that were so rotten that drastic action had to be taken. Were the Mafia implicated? We asked an Irish friend who had married a local and had lived on a small vineyard for many years, without high walls or gates.

'No, I don't think it is the Mafia. Our house has been broken into on a couple of occasions when we have been away, and we have had offers of help with security from local villagers, but we have not yet succumbed to paying for this.'

We had heard of an English friend of a friend who had become so tired of paying exorbitant 'protection' money for his Italian holiday home that he had sold it. However, these reasons, along with the desire to keep teenage daughters firmly ensconced at home during the night, hardly seemed sufficient to warrant the lengths that were being taken to ensure domestic privacy.

Finally, it was a helpful vigneron who shed light on the mystery.

'You see, Italian property law is quite different from Anglo-Saxon law. It's very old and dates back to Roman times. When you buy a piece of land in Italy, what you purchase is the exclusive right to use it. You can plant a garden, grow crops, farm, run a vineyard and the like, but you cannot stop other people from walking through the property.'

'But that sounds dreadful!' Chris exclaimed. 'They might interfere with what you're doing, break things or steal.'

'That is the risk. It is not so much a matter of personal security but one of privacy and avoiding damage to things. Should they steal your fruit, smash your equipment or in any other way interfere with your property, then you can report them to the police or take legal action. However, if they can gain access to your property without damaging your fence, wall or gates, then they are entitled to do just that. But the worst things are the cinghiale.'

'Cinghiale?' echoed Chris. 'What are they?'

'Cinghiale are wild boar and, as they are wild, they don't belong to anyone in particular and can be hunted by any Italian. Italian males are very macho and consider themselves to be romantic, swashbuckling figures, especially when it comes to guns. They believe they have a God-given right to hunt with guns. They will shoot at anything that moves and often take pot-shots at objects they are uncertain about. The philosophy is that it is better to shoot at an uncertain or mysterious target rather than miss a potential game animal. They especially come at dawn to hunt cinghiale, creeping through the vineyard and firing willy-nilly.

'They can come right beside your house and shoot. As it is half-light they are often blasting off at things that aren't cinghiale. I can tell you it is not very nice for you and your family to be suddenly woken up by gunfire right outside your window. In the hunting season it is dreadful around here. It seems just like the Third World War. A lot of country houses have high walls and gates in order to keep people, especially hunters, from just wandering through their property. Naturally, they can't get in without damaging this ring of security, which would be illegal. If I could afford it I would also build a high wall right around our home and winery. At least it would make it safe, even if we still got woken up by the noise.'

We have frequently thought of these words when hiking through the Italian countryside. So often the path on which you are directed goes through private property, including vineyards, orchards, olive groves, crops and cultivated fields. It may even go so embarrassingly close to dwellings that it is possible to see the farmers and their families having a meal or watching television. The 'owners' seem to be unconcerned and take it in their stride, but their dogs usually protest noisily, although never as savagely as our old friend Cerberus.

**I FIRST REMEMBER SPANISH WINES** appearing on the shelves of Kiwi wine merchants in the late 1960s and early 1970s. Due to the Spanish regulations regarding terms such as *reserva* and *gran reserva*, these wines had had many years of barrel- and bottle-ageing before reaching us. Thus, they seemed harmonious, mellow and sophisticated compared with the rather rough young plonk that was being turned out by the majority of New Zealand vineyards at that time. In addition, there was the novelty of having lashings of toasted coconut and vanilla in the aroma and flavour, the result of the Spanish favouring American oak barrels that seemed to suit their red wines. Another advantage for the penurious was that they were stunningly cheap. As a result of this we had thoroughly done our homework, both in New Zealand and in England, before our campervan turned its nose towards the Spanish border. Chris had also learnt Spanish for three years because we had correctly assumed that English was not high on the list of educational priorities south of the Pyrénées at that time.

As we had come from Italy, we had chosen to enter Spain not far from the picturesque little French town of Banyuls-sur-Mer, famous for its alcoholic sweet red wine, a little like a light style of port. The passport control and customs facilities were as rustic as the view, which we had plenty of time to admire as we patiently queued for the privilege of being processed. What both countries had saved on buildings and amenities they had clearly invested in the arms industry, which was doubtless more profitable than the real estate business. The tired, bored and sweating officers were all sporting handguns, and more than a few carried vicious-looking automatic weapons. We certainly were not tempted to start a riot, or even drop a sweet wrapper on the ground.

After what seemed an interminable wait in the scorching sun, we were halted just one car short of the immigration booth. At the same time the motor of a truck coming from the Spanish side, which had no doubt waited for a similar age, began to smoke. Vapour started to pour from under its bonnet. The owners made no move to take corrective action and suddenly became fixated on a point in the distance, which they seemed to be discussing volubly. Chris and I glanced in the same direction, but we could not see anything that looked remotely interesting. At this point two guards descended on the driver and told him to pull the truck over to one side, where they indicated that he should lift the bonnet. He started to argue, but a third officer, one of those shouldering an automatic weapon, seemed to be prepared to lend a helping hand and sauntered over towards the group. The driver half raised his arms, shrugged his shoulders and acquiesced.

As the bonnet was raised, a cloud of smoke obscured the view, but as it cleared a revolutionary new design of motor was revealed. It seemed to be made entirely of bottles of Spanish brandy. It must have been a very large motor because it filled every available centimetre of space under the bonnet and there was no sign of anything else that might have been capable of propelling the vehicle. What seemed even more of an engineering marvel was that these bottles of brandy were packed in cardboard boxes. The sole design fault was the fragility of the bottles, one of which had broken or exploded, and presumably the brandy had ignited. It looked just like a giant Christmas pudding being flambéed and it cried out for a good helping of custard. Presumably the rather depressed-looking driver had overlooked the *crème anglaise*, but it was rapidly applied by yet another guard wielding a foaming fire extinguisher. It seemed to us that with the heat more bottles could burst and that the whole truck might explode.

While all this was going on we had not really been paying a lot of attention to the officer inspecting our passports but he suddenly indicated that we were free to go. We did not need a second invitation and limped away from the border as fast as our ancient campervan could go. That evening, when I went to a shop to buy a bottle of wine, I checked the price of Spanish brandy. As I suspected, it was only a small fraction of the price of French brandy. Perhaps our Don José might have been more successful if he had taken along his Carmen to lend a helping hand or leg.

**IT WAS SIESTA IN MADRID,** a time when all self-respecting Spaniards should be indoors, attending to their stomachs, beauty sleep or love lives. We were like mad dogs and were still out in the midday, or to be more precise, early afternoon, sun. We were sitting in a roadside public park, having that morning dragged our long-suffering kids around the extensive Goya display in the Prado. We were just starting to enjoy a picnic lunch when we saw a tall middle-aged man dressed in black, wearing a matching wide-brimmed hat, come strolling down the street. He looked rather like the bad guy from a cheap 1950s cowboy movie. The rustler stopped beside an enormously long black convertible, which had been fully converted to suit the weather. He then walked to the back of the car and eyed up the vehicle behind before doing the same thing at the front of the car. We could hear what seemed to be an expletive. It seemed to us that the other motorists had been very respectful, were well inside their parking spaces and that the *hombre* had plenty of room. Suddenly, he sprinted towards the convertible and leapt over the door onto the front seat. He then gunned the motor to life, reversing into the car at the rear. When the bumpers were in contact he accelerated wildly so that the other vehicle was forced back against the car behind it. He then repeated the manoeuvre on the car in front before reversing once more and then casually driving away.

'A bullfighter on wheels,' commented Chris drily. 'No doubt it is Escamillo on his way to pick up Carmen.'

Although the day had been laden down with hours of heavy, oppressive sunshine, the sky had now darkened and there was the smell of a refreshing thunderstorm in the air. As we stopped at the roadside pottery stall, a little out of Toledo, the scene resembled an El Greco painting, full of splashes of blue, grey, black and white. As these things go, it was a large stall, with several horizontal trestles in front that were attached to a big wooden vertical backdrop. This grand display space was crammed with all sorts of pottery gems, ranging from the utilitarian and rustic to the obscenely ornamental and gaudy. We had not really intended to buy, but we were all in need of stretching our legs and having a break. We had been driving for a long time and the boys had been excellent. However, they and their parents were all beginning to get a bit restless.

'Look at that!' exclaimed Chris. 'It's such a beautiful shape, so traditional and functional. It just pokes its chest out and says "I am Spanish, Spanish, Spanish", but in a humble rather than a flamboyant way.'

'Yes,' I agreed, 'and we could use it on this trip. It would keep our drinking water cool.'

The object of our attentions was a squat jar with a single handle opposite a neat little spout, and a short neck at the top where it could be filled with water. We had seen workers in the fields and vineyards drinking from such jars. They were made of grey clay and, although fired, they were not glazed. With time a little water soaked through the vessel to the outside and its evaporation kept the contents cool, even in the blistering noonday heat.

'Cuánto cuesta?' asked Chris. The lean, swarthy woman behind the stall mumbled a price and held up some digits as translation aids. The amount seemed quite reasonable, but we were highly experienced travellers and we knew it was an inviolate law that all tourists get ripped off by the locals in continental Europe, especially English-speakers in exotic destinations like Spain.

'Bargain her down,' I commanded imperiously, feeling secure that she wouldn't understand English. Chris then offered the vendor 20 per cent of the price she had quoted but the woman vigorously shook her grey but wise head and made a counter-offer. Eventually, we settled on half the original price. Although the amount that we had saved by bargaining was, in our terms, a mere pittance we felt extremely smug and self-satisfied as we turned back towards the campervan.

A sudden crash caused us to freeze in our tracks. My first thought was that there must have been a motor vehicle accident behind us but then I realised that this was impossible. Chris and I turned to see that the entire back of the stall, which had been covered with hanging items of pottery, had fallen forwards onto its front and that the ground was littered with broken items. What a disaster! But before we could start to feel sorry for the elderly proprietor we were horrified by another sight. There, revealed by the now collapsed back of the stall, stood a small, frightened little boy whose hand was outstretched towards where the back had been. It was our own Matthew, and it was clear that his side of the vertical back had also been covered in tempting pottery animals. He seemed to have been reaching for a cute little rabbit, whose pottery body he still clutched but whose ears were now sadly detached from its head. The ancient one, who a moment before had seemed reasonably happy when we had miserably ground a few pesos off her profit, was now contorted with grief and started to wail most lamentably. She may well have been keening, for she had indeed lost a beloved, who was probably her sole means of support, and it was clear that the Donaldson family had killed him.

'Vamos a pagar por todo esto,' Chris said consolingly, going up to the broken woman and putting her arm around her. We would pay for it. The screaming immediately ceased and the wretch brightened visibly, even managing a slight smile. We all set about gathering up the smashed items and piling them in a heap on one side. The children helped, regarding it as a jolly game. There was no point in blaming Matthew, as he had been merely 'looking' with his fingers and the stall must have been excessively rickety for the back to have collapsed. There were pink flamingos, whose delicate legs had been fractured in a dozen places, red and green parrots without heads, trunkless elephants, assorted virgins and children, cheerful pigs, who had been untimely cracked open, pawless dogs and many other equally obscene objects, not to mention the cheerful rabbit.

'Why on earth did we bother to bargain her down a stupid little peso or two? Now she has got us over a barrel and can charge us anything she likes,' I whispered to Chris in a wave of self-pity.

I had begun to feel my wallet aching with the lightness of being, or perhaps more appropriately not being, for at that moment it seemed in danger of disappearing into thin air.

'Because we had to,' my wife replied. 'It's our natures. We are miserable!'

The heap of broken pottery had to be sorted through and laid out in state in order to do the final roll-call and assemble for the last post. The now happy proprietor flattened out a crumpled brown paper bag and, with a very blunt pencil, which she had to suck in order to make it write in a watery purple colour, began to make a list of the prices of all the smashed items. She then started to add them up, assisted by much frowning, pursing of lips and counting on digits. Finally, she looked up with an expression of triumph and nominated what seemed to be a staggering sum, a number of pesos ending in multiple zeros. Chris told me in English the total cost and I calculated it back to pounds sterling.

'There must be a mistake,' I whispered. 'That's only £6.'

Even during the 1970s this was not a huge amount. Chris asked the old lady to recheck, which she did, coming back with the same total cost. We paid up very happily, and the vendor looked even more pleased. She had no doubt had a very profitable day and might even be able to go on holiday for the rest of the week. We would not have blamed her if she had ripped us off, given our misplaced display of bargaining prowess, but she seemed to have resisted the temptation. We had just started to troop back towards our campervan when the woman emitted an agitated cry. My heart sank and I was tempted to jump into the vehicle and speed away. She had clearly found some fault in her addition. We turned around to find her running after us and waving her arms.

'What does she want?' I asked Chris.

'She says that now we have paid for the ornaments they are ours and we are welcome to take them. We only need to glue them together and they'll be as good as new. She believes that we will get a good price for them.'

We both burst out laughing and waved the stall-holder a cheery goodbye. Chris called out that she was welcome to do it, and that it would be extra profit for the day. Our Lady of the Shards seemed doubly grateful.

We have a saying in medicine that 'a little spilt blood goes a long way', meaning that you do not have to have much bleeding before the scene looks like a dreadful massacre. I now knew that this sentiment could equally be applied to broken pottery.

**WE WERE MOVING FURTHER** west in Spain and had our sights set on entering Portugal through the Douro Valley, after first visiting the ancient spanish university town of Salamanca. The countryside through which we were passing looked increasingly parched, dusty and barren, with stunted crops, gnarled old grapevines, occasional olive trees, and a few goats. The farmhouses were small, whitewashed, simple buildings with few windows and no electricity. Donkeys were not only the basis of a lot of local transport but were also the powerhouse for much other activity. We saw them patiently walking in circles, drawing well water for irrigation or grinding grain by turning millstones. Everything seemed primitive and picturesque.

Before long the mercury started to climb steeply. Our old Bedford campervan either dated from an era before the advent of air-conditioning or had spent its life entirely in Britain where such equipment was regarded as obscene luxury. It became so hot that we thought of travelling by night and sleeping somewhere cool and shady during the day.

'It wouldn't be practical, Ivan. We couldn't reset the boys' diurnal rhythms. They would sleep at night while we were driving and then keep us awake when we wanted to snooze in the daytime. Plus, we would miss out on seeing all this fascinating country.'

'But even with the windows open to their maximum you can't get enough air circulating through the vehicle to keep it cool.'

'Why don't we just drive with the doors open?' Chris suggested.

And that is what we did. Our campervan had sliding doors on each side so we hitched them wide open and off we drove. Such a thing would doubtless be prohibited today, being regarded as too dangerous, and even then it gave us a certain nervous thrill, but it worked a treat. The air was still hot, but its close-to-zero moisture content meant that it was very drying as it whistled around our bodies. As liquid evaporates it conveniently sucks out heat. Our rapidly sweating, nearly naked bodies were thus kept nicely cool. We just had to remember to keep up the fluid intake in order to keep our kidneys ticking over.

**AS THE WEATHER BECAME HOTTER** our campervan began to lose increasing amounts of oil. It seemed to well up from the bowels of the motor and weep its way over the head before running down its sides and finally trickling onto the road. We told the kids that our motor was sad and crying from having to do so much hard work in the heat. Perhaps this was a mistake, as they asked us to go slower and give it more rests. If it had been going much slower we would have been stationary. The leak had become so obvious that cars would pass us while we were motoring along the road and then stop some way ahead, flagging us down in order to tell us we had a problem. Our motor seemed not just a bit dispirited but frankly depressed, and Chris and I wondered whether it might be suicidal. In order to jolly it along we were administering our patient an antidepressive dose of 1–2 litres of oil daily. When the motor was not going, there was no oil leak.

Top of my list of differential diagnoses was a leaking head-gasket, but I could not get a Spanish car psychiatrist, physician or surgeon interested. While the rate of replacement meant that the campervan clearly did not require a change of oil, I felt that it needed to be greased because we had travelled a long way. But it was impossible to find a Spanish mechanic who would lower himself to look at a British vehicle. Were we too close to Gibraltar, or were the post-Armada wounds still raw? It was impossible to tell. There was nothing for it but to keep lumbering forwards.

The oil saga had started a year or so earlier when we had been looking for another campervan. Chris had answered an advertisement in a second-hand-vehicle magazine and we had been lured to a small village on the outskirts of south London. We got off the train in bright sunshine and walked to the local Anglican vicarage, just next door to a small but solid-looking old stone church. The vicar was unduly pallid, even allowing for it being early spring, and he had an unnerving habit of not looking at you when he spoke. Perhaps his forte rested in his sermons and not in ministering to the needy.

He proudly displayed his mechanical treasure and gave us an enthusiastic appraisal that would have brought tears to the eyes of the most professional of second-hand-car dealers. It had given him loyal service and he felt absolutely wretched at having to part with it, but his wife needed an operation and his stipend was meagre. He lifted the bonnet and displayed the motor, which shone like a new pin. When I exclaimed that it was remarkably clean, he confessed to having had it steam-cleaned, being a meticulous person who wanted to do the best by the new owner, whoever that lucky person might be. We took his pride and joy for a little spin down by the village green, past the local pub and along the high street. There were no hills where I could give it a more serious and stressful testing, but it seemed to putter along quite satisfactorily.

'It has got quite an oily smell, hasn't it?' I commented to the vicar.

'Yes, I thought so too,' Chris agreed.

'I don't smell anything,' said our man of the cloth, looking upwards. 'I've never had any trouble with the oil. Oh, I remember now. I did wipe the dashboard with an oily cloth just to get rid of any dust and grime. That must be what you smell.'

And so we proudly drove our new second-hand campervan back to central London and thought no more about the oil. No more, that is, until we pulled into a garage in France to get some *essence*. More out of habit than suspicion, I checked the oil. The dipstick was completely dry! Panic stations! I broke out in a cold sweat and started to pour oil into the motor. It took 2–3 litres before it even started to register on the bottom of the dipstick! From that time onwards I always checked the oil when buying petrol and I carried a can of oil in the back of the van. So while I cannot say that I was completely surprised when our motor began to gush oil, I was worried. It wasn't that I did not like supporting our Arab brethren; it was just that I had not planned to support their economic development to such a large extent.

**EVENTUALLY WE LIMPED OVER** the Portuguese border. It was higher here and hence somewhat cooler. We had not gone far before I noticed that a red light had come on, indicating that the battery was losing its charge. Hence it would not be long before we would either stop involuntarily or be unable to restart. We decided to call into the next garage that we saw and plead for their help. Imagine our surprise when they welcomed us with open arms. Yes, they could fix any British car. Did we not know that every third car in Portugal was British-made? I then vaguely recalled the Treaty of Windsor, which is the oldest alliance in the world that is still in force and dates back to the Middle Ages. It had served as the basis for much trade and political/military manoeuvring over many centuries.

So while the happy mechanics attacked our sad old friend, we took the children for a walk around the local park. They had told us that we would have to stay for several days in order for them to fix the oil haemorrhage. Instead we had opted for a grease and having the generator fixed, which they assured us would deal with the discharging battery. We returned two hours later to find the work had been completed.

'How much does this work out at?' Chris asked me after she had taken possession of an imposing invoice in escudos, which was the Portuguese currency at that time.

'Good grief. That's only five quid!' I exclaimed. 'Let's pay up and get on the road before they change their minds.'

That night we parked a little off a dirt track high up in the mountains. It was a slice of pure rustic paradise; cool but not cold, with not a cloud in the sky and not a breath of wind to ruffle the tranquil scene. The ground in front of us sloped gently downwards for quite a way before descending more steeply into a distant valley. Scattered trees enhanced the view. We felt completely isolated, with no sign of fellow human existence. If it had not been for the track, which suggested the contrary, we might have been the first to have set foot in the place, but then perhaps it was just an animal trail.

We were musing about this while sitting outside around a small table and enjoying our dinner. Then we heard the faintest of sounds somewhere in the far distance. We could not be certain what it was: animal, human, mechanical or just a trick of nature? Was it music and, if so, was it played by mountain spirits? Very gradually it swam into focus and became more discernible. There were two quite separate but intertwined sounds. The first was caused by myriad little tinkles, which rose and fell and intermingled seemingly haphazardly. The second was anything but random. It was marvellously put together, with an enticing pattern and a palette of simple but strikingly translucent colours. It gradually emerged as a clear but delicate little voice, completely incomprehensible but unmistakably full of hope, joy and love.

Well below us, around a corner of the hillside, came a small boy with a herd of goats. He was not leading them and he was not driving them, but merely walking amongst his charges and encouraging them upwards towards greener pastures. The goats bleated frequently, seemingly in response to their little master's care and concern. Slowly this magical and traditional mélange of human and animal sounds came closer as the troop wound its way up the track, near which we were parked. Eventually we were surrounded by the inquisitive flock, which ate the grass around us and even under our table. A few of the goats were happy to try other things, including our tablecloth, shoes and clothes, but they could easily be bribed away with a little bread. The lad, who could not have been more than eight or nine years old, was equally friendly and curious. We could not understand a word of each other's language and communicated with international smiles and gestures. He was delighted to accept a large slice of watermelon before he and his assembled tribe continued on their way to higher things, his pure and innocent soprano voice leading the charge.

A few minutes later Chris said, 'This is becoming a bit like Piccadilly Circus. I thought this was meant to be the middle of nowhere.'

I followed the direction indicated by her outstretched index. In the distance, coming up the same track, was a small blob that gradually morphed into a couple and a donkey. As they got closer it was apparent that they were elderly. The woman was riding side-saddle on the faithful beast while the man walked alongside, holding the lead and resting one hand on the animal's neck. Their clothes were a little threadbare but clean, and the pair seemed dignified and friendly. We waved and they veered from their path, coming over to our table. We also offered them watermelon, which they gratefully accepted. The old man reached inside one of two sacks that had been tied together and slung across the donkey's back. From it he withdrew a couple of onions, which he placed on our table. We nodded our acceptance and expressed our gratitude. The trio then made a stately exit over the brow of the hill and down into the next valley where presumably they resided.

'That was one of the most memorable and beautiful evenings that I have ever experienced,' Chris pronounced as she put the light out and we settled down in bed.

'That doesn't say much for our honeymoon!' I replied.

'Don't be like that. You know what I mean.'

'I do, and as a romantic evening it was certainly right up there!' I mumbled sleepily.

The next day we went down into the Douro Valley, the home of the internationally renowned port wine. As we descended the temperature ascended, and before long the boys forced us to stop by a shallow pond where there were many locals wallowing in an attempt to cool off.

'I'll go over and make certain it's safe,' Chris volunteered. 'We can have lunch here when they have had a bit of fun.'

They all donned their bathing costumes and headed off, Chris returning a little later.

'It's fine. The natives are friendly and there are lots of other kids in the pool, which is quite shallow. The boys can't get into any trouble and we can keep an eye on them from here in the shade. Let's get our books and have a read.'

We had only just settled down in our chairs and knocked off one or two pages when there was a loud screaming and the children came belting back.

'Snakes! Snakes!' they shouted in unison. 'There are snakes in the water.'

Their eyes were as large as saucers, but they looked excited rather than terrified. We glanced over at the pool where the locals were still lounging. They seemed totally unperturbed.

'They must be small eels,' I said hopefully.

'No! No! They are snakes and they are swimming in the pond over there.'

'I'll go over and see,' Chris said, getting up. 'There's someone over there who speaks English.'

She returned almost immediately, saying, 'The woman confirmed that they are snakes but they are not poisonous. It is evidently quite safe in the pool. Do you want to go back, boys?'

The boys all shook their heads and refused the invitation. Secretly we were rather relieved; being Kiwis we were uncomfortable in the company of serpents, unless they were well and truly dead. Fortunately, it was not long before the kids' attention was diverted. Lumbering down the road was an old cart, pulled by a tired and hot-looking ox. The boys rushed over to see it and were ecstatic to be given a ride in the cart by the friendly driver.

We slowly made our way down the Douro Valley, the steep sides of which were covered in terraced vineyards. We marvelled at what is among the most picturesque of viticultural scenes in the world, with its famous *Quinta* or wine estates. We eventually arrived at the fascinating old city of Oporto, which gives its name to the region's wine and is the home of the port shippers' 'houses', where the lusciously fruity, purple young wine is matured before being blended and dispatched to thirsty *bon vivants* all over the globe.

**THE COMPARATIVELY TINY COASTAL** wine district of Colares, situated a little out of Lisbon, is not well known and I am now uncertain why we had a hankering to see it. While today it is little more than a dormitory suburb of the capital, in those days it was quite bucolic. We were enjoying our visit to the region on a sunny Saturday afternoon when we had reason to be grateful to the magnificent institution of the Royal Automobile Club (RAC UK). I suspect the Royals do not use it quite as often as we did, because on that particular continental jaunt we called upon its extended services on five occasions. One of the best things about the club was the reciprocal arrangements it had with like-minded organisations in other countries, including Portugal. Call us skinflints, but if we had to choose between, on the one hand, buying an expensive, reliable car and forgoing RAC (or Automobile Association) membership, and on the other purchasing a cheap, clapped-out old heap and taking out a subscription, then we would opt for the latter option any time. In those days we did not have a choice.

So, here we were in Colares, taking a tight right-hand curve while motoring up a steep hill, when our campervan abruptly stopped. It did not putter to a graceful halt but just froze, jerking us all forwards, fortunately rather gently because our upward progression had been fairly leisurely. Even though it was not a busy road the situation was decidedly dangerous, as a following motorist could have unintentionally rear-ended us at any moment. I left the vehicle in first gear and applied the handbrake while Chris put a couple of large stones behind the wheels to ensure it would not run backwards. She then put an emergency triangle around the corner behind us while I flipped the bonnet and peered inside.

I have never claimed to be mechanically inclined, but I knew that an unheralded cardiac arrest was almost certain to be the result of an electrical disturbance of the heart. The other option, running out of blood, could be expected to give some sort of a warning, and a glance at the fuel gauge told me this diagnosis was incorrect. Nonetheless, I would check the carburettor as well as the electrics, just to be sure. The battery terminals looked fine and a screwdriver touching between them elicited a healthy spark. The generator leads were correctly attached, so I turned my attention to the distributor. There I found that a plug, leading from the distributor to the spark plugs, had come loose. This was clearly the problem. I pushed the plug back into the socket and tried to restart the vehicle, but it was obviously in a bloody mood and stubbornly refused to oblige. I took the plug out again. Yes, there was only one way it could fit into the socket so I reinserted it, vexingly with the same negative result. After repeating this manoeuvre a couple more times I had to admit I was completely foxed.

'We'll have to call the local equivalent of the RAC,' I told Chris dejectedly. 'Where's the booklet with the list of telephone numbers?'

'You'll have to try and find a house with a telephone. You had better go up the hill; we haven't passed a house lower down.'

I headed up the road while Chris entertained the boys under the shade of a tree. Eventually I found what seemed to be an old holiday house, and after braving an unpleasant-looking hound I made it to the front door. The elderly couple were very helpful and spoke enough English to be able to understand our predicament.

'He come Monday,' said the husband, holding the telephone to one side.

'No! Tell him it is dangerous. He needs to come now.'

Finally, it was agreed. He would arrive in about an hour. I went back to tell Chris that there was a glimmer of hope. After about two hours, much to our surprise, a large truck arrived. We had been expecting a small van, of the type that would attend a breakdown in the UK or New Zealand. The driver proceeded to attach a large hook and chain to the front of the campervan with the clear intention of hauling it up onto the deck of the truck. I remonstrated with him and tried to explain that the problem was likely to be simple and easily fixed, but there was no way he was going to look at anything under the bonnet. He was not a mechanic but a driver. He had to take our campervan back to the workshop.

We watched in dismay as our horse and home were wound up onto the sloping back of the truck, where it rested at quite a steep angle, while the driver prepared to leave, clearly solo. We all surged forward with the intention of getting into the truck's cab but our rescuer would have none of it. He was not permitted to carry passengers.

As on many occasions before and since I had reason to be impressed by Chris's singular powers of persuasion. Our saviour knight in now dull armour did not stand a chance as she strutted her calm mixture of charm, flattery, common sense, reason, insistence and feminine *force fatale*. Before he knew what had hit him, Chris had installed herself and the younger boys in the cab while the hapless driver instructed Matthew and me to get into the campervan. He indicated that we would have to lie flat on the floor for the entire journey as it was highly illegal for us to be there. This was easier said than done because as we swayed along the rough road we had to hold onto the legs of the seats to stop ourselves from sliding backwards and out of the dubiously secured rear doors. The driver stressed to us that we must not show ourselves until we were inside the garage and its outer doors were closed. He would bang on the van when it was safe to get up. While I did not find it to be one of the most comfortable, interesting or scenic trips that I had ever undertaken, it was one of the more soothing and settling. I had found the alternative possibility, that of being stranded in foreign countryside with nothing but our clothes, distinctly unnerving. Sure, we might have been able to get a taxi, catch a local bus or thumb a lift but, given the time and the circumstances, this all seemed rather unlikely.

As the gloom descended there was a sharp rapping on the campervan and one of the side doors was slid back. Matthew and I unfolded our stiff limbs and emerged to rejoin the rest of our little clan. It was nearly pitch-black inside the garage, but a moment later our driver flicked a switch and a fluorescent light high above spluttered into life, casting a pale glimmer over the scene. We were in a cavernous barn, or rather barns, as there seemed to be a second one immediately adjacent to ours and they were interconnected by large doors. There were a number of vehicles scattered about in various states of disrepair and repair. A strong 'garagey' smell filled the air, that indefinable but oily, minerally aroma that is exuded by all motor mechanics, their clothes and their workplaces. It inspired us and gave us a sense of confidence. The people here were clearly experts in the honourable art of tinkering with the inner parts of engines. We could trust our delicate beast to them, with the same degree of surety that one might place in one's gynaecologist, if one had a private matter that needed attention.

'Where is the mechanic?' I asked.

'No mechanic. He come Monday,' said our friendly driver with a smile. We remonstrated with him but to no avail. 'Mechanic not work weekend.'

'But we can't wait that long,' Chris chipped in. 'What will we do? Where will we stay? All our things are in the campervan. We will pay to have a mechanic come and look at our car now.'

'Mechanic not come. You stay here in garage until Monday.'

'Is there a hotel nearby?' I enquired in desperation.

'No hotels. Big festival. Hotels full.'

'But we will need to cook and it would be dangerous to turn on our gas in here,' I argued, hoping he would see sense and call a mechanic.

'I show you cooking.'

He took us to a little room at the back, still inside the garage, which we accessed by a short flight of stairs. Here there was a staffroom, its interior as spotless as a mechanic's overalls, with a single food-encrusted electric hotplate, an electric kettle, a dripping tap suspended above a rusty old sink, a motley collection of mugs and battered canisters of tea, coffee and sugar. A proud display of darkly streaked grey rags, which clearly served as hand towels, was suspended at various levels around the sink. It would have made a popular work of art at the Tate Modern. A battle-scarred wooden table, an assemblage of ancient chairs and a dying, once-red couch, its vital organs herniating through multiple wounds, completed the scene. The windows of our new home-away-from-home looked over the dimly lit interior of the garage, and in the distance we could just make out the form of our forlorn campervan.

'This looks just perfect,' Chris said semi-enthusiastically, and our helpful rescuer burst into a broad smile.

'Let's go and see if we can find a hotel and a decent restaurant,' I suggested after he had given us a key to the garage door and left us to our own devices.

Blindingly bright sunlight and a wave of searing heat overpowered us when we emerged onto the street. We had no idea where we were, but it was clearly a fairly industrial part of Lisbon. The streets were deserted. We walked around looking for anything that had a retail appearance but we were disappointed. No hotels, restaurants or shops could be seen. No pedestrians or vehicles came by. After an hour of fruitless searching we dispiritedly retraced our steps and gladly sought the shade and relative coolness of the garage. The place was deserted. We were trapped there alone and we would just have to make the most of it.

'How about a story, boys?' Chris asked, trying to sound enthusiastic. And so we passed the rest of the afternoon reading and playing games in the fumy gloom. Because there was no daylight we were thrown back on nature's gastric clock to tell us when to eat. As our stomachs chimed six o'clock we trooped back to the staffroom to cook our evening meal. We had put out the light when we left, so that as we entered the room was dark. The flick of the switch produced a nauseating sensation of disorientation. The bench between the sink and the hotplate seemed to be swaying erratically but then it swam into sharp focus. It was merely swarming with cockroaches. While we stood there gaping, the brown tablecloth of insects evaporated like a mirage, scuttling off to their multiple nooks, crannies and other hidey-holes.

'Ugh! Disgusting!' exclaimed Chris.

'Yes, but just remember, they are not like flies, which feed on filth and can come from a long distance away. These cockroaches just live around the bench, only feeding on leftover food and the like. They look horrible but they are pretty harmless,' I said, trying to sound reassuring.

'Can we biff them with our sandals next time we come,' asked one of the boys.

'Yes! Yes!' yelled the others.

We had had plenty of experiences with cockroach infestations in our London flats, and had dramatically reduced their numbers by pounding them with old shoes as soon as we had switched on the electric light at night. It was not a sport for the faint-hearted, but one that our battle-hardened children really enjoyed. Using our own pots we hurriedly cooked our dinner and retreated to the safety of the campervan to share our meal before settling down for the night.

'Great view from our camping spot tonight. It almost matches the one in the Douro mountains, where we met the goatherd,' I commented as we settled down to sleep.

'Yes, but the scene will look much better in the sunrise tomorrow morning,' was the sarcastic reply.

Because of the dark the boys did not stir quite so early in the morning, but if we had been expecting a Sunday sleep-in we would have been disappointed. A tow truck arrived at about 7 a.m. proudly dragging another salvage job. We were ready with a barrage of questions for the driver, and we established that there was a stop nearby where we could catch a bus to the beach. We opted for a jaunt to the seaside rather than crouching in the garage for another day. It was a beautiful beach, spoiled only by the teeming mass of humanity, all of whom seemed determined to turn themselves into beefsteak. They catered for all tastes, rare, medium and well done.

'Just move a little to the left, dear. No, that's too far. Take another step to the right.'

'You seem to be very fussy taking your photographs today, Ivan. Why is that?'

'It's just the light. It's difficult to get it right. The sunlight makes the sand so bright.'

It was not until we got back to London and were looking through our prints that Chris made a quite unjust accusation.

'You bastard! In each one of these shots you have deliberately placed me or the children so that there is a bare-breasted woman in the picture. They are full of tits.'

It is true that at that time I had never seen such a profusion of what comparative zoologists tell us are merely sweat glands, which have been modified in mammals to feed the young of the species. Even the French Riviera seemed prudish in comparison. Nevertheless, I protested my innocence and insisted that, while it might seem freaky, it was pure chance. Whatever the truth of the matter, there is no doubt that we all had a great day. It was with reluctance that we boarded the overcrowded, battered old Lisbon municipal bus to take us back to our dark cockroach lair.

Come Monday morning we were up with the larks, chirping and chattering with excitement. Today our saviour would come and release us from our black prison. The children, who were usually reluctant to move on, were refreshingly keen to be on the road again and to put kilometres between us and the garage. At 8.30 a.m. an unlikely looking messiah — middle-aged, unshaven, with tousled hair and a cigarette dangling from his lower lip — strolled into the garage and sauntered over to our campervan. His holey robe was a heavenly sky-blue, liberally anointed with oil that looked like numerous black clouds.

As best I could, I explained our problem, how it had started, what I had found and my unsuccessful, amateurish attempts at correcting the situation. He nodded sagely while enveloping us in an eye-watering cloud of smoke, thus largely concealing himself in much the same way that deities are reported to do when communicating with mere mortals on high mountain tops. He then took the plug out of the distributor, gave it a cursory inspection and reinserted it in the socket. He turned the ignition key and the motor started without hesitation. It was clear he was blessed with a divine healing touch, for the manoeuvre he had just carried out was seemingly exactly what I had done on that fateful uphill curve in Colares. This was truly a miracle. We all looked on dumbfounded, as if we were seeing Lazarus rise from the dead.

'I tape plug in place. No money. You go. Maybe generator faulty. I replace. Front tyre on right side badly worn. Dangerous. I replace with good old one.' He named what sounded like an outrageous price.

'How much is that?' I asked Chris as we both started our mental calculations.

‘Nine pounds,’ she replied, clearly having newer batteries in her calculator.

‘Yes, please do it,’ I happily acquiesced, and then asked him if he could fix the oil leak.

‘Perhaps, but take three days for head-gasket to arrive.’

We looked at our sons, who were excitedly expecting to leave any moment.

‘Forget it. How long will the new distributor and tyre change take?’

‘Come back two hours.’

And so before lunchtime we crossed the Tragus River on the Ponte 25 de Abril (Ponte Salazar) and merrily continued south on our way out of Lisbon and into the Portuguese countryside.

**LIKE OTHER MOTORISTS FROM THE UK**, we always cross the frontier from Portugal into Spain with sadness, not because we are entering Spain, but because it signals the start of the homeward leg of our journey. In those days, however, the sights were so novel, exciting and extraordinary that it was not long before our spirits were on the rise. On this occasion we had decided to keep away from the tourist trap of the Mediterranean coastline and to return via a more inland route, which was where our ‘true’ Spain resided: towns, villages and countryside that seemed to have been left untouched by the passing centuries. So it was that we came to Valdepeñas, in the small province of Ciudad Real, which is almost completely surrounded by that of the much bigger and better known La Mancha. While not the most famous of Spanish wine regions, Valdepeñas is known for good, solid, no-nonsense reds.

The vines of that region, like virtually all those of the Iberian Peninsula and southern Europe, were grown as unsupported vase- or goblet-shaped bushes. The French call this type of vine training *gobelet*, and this has become the internationally accepted adjective. We were searching for vineyards in which such *gobelet* vines appeared very old and yet in good condition. The fruit from such plants tends to produce the best wine. We were especially impressed by the wine from one such small-holding. It was unpretentious, robust and full of character. This red had no makeup and needed none, simply proclaiming to the world that it was bottled sunshine.

Like many of the region’s wines in those days it was fermented in huge, picturesque earthenware pots called *tinajas*, which stood several metres high and held about 7000 litres. These were a special feature of La Mancha, constructed, rather than turned on a wheel. The potter stood inside the pot while slowly building it with coils of clay, and when the vessel reached head-height a previously moulded top half was lowered into position before being sealed onto the bottom. Claustrophobia was evidently not a strong feature of the La Mancha personality. The tops of the *tinajas* were simply covered with conical straw 'coolie hats' and accessed by a stairway leading up to a separate floor or catwalk above. We stood on this elevated wooden floor, breathing in the heady vinous atmosphere while sampling the wine. Our smiles said it all.

'*Cuanto cuesta?*' enquired Chris. After hearing the peso price and doing her mental exercises she turned to me and said, 'Ninepence a litre.' It was then and there that an unwanted thought began to worm its way into my brain, like a nasty little parasite, and although I could suppress it temporarily it kept popping up again when I had my attention elsewhere. We had really been asking about bottled wine, but the winemaker clearly thought our enquiry was about the best of his unbottled product. Then the worm of a thought began to articulate something like this.

'Why don't you buy a few bottles to drink on the way back to London?' it asked in a perfectly reasonable voice.

'I would like to,' I thought, 'but I don't have any bottles. We throw them away when they are empty.'

'They must have some empty bottles here at the winery and they would be only too happy to give them to you,' whispered the little voice.

'Okay. That's a good thought,' and so I turned to Chris, who translated my worm's request to the proprietor. He had no sooner disappeared to get half a dozen bottles than the wheedling little parasite's voice reappeared.

'You need to buy more than that. It's such a bargain. Why, you could use it for your house wine in London.'

'I don't have room in the vehicle for more bottles. All of the cupboards, nooks and crannies are crammed with bottles of wine from the various regions we have visited.'

'You need some big container. You could put it outside when you camp. Then it wouldn't be in anybody's way.'

'I don't have any room for a big container full of wine in the campervan, even if we could lug it in and out of the van each time we stop.'

Just then our obliging winemaker returned with his half-dozen empties. He was just about to start filling them when I heard the voice again.

'Wait! Why don't you fill the campervan's water tanks with wine?'

'From where would we get our water? Silly, dumb worm!'

'Fill the six wine bottles with water. You can replenish those each time you stop. After all, you are on your way back to England and you will be there within the week. It is not much of an inconvenience for such a grand supply of good wine.'

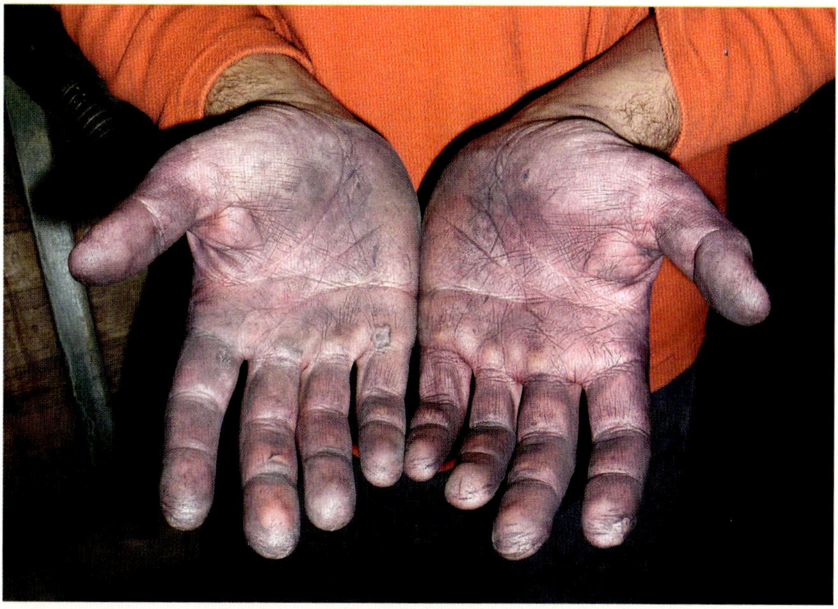

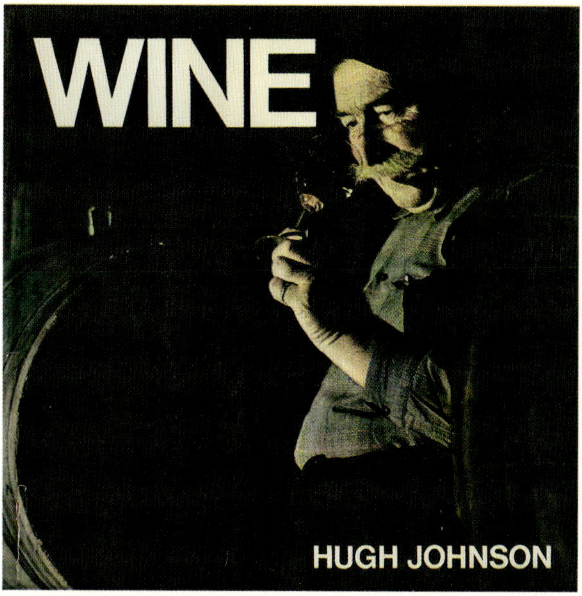


**ABOVE**
The evil-looking purple-black hands of a real winemaker.

**LEFT**
The cover of Chris's seductive Christmas gift, 1966.

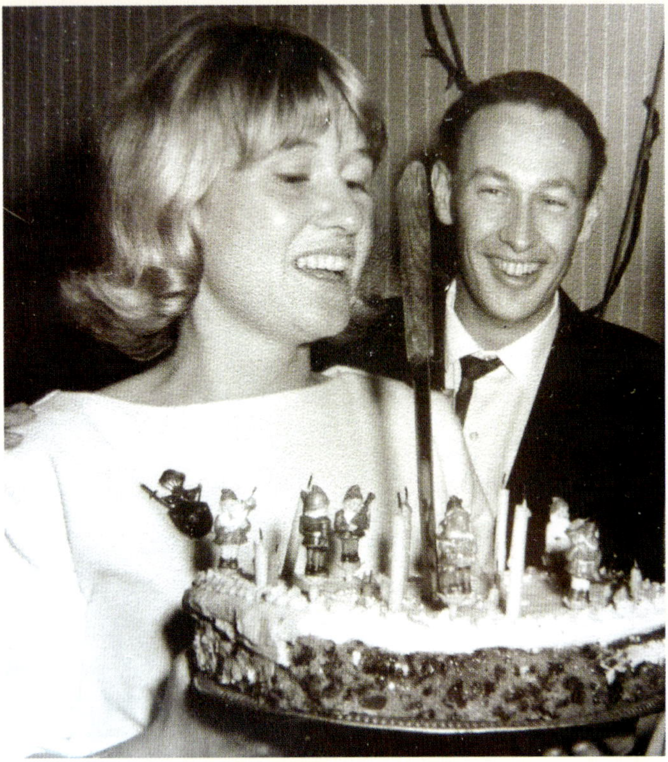

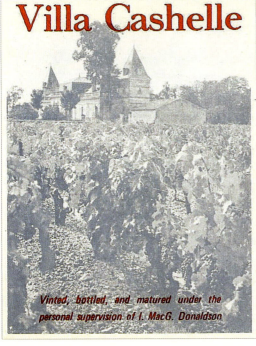


**ABOVE**
A fairytale cake guarded by gnomes and candles: Chris and Ivan at Chris's 21st birthday, 1967.

**LEFT**
Chris and Ivan's first amateur wine label (1968) showing Chateau Tronquoy-Lalande of Bordeaux, filched from Hugh Johnson's book and named after Cashel Street, where they lived.

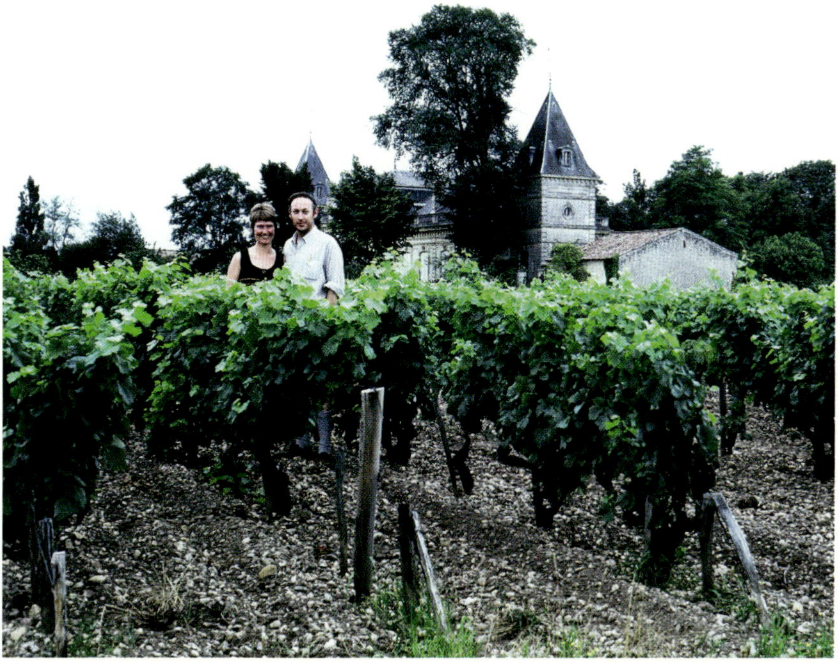

**ABOVE**
Chris and Ivan visit Chateaux Tronquoy-Lalande,
Medoc, Bordeaux, 1984.

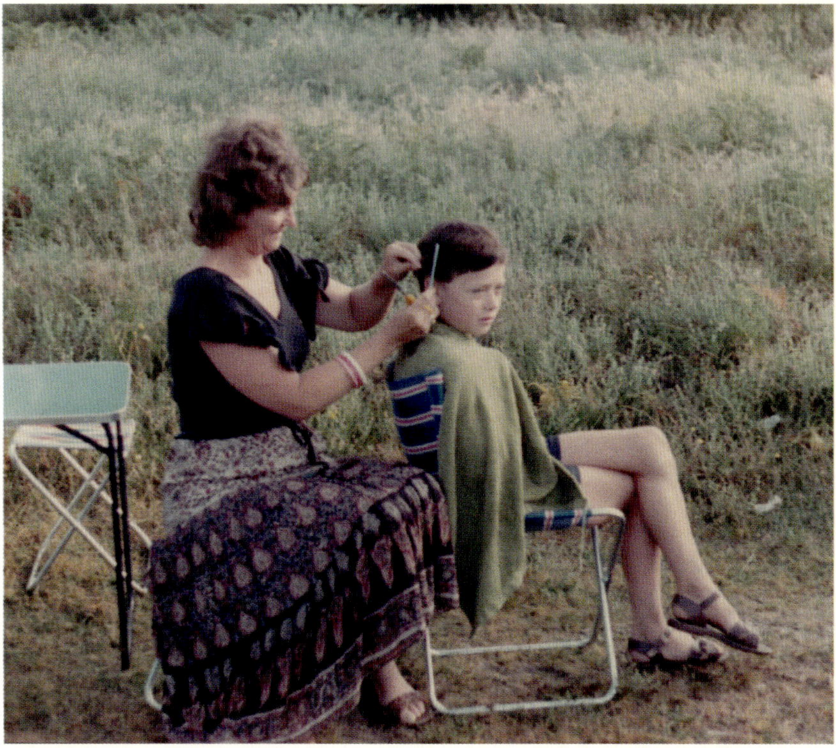

**ABOVE**
Chris cutting Edward's hair while camping in the Italian countryside, 1984.

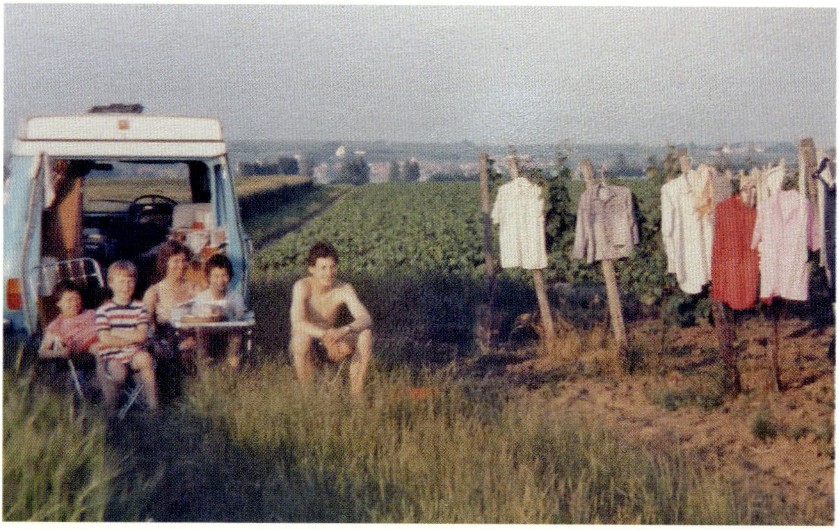

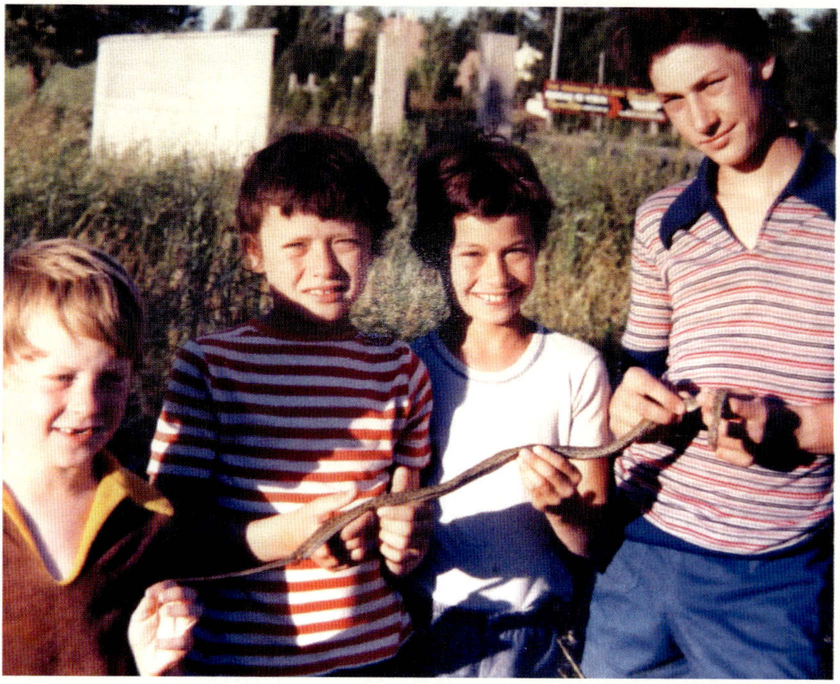

**ABOVE**
Camping in a German vineyard (from left: Edward, Paul, Chris, Michael and Matthew), 1984.

**BELOW**
The deadly but very dead serpent in the south of France (from left: Paul, Edward, Michael and Matthew), 1984.

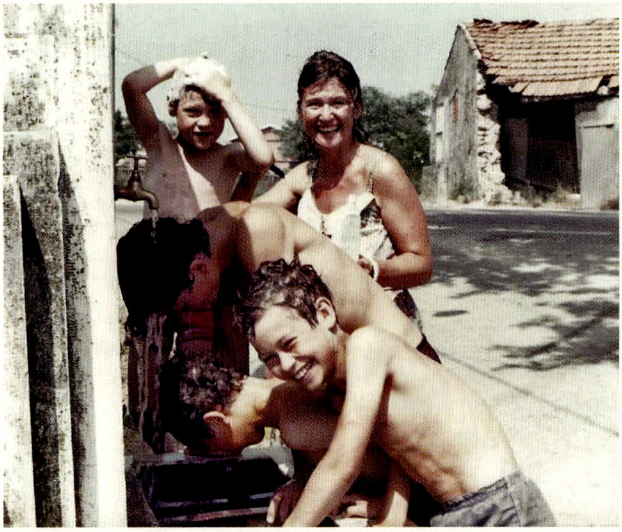

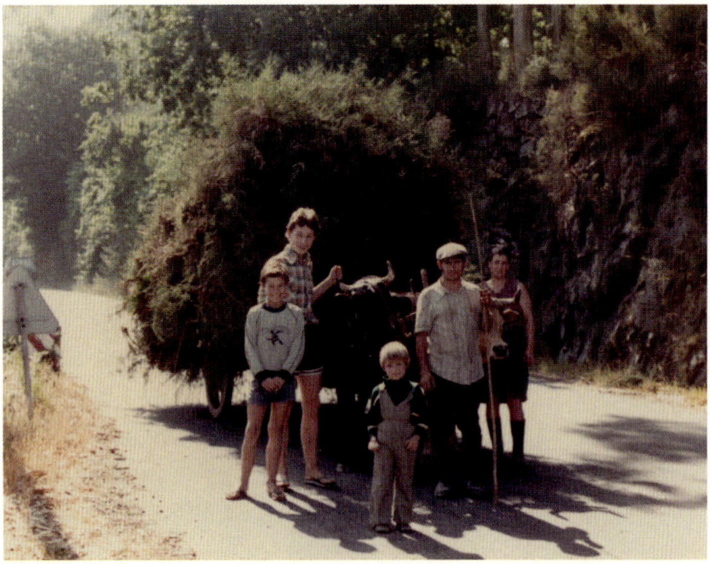

**ABOVE**
Hair washing at a wayside tap, (heads from above down: Paul, Chris, Matthew, Michael and Edward) Spain, 1984.

**BELOW**
Matthew and Michael (on the left) with farming couple and their son, Portugal, 1984.

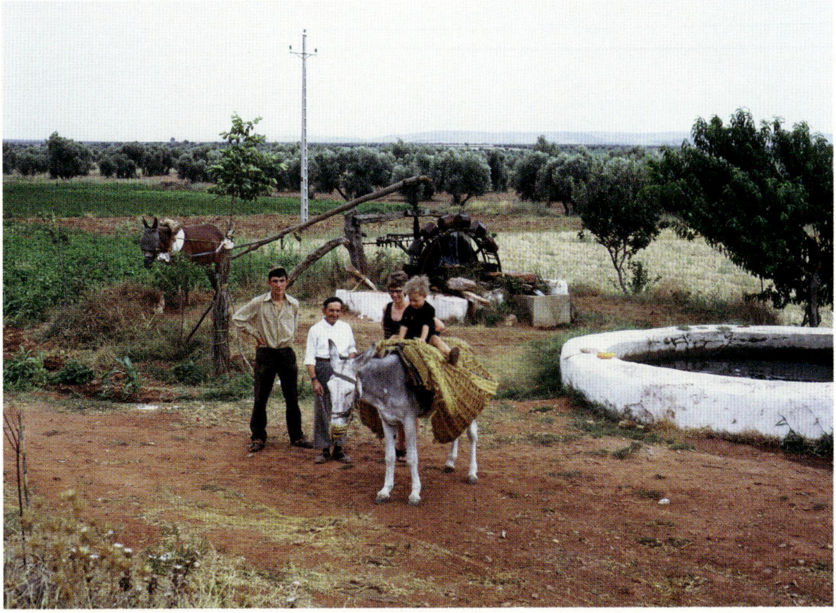

**ABOVE**
Chris helping Matthew ride a donkey on a Spanish farm while the second donkey patiently draws the water, 1973.

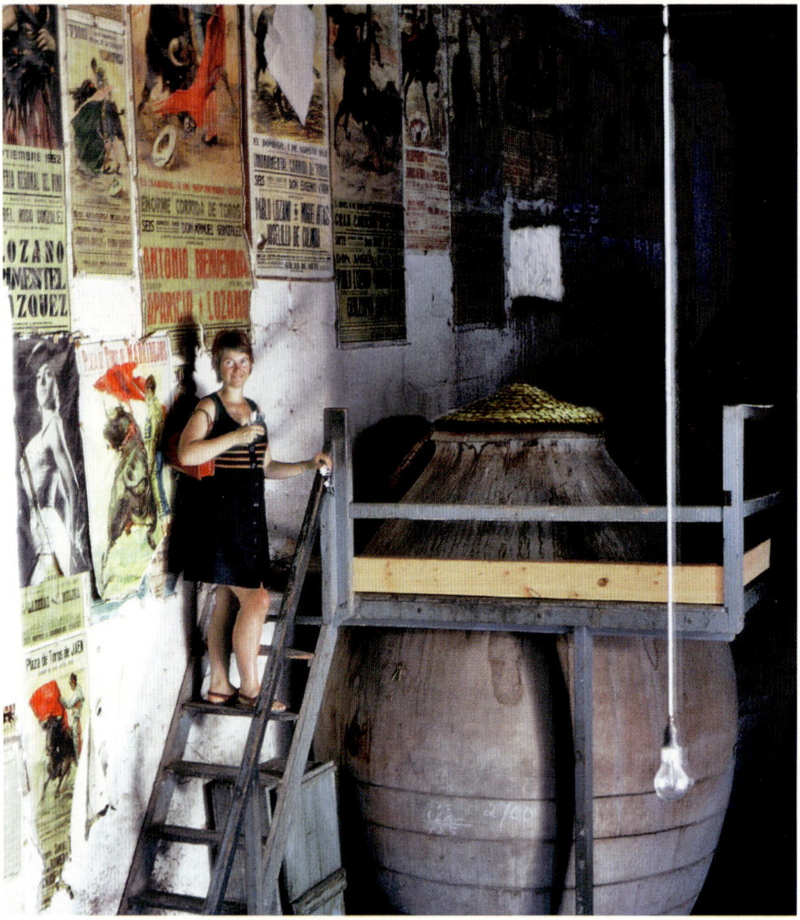


**ABOVE**

Chris with large earthenware pots (tinajas) full of wine and 'sealed' with straw lids to keep out the dust, Valdepenas, Spain, 1973.

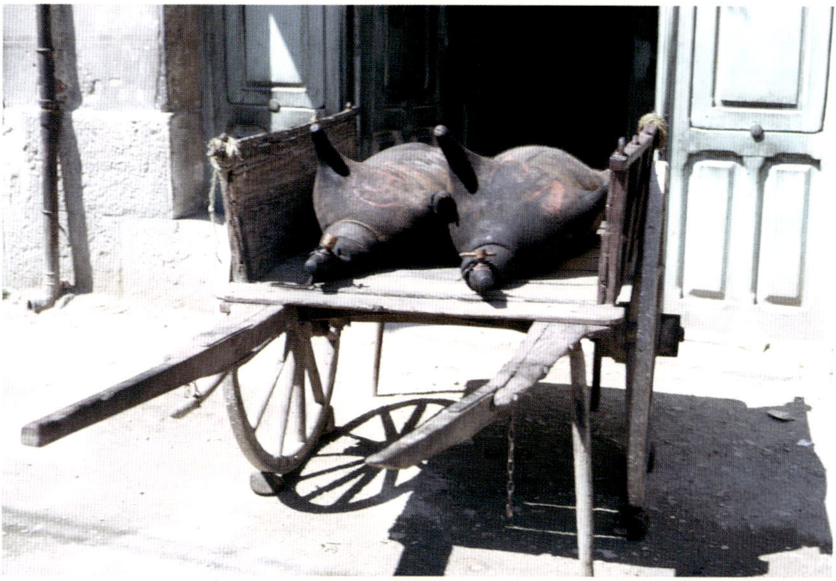

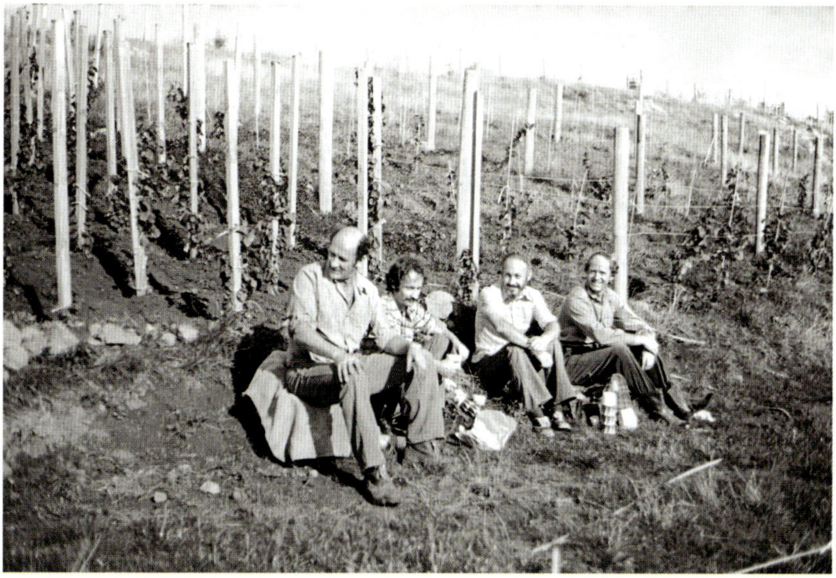

**ABOVE**
Pig skins (pellejos) full of wine. Valdepeñas, Spain, 1973.

**BELOW**
Morning tea break in a corner of Mountain View vineyard (from left: Brian Hearfield, Graham Watson, Ivan, and Paul Straubel), 1978.

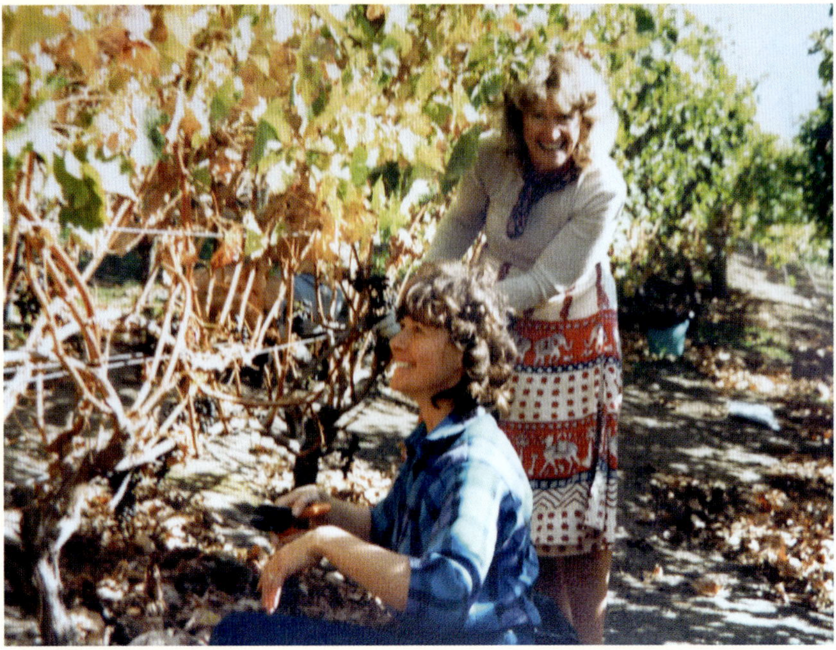

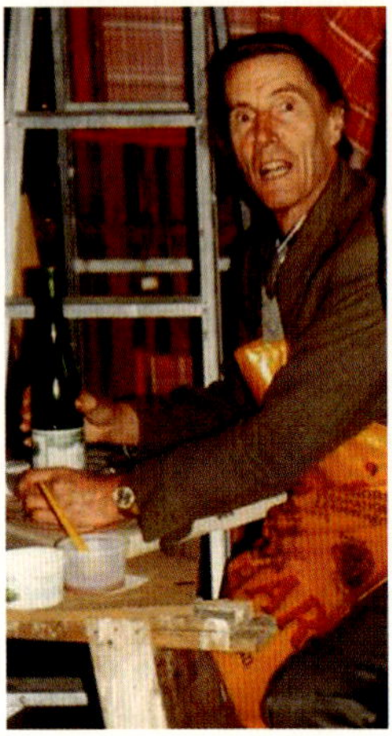

**ABOVE**

Chris (upper) and Paula Watson (lower) at Mountain View Vineyard, 1985.

**LEFT**

Don Beaven labelling Mountain View Vineyard wine, 1983.

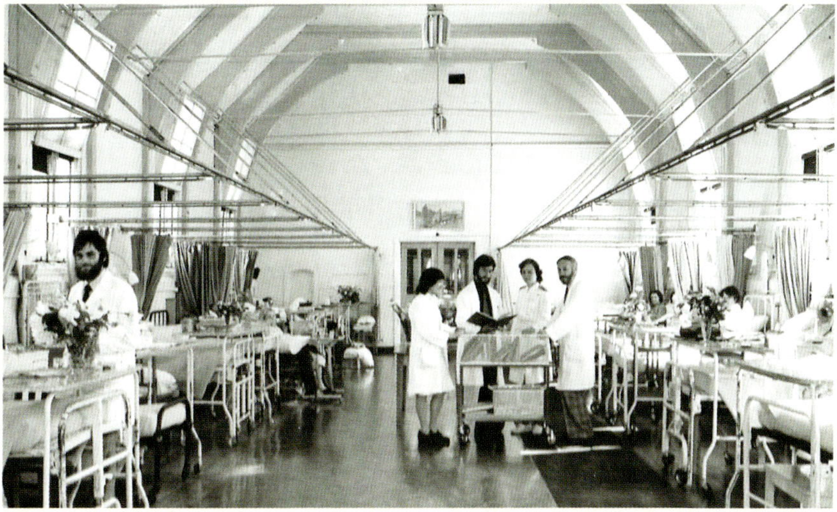

**ABOVE**

Ivan (right) with junior medical staff and charge nurse carrying out the last ward round in ward 4 at Christchurch Hospital prior to its demolition, 1977.

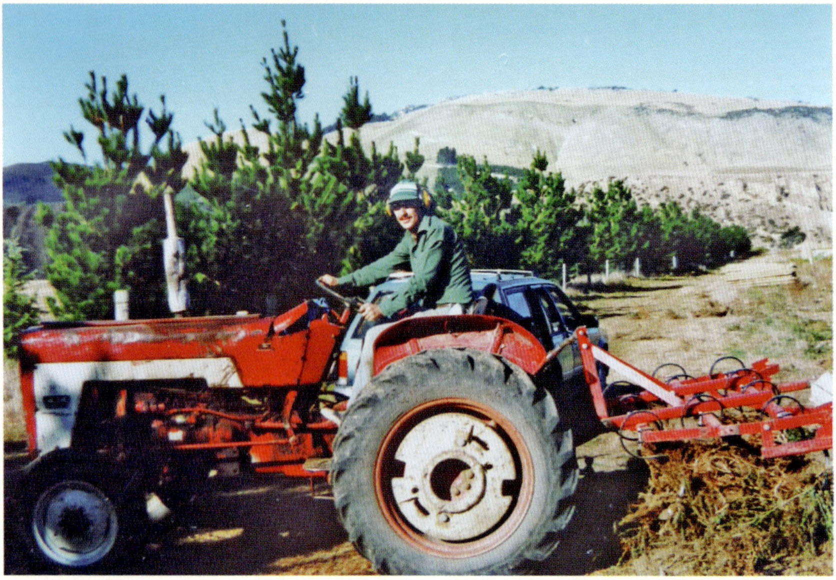

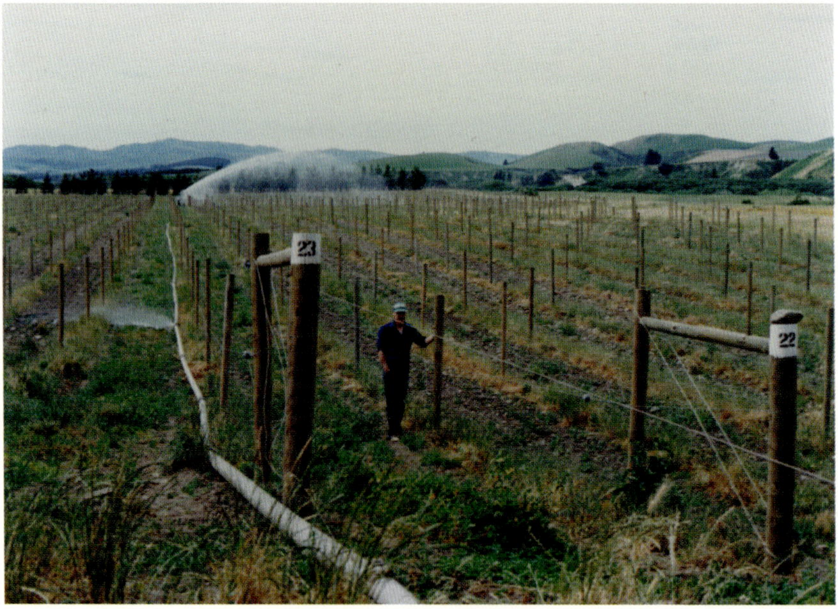


**ABOVE**
Ivan getting rid of the weeds with Chris's Christmas present (the roto crumbler). Pegasus Bay Vineyard, 1988.

**BELOW**
Ivan growing weeds while trying to water grapes with the mobile irrigator. Pegasus Bay Vineyard, 1989.

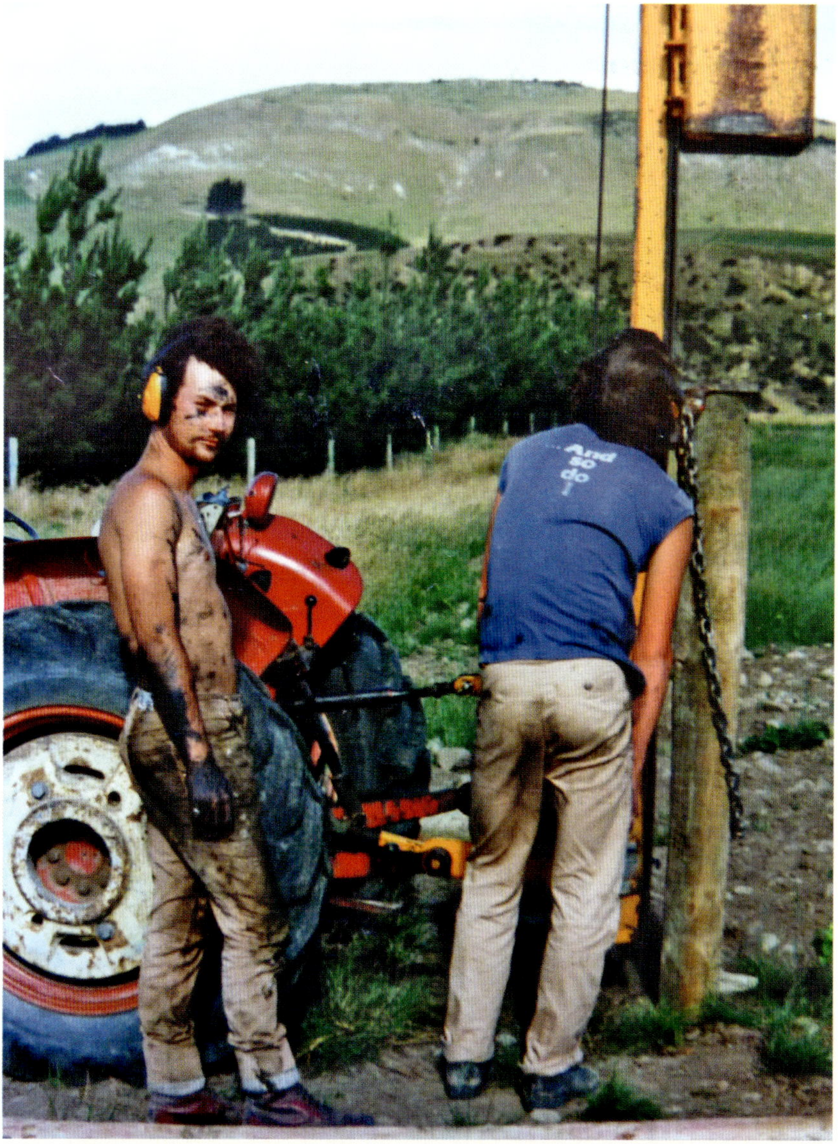


**ABOVE**

Grease monkey Matthew (left) and his school friend Shaun Harper post-driving the first of the trellis for the grapes at Pegasus Bay Vineyard, 1987.

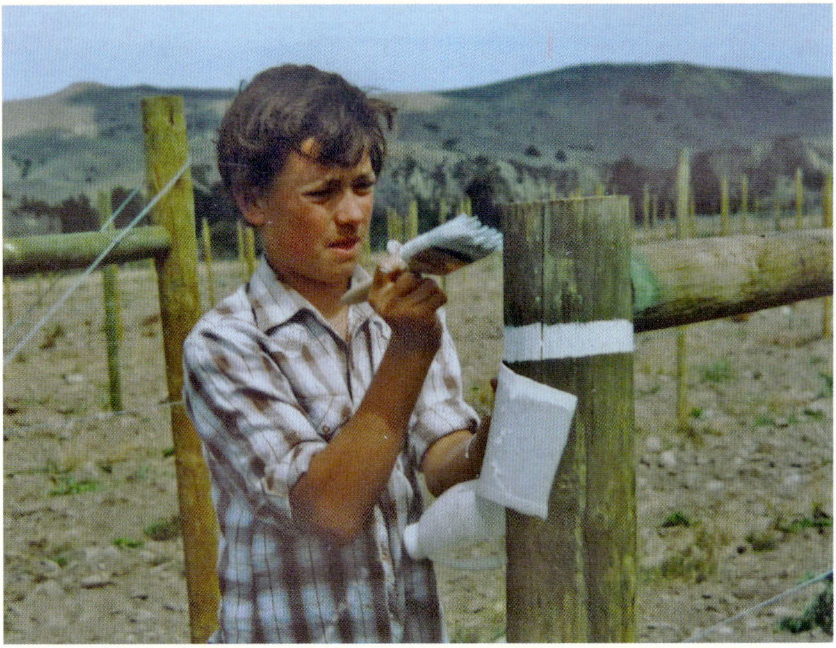

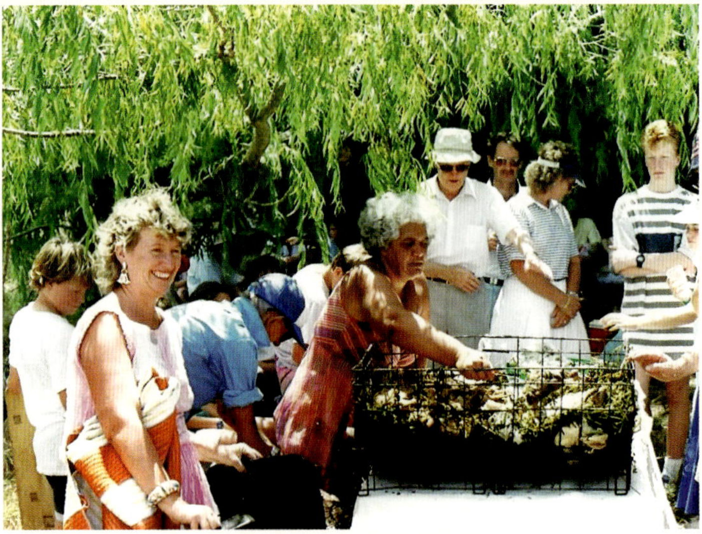

**ABOVE**
The concentration of a true artist. Edward paints the tops of the trellis ends. Pegasus Bay Vineyard, 1989.

**BELOW**
Chris supervising the serving of a hangi to vineyard staff and friends (Paul is to her left), 1988.

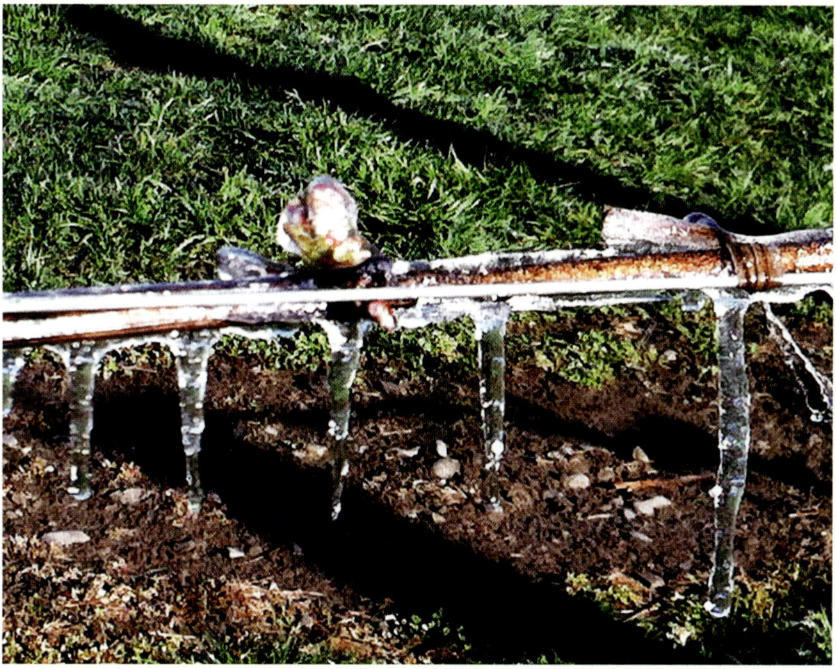

**ABOVE**
A tender bud in a cocoon of protective ice after using waterfrost protection, spring, 2010.

**OVERLEAF ABOVE**
The magic of bud burst in the vineyard, spring, 2013.

**OVERLEAF BELOW**
A wind machine is used to fight frost, 2012.

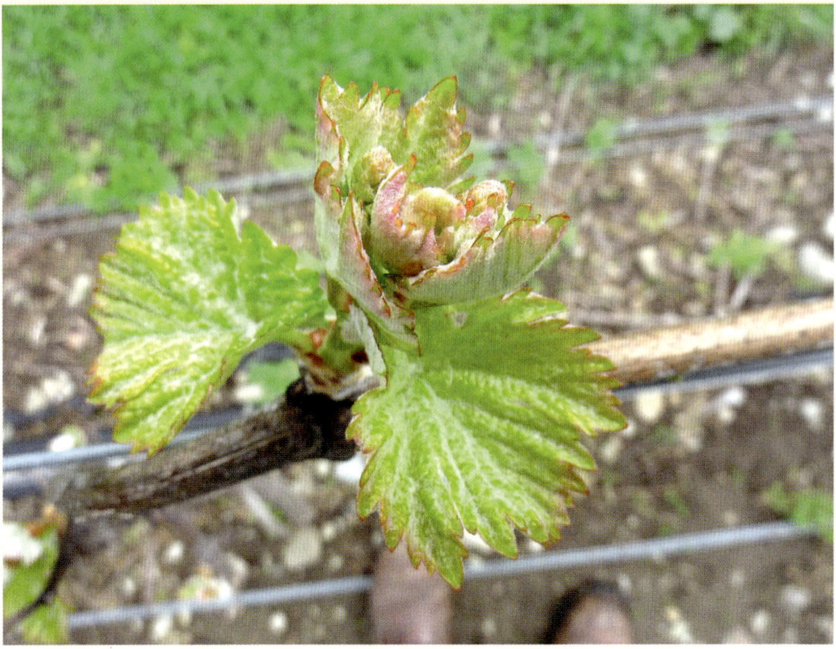

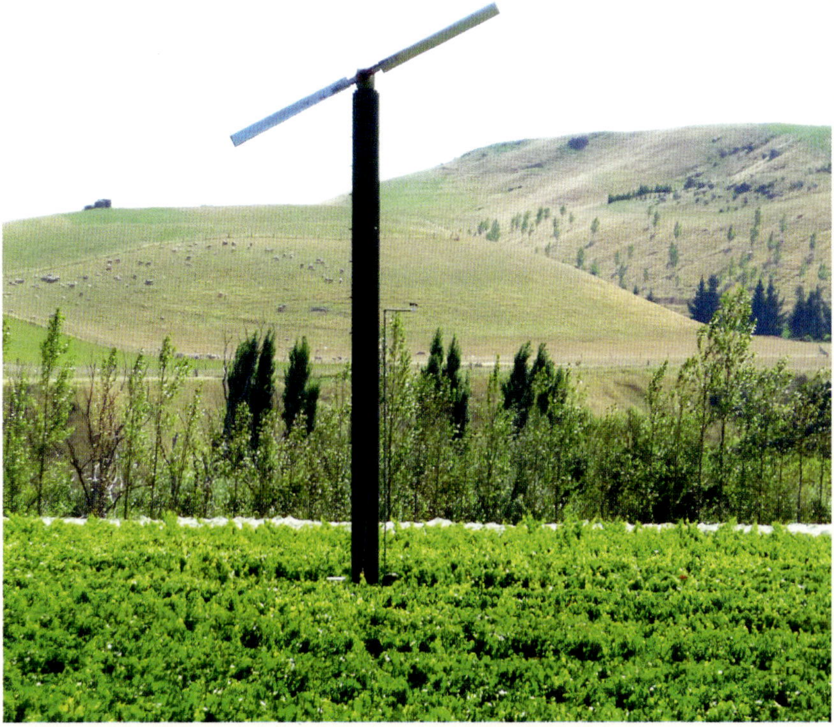

And that is how I was tempted into sin by a mere worm of a thought, or perhaps it really was Eve's snake. Whatever the explanation, it is a fact that we then and there filled our campervan's generous water tanks with wine and sealed them tightly to keep out the air, thus preventing spoilage. As we were leaving the winery we noticed several gristly-looking *pellejos* lying in a rough wooden cart. These so-called 'wine skins' were made from the hide of a single pig and retained the unfortunate animal's shape, including the legs and the neck, which stuck out proudly and stiffly. They were said to each hold about 150 litres of wine but I guess it depended on the size of the original owner. They were an uncommon sight, even back then, but they reassured us that our winemaker was a true traditionalist and not some fly-by-night novice.

'Nice meeting you,' said Chris, shaking a turgid foreleg. 'Don't bother to get up, we can see our own way out.'

When we returned *chez nous*, our little London flat was turned into a bottling factory. Because of my amateur winemaking I had all the equipment and the corks to hand, but I had to scrounge about to get enough empties to do the job. It was with satisfaction that I filled all of our spare storage space with bottles of wine. Those looming cold, dark winter months would clamour loudly to be lightened and warmed by an occasional sip of our bottled sunshine. We had more than enough wine to see us through the year until we could take our next annual jaunt around the vineyards of Europe.

## CHAPTER 5

# Virgin Territory *and the* Grapes *of* Wrath

1975–1983

**'I WOULD PREFER TO GO TO AUCKLAND,'** I said, trying to sound decisive and positive. 'There's an established neuroscience service there, with excellent clinical neurology, neurosurgery and neuroradiology. I like the people, they know me, and I'm sure I could happily become a useful player in that team. It's a vibrant and exciting city and I know we would all enjoy living there.'

'We' had become five, as our little family had somehow mysteriously expanded to include three sons, Matthew, Michael and Edward, the last-mentioned being only weeks old at this point.

'Besides,' I added, almost as though it was an afterthought, 'it's the only place in New Zealand where I could work as a neurologist and we could own a vineyard and winery. Think how exciting and wonderful that would be.' Then, with finality, I pronounced, 'That settles it for me. I'm going to take the neurology position I've been offered at Auckland Hospital.'

'You must do exactly what you feel is best, and the choice is yours, but I would prefer to go to Christchurch,' Chris replied, marshalling her counter-offensive. 'My family is there and I would enjoy being close to them. I think it would be good for the boys to be brought up close to their relatives.

'Besides,' she continued, 'the Christchurch job is a university one and you'll be able to do research, whereas the Auckland position is as a hospital neurologist and there won't be a research component. And no, there isn't a proper neurology department or any neurosurgery in Christchurch, and there is only one physician looking after patients with neurological disorders. Think of the opportunity to build up your own department and possibly get neurosurgery established in the city — wouldn't that be exciting! I'm sure you could do it.'

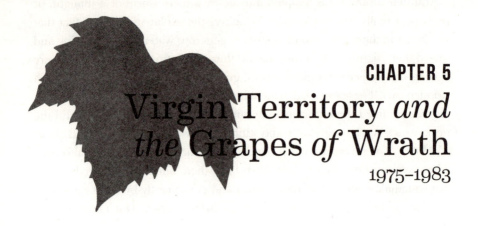

Then she added, 'It wouldn't be the end of the world not to have a vineyard and winery. It's your idea and I think it would just be a lot of work, especially for me.' As an afterthought, she casually let drop, 'Besides, I don't like the weather in Auckland. It may be warmer than Christchurch but it rains all the time. I would forever be having to rescue drying washing from passing showers. I could never get Matthew's nappies dry when we lived there before.'

And so that is how the uneven, age-old battle of the sexes began in our little family. I should have known right from the start that mine was a lost cause, but I was not sufficiently sage or experienced to recognise the tender trap that had been set for me: the 'You make the final decision, but I prefer …' touch.

I had applied for and been lucky enough to be offered neurology positions in both Auckland and Christchurch, and I had naïvely thought that I had a choice about where we would go. My decision was definite and final. We would go to Auckland! But then I began to ponder the situation. Ever since we had become an item Chris had subjugated her interests to mine — well, sometimes. She had followed me across the globe, scrimped and saved to make ends meet, lived in basic accommodation and sacrificed her holidays to my vinous whims, and not once had I heard a serious gripe. Now she would do the same thing again, but not without letting me know that it was against her wishes.

I took the coward's way out and delayed making a decision. It was not that I put it out of my mind — in fact, I thought about little else — but I could not stop vacillating. One day I would make the decision for Auckland and the next it would be for Christchurch. It was getting dangerously close to the final acceptance dates when I finally made up my mind, returning to our flat one evening after dragging my confused thoughts around and around the back streets of London, not to mention the inside of my head.

'We will go to Christchurch,' I said with finality as the front door clicked shut behind me, 'just for you. Perhaps I'll be able to build up decent neurology and neurosurgery services, but we will never be able to have a vineyard and winery.'

And so the die was cast.

**'WE SHOULD FIRST LOOK FOR A PIECE** of sloping ground that is facing north so that we'll get the maximum amount of sunlight,' Don asserted enthusiastically.

This slightly built ball of energy was in the habit of co-expressing and emphasising his words with gestures, and now he appeared in need of a straitjacket to prevent him from unconsciously injuring his upper limbs.

'I know somebody who can probably supply us with vine cuttings, but who could we get to make the wine?' he asked pointedly.

All the eyes in the room turned towards me.

'I would be happy to try,' I volunteered, 'but you must realise that I have had very limited experience with grape wine. Most of what I have produced has been made from other fruits, so-called country wines.'

'There can't be much difference. At any rate, any grapes that we produce will be so green that even if you don't stuff up the winemaking the plonk will be undrinkable. The whole idea is bloody stupid and we are a bunch of idiots, but we might as well do it.' The interjection came from Brian Hearfield, a good-natured but rough diamond of an engineer.

It was the first meeting of a motley group of wine enthusiasts who had been rounded up by Don Beaven in order to explore the possibility of establishing a small vineyard in Canterbury.

When, at the start of 1972, I had left to undertake postgraduate medical training in London, all of New Zealand's vineyards were sited from Hawke's Bay northwards; in other words, in the upper half of the North Island. In the first half of the twentieth century the sum of New Zealand's fledgling wine industry had been based around Auckland, from where it merrily churned out unexciting, sweet, fortified wines from low-maintenance American, rather than European (*Vitis vinifera*), grapevines. It was only during the late 1950s and 1960s that vineyards planted with *Vitis vinifera* started to march southwards into cooler and drier regions.

As so often occurs in life, I had imagined things remaining the same as when I had last seen them. My picture of New Zealand's wine map had been frozen in time at the point when I had gone away. When I returned I was unaware that two years earlier Montana, the biggest New Zealand wine company of the day, had taken the bold and exciting move of planting the South Island's first vineyard in Marlborough. Now here we were, three years later, planning to plant the first vineyard of modern times in Canterbury. Early French settlers who had arrived at the little port of Akaroa, near Christchurch, in 1840 had established small vineyards and made wine. These pioneering attempts had died out, however.

A small plot of vines had just been established at Lincoln College (now Lincoln University) by the visionary Dr David Jackson, in order to assess the potential of Canterbury for winemaking. However, our disparate little group of nutters had decided not to await the results of these experiments. Rather, we were going to put our toes in the water and learn on the job. We did not have the spunk to go commercial, and we were only intending to plant a hobby vineyard because we were all fully employed in other professions. There was my immediate boss, Don Beaven, a professor of medicine; Graham Watson, a radiologist; Alan Cookson, a dentist; Neville (Nev) Ackroyd, another dentist; Paul Straubel, a solicitor; Brian Hearfield, and me. We were all hopeless dreamers apart from Brian, who was a practical 'bloke's bloke'.

**'MY BACK'S KILLING ME,' I COMPLAINED**, holding my hand on my lower lumbar spine and trying to straighten up.

'I'm starting to get blisters on my hands,' said Graham. 'I should have thought to bring gloves.'

'Why don't I take a photograph of you all working?' Paul suggested, quickly detaching himself from the line of stooped men and making a beeline for his camera. Even in the short time our group had been going Paul had earned himself the soubriquet 'Official Photographer of Mountain View Vineyard'.

Alan and Nev had their heads down, working doggedly and silently but at a visibly decreasing pace.

'I think we should stop and have lunch,' Don chipped in hopefully, but he was cut short by Brian.

'Keep working, you bloody lazy academics. You're soft and bloated from your desk jobs. You've only just had morning tea and we have hardly done any work today. You all need to spend a month or two working in the paddy fields!'

We were learning the hard way what had been self-evident to the peasants of Europe for over a thousand years, i.e. that vineyards are a lot of arduous physical work. What was also becoming clear was that the easiest job of a vigneron is *planting* the vineyard. It is the subsequent training of the vines and their ongoing maintenance that is the difficult part.

As a group we had passed a splendid weekend in Marlborough, four hours' drive to the north of Christchurch, where we had wined and dined with Danny Schuster, a German-speaking Czech viticulturalist and winemaker. He had provided us with most of the vine cuttings for our vineyard and was the fount of all our meagre knowledge on viticulture. It had been a fun-filled, romantic trip, packed with balmy early spring weather, fine wines, splendid food and great company. If this was the life of a vigneron, we could not wait to embrace it to the full.

We were soon in for a dose of harsh reality. The vine cuttings, which we had planted into a north-facing hillside in the Halswell district of Christchurch, demanded a regular supply of water. Being on a slope, the infrequent rain just seemed to chuckle at us as it ran away to the bottom of the hill without really penetrating the soil. We had to mound up the earth and build a water-retaining bowl around each potential vine. As spring marched into early summer even the meagre showers went on holiday and we were reduced to hand-watering each dusty little depression in the ground. The weeds, however, had not heard that there was a drought and they just continued to grow. Not only were they preparing to shower their wretched seeds all over our land, but like an army of leeches they were also sucking the very lifeblood, the little bit of moisture that was left, from the soil for their own malign purposes. Most surely they were a creation of the Devil.

We had all seen the pristine bare-earth vineyards of Europe, so we knew how to deal with the problem. The ground had to be cultivated and left bare. Our slope, however, was too steep to be cultivated by machine, so we would have to mimic what was done in places like the Mosel Valley in Germany; just hoe out the weeds. If German workers could do it then so could we! Simple, was it not? No, it was not!

This was our first morning at attempting to control the weeds, and it was rapidly and demoralisingly apparent that our performance was only in the poor to hopeless range. As it was a hot sunny day we were all sweating profusely and we were covered in dust. To make matters worse, by the end of the day the six of us had covered only a very tiny area, perhaps 10 per cent, of our small vineyard.

'This is hopeless,' Don said, verbalising the self-evident. 'We need to explore other options. There has to be an easier way.'

'We need another meeting,' someone suggested.

'If we are going to waste our time sitting around having a talkfest then make sure the wine is better than last time. It was bloody disgusting.' Brian had a particular weakness for chardonnay, especially from Burgundy and naturally the most expensive, Le Montrachet. In spite of his macho appearance and provocative manner of speech he was not a man of simple tastes.

After some discussion we decided to clear a number of rocks, flatten out certain areas and sow grass in our vineyard. Then, with the aid of a mower we could cut the grass relatively easily and we would only have to maintain a small weed-free patch around each vine. It was still a considerable amount of work but only a fraction of the back-breaking, callous-forming effort that grubbing had required. Nevertheless, our former leisure time was more than fully occupied by the hundred and one other tasks the vines demanded, including pruning, training, tying, spraying and the like.

Never in our wildest dreams had any of us considered just how much ongoing work, most of it repetitive, boring and tiring, even a small vineyard like ours required. For the first three and a half years our only rewards were the satisfaction of seeing the vines grow and the vineyard becoming established, and in the fellowship of the ring, our little cooperative ring of vignerons. Then we had our first tiny harvest, which I made into wine in the empty half of our double garage. At the best the vintage could be called a very modest, qualified success. At least it was drinkable, but only just.

**'HELLO, IVAN SPEAKING.'**

'Ivan, thank goodness we've found you. You need to come back. We are picking the pinot noir tomorrow.' The voice sounded stressed and irritable.

'You can't do that, the grapes are not ripe enough. The wine will be thin, weedy, green, acidic and completely undrinkable. We need to leave them to ripen for a further fortnight at least.'

'But the birds are eating the grapes. In another fortnight we will have lost a fair portion of the crop.'

'I think we would all prefer to have a smaller quantity of better wine than a larger amount of inferior plonk. Can't you think of any way to keep the birds away from the grapes? Isn't it possible to have a roster and just scare them away more frequently? After all, the vines are netted.'

'Yes, they may be netted but the birds are just perching on the nets and pecking through the holes.'

'They will only be able to get the few berries that are closest to the netting, which won't be a big proportion of the crop. I really think we are best to wait until the grapes are fully ripe rather than letting bird brains decide the harvest date. Anyway, I can't come back to Christchurch until next weekend, and because I'll be working at the hospital during the week the first time the grapes could be processed will be the following weekend.'

'I'm not sure that Nev will be happy with waiting that long. We might just pick them and get him to make them into wine. He has made home-brew before.' The voice was now sounding decidedly tetchy and challenging.

'I'll get Don to come and see the grapes with you, and feel free to involve all the others if necessary. Then we can make a decision that will suit everybody. Would that be okay?'

'All right …' the speaker conceded reluctantly, 'but it would be much better if you could manage to come earlier so that we can start harvesting.'

'I'll do my best but I think it's unlikely. Good luck.'

I hung up with a sigh and then telephoned Don, explaining the situation and asking him to act as a mediator, as he had done during previous vintages.

'No problem,' he said. 'I'll go and look at the vineyard with the others. I'm sure I will be able to talk them round.'

I had attempted to make myself uncontactable by taking the family to the thermal springs mountain resort of Hanmer for the May school holidays. I had purposely not said that I was leaving Christchurch or where I was going, and I had not left the telephone number of the house that we were renting. In those pre-mobile-phone days such a sly manoeuvre guaranteed — well, almost guaranteed — being undisturbed. It had worked a treat in earlier years. Now I had been outsmarted. How I had been discovered was, and still is, a mystery, but clearly attempts were being made to flush me out of my lair. I could feel the hounds baying for blood, even if the blood in question turned out to be a wishy-washy pink, rather than the generous red of a well-ripened pinot.

Our little co-operative had developed the habit of being somewhat uncooperative at vintage, that time of the vinous calendar when all of the year's hard effort should come to a satisfying and delicious conclusion. Those mellow, golden days of autumn, when ripe fruits lie temptingly within grasp, should be the happiest of seasons. Yet a disagreeable little schism seemed to open up regularly at this time, only to disappear again once vintage was over. Our group would become divided into two camps, *the premature* and *the retarded*. The former, not unreasonably, did not want to see their hard work being lost to birds, rain damage and rot caused by fungus. The latter, quite understandably, wanted to get the grapes optimally ripe in order to make the best wine possible, even if it meant losing some of the crop. Debates would rage and telephone calls would be made virtually daily.

Being the winemaker I would cop most of the flak. It was not that I alone had the right to decide when to pick — after all, it was a co-operative — but because I had to process the fruit my availability was crucial in deciding the harvest dates. Each vintage time, those in the *premature* camp became convinced that I was not only *retarded* but also obstructive. Because this annual group intercourse had become increasingly passionate, without ever reaching a mutually satisfactory conclusion, I took the coward's way out. By multiple strange quirks of fate my timetable allowed me to be available only when the sugar and acid levels in each of the different varieties of grape reached optimal levels. It was a ruse that might have worked the first few times, but I was fairly sure that now the *prematures* only pretended to be fooled.

It was not hard to assemble a team of happy volunteer pickers in those days, our vineyard being such a novelty. The most productive work was done in the mornings, because the lunchtime picnics, with the inevitable sampling of previous vintages, mysteriously slowed progress in the afternoons. Lying in the sunshine on the grass between the rows was an amazingly warm and soporific experience, even in the late autumn. Very often, however, you felt a cool breeze when you stood up out of the shelter of the vines. We swore that our particular patch of dirt caught every breath of wind that emanated from the four corners of the earth or came from any one of its seven seas. It was on a little knoll that formed a type of corner, around which every little zephyr loved to dance and hurricanes regularly fought battles. Although it officially gloried in the name Mountain View Vineyard, we nicknamed it Pleurisy Point.

When our pickers had finished for the day we would start processing the fruit. The black grapes, to be made into the red wines, would be taken to a small winery and laboratory that I had now built onto the back of my garage. There, the stems would be removed and the grapes crushed before being put into small fermenting vats. The white grapes, however, were taken to the Princess Margaret Hospital where Don had access to a laboratory. Here we would press them to extract the juice, which would then be put into large glass carboys and left in a refrigerated room for a couple of days to allow the sediment to settle. The low temperature prevented fermentation from starting spontaneously. The clear juice would then be siphoned (racked) off the top and the remaining sediment discarded, because we only wanted the clarified liquid (must) to ferment into wine. It was felt politic to do this work in the absence of curious eyes, usually at night or during the weekend. Once processed, the must was transported to my makeshift little winery across town, where I would start the fermentation after the juice had warmed up to ambient temperature.

Coming to the end of a particularly busy afternoon doing neurological consultations on inpatients at this particular hospital, I was aware that there were two 12-gallon (48-litre) carboys of clarified grape juice sitting in the refrigerated room, ready to be carted back to my little winery. It would be extremely convenient if I could put them in the back of my station wagon and take them home with me. Unfortunately I had taken my registrar with me that afternoon in order to give him additional teaching and experience, and I now had to take him back to Christchurch Hospital, where neurology was based. I hesitated to involve him in our nefarious vinous activities.

'What the hell,' I thought, 'he's a sensible chap and strong to boot. He would come in handy helping me to lift those heavy carboys into the back of the vehicle. I can't do it by myself at any rate. I'll ask him to help me.'

It was a decision that I was to regret.

We had just put the two huge glass jars into the back of my pride and joy, my new Burgundy-red Peugeot estate. I was leaning forward adjusting their positions in preparation to separating them with pillows and strapping them in place when suddenly a mighty blow struck me high on my forehead. Everything went black and I staggered forward, fearing that I might lose consciousness. There was a sharp shattering sound combined with a type of dull explosion, then a wave struck me amidships, causing me to recoil sharply.

A blurred scene of horror swam into view. The blow had caused me to lose my grip on the carboy that I had been moving, it had slipped against its twin and they had both shattered. The best part of 100 litres of precious chardonnay juice had merrily cascaded forwards over the floor and now lay, looking somewhat like a grubby fish pond, in the footwell of my vehicle. A portion of the juice had splashed backwards and soaked me from mid-chest to shoes. I looked like a ridiculous scarecrow that had fought its way through a thunderstorm in an old black pinstripe suit. Then the scarecrow began to taste blood, its own blood, which was trickling down its face, seeping into its mouth and dripping off its chin. In a dazed state it stupidly raised a hand to its forehead and felt a gaping gash. It still did not know what had hit it. It looked around but there was nothing out of the ordinary; nothing, that is, apart from a terrified-looking, very pale junior medical officer.

'I'm sorry, sir. Dreadfully, dreadfully sorry!' the apparition stammered. 'I thought you had finished with the carboys and I was just slamming the back door shut.'

I now saw that he had hit my head with the sharp right-angled corner of the door, to which a little piece of flesh was still attached. I mumbled something about it being a mere trifle and not to think anything more about it, while inwardly seething with rage at my stupidity in involving him. Our mood during the trip back to the main hospital was rather subdued, in spite of me trying to make small talk. Perhaps my junior colleague was inhibited by the ignominy of being required to adopt the lithotomy or gynaecological examination position. He had been forced to tilt his seat back and put his feet up on the dashboard to avoid getting his fancy shoes soaked by the juice, which was still sloshing backwards and forwards beneath him.

Call it my paranoia, but in spite of taking the mats out of the car and washing everything with soapy water a number of times, I remained convinced that the vehicle still smelt like a winery when I sold it several years later.

**PERHAPS YOU SOMETIMES PLAY** Chinese Whispers. I am not sure why the Chinese should be accredited with or accused of involvement in this game, in which a story is whispered in the ear of one person, who then whispers it to another and so on around a group of people. The last person's version is generally radically different from the original. It shows how we like to embellish things and how truth can become completely distorted by rumour. I suspect it applies equally to all cultures, and I certainly now know that the Chinese do not have a monopoly on such behaviour. I blame the phenomenon of Chinese Whispers for the rumour that Mountain View Vineyard wines were made in a hospital morgue in the dead of night. It is true that I felt dead that night after I had been caught up in the tsunami of grape juice, and that some of our little group had a mawkish view of our wines, but I wish to put it on record that none of our fine bottles had a morguish association.

Our first years at Pleurisy Point proved to involve a very steep learning curve. We gradually mastered the theories and practices of vineyard management, discovered by trial and error which grape varieties were best suited to our soil and climate, and learnt the rudiments of making something drinkable from real wine grapes. In this we were aided — no, led and encouraged — by Danny Schuster, who had taken a position in the newly formed grape-growing and winemaking (viticulture and oenology) department at Lincoln College and made the experimental wines from the college's little vineyard plot.

The department also aimed to find which grape varieties had most potential for making wine in the South Island. Thus, small experimental batches of wines were fermented (vinted) to dryness as simply as possible, without any adjustment of parameters such as acid or sugar levels. Such adjustments would commonly have been employed in a normal commercial situation. This lack of intervention was so that the attributes of each variety could be clearly seen and compared, without being obscured or 'dolled up'. It was as though entrants in a beauty contest had to parade nude, without makeup or fancy hairstyles. The intention was to assess scientifically what the candidates had to offer, warts and all, without the distraction of any coquettish device. David Jackson and Danny Schuster established a panel of so-called experts to judge the line-up.

Given the circumstances, most of us would have preferred to cast our eyes over a parade of real beauty queens. I am sure we would have felt more qualified and confident of our results and it would have been eminently more pleasurable, at least for the males. Nonetheless, our panel dutifully met on a regular basis over a number of years in order to do blind assessments and scoring of these experimental wines. On occasions, we even drank out of black wine glasses so that we would not be biased by the wine's colour.

These were not exactly festive events, given the standard of the wines and the need for silence to avoid influencing other judges before the serious pronouncements were made. In the discussions that followed, terms like 'battery acid', 'green pickle', 'cow manure', 'stale sweat', 'cat's piss', ' baby spew' and 'dog's droppings' were heard intermittently and were generally taken to be a negative. Words such as 'thin', 'mean', 'harsh', 'bitter', 'astringent', 'wishy-washy' and 'coarse' were more frequent and almost encouraging. The descriptors 'light', 'subdued', 'grippy', 'spine tingling', 'lacking direction', 'unfocused' and 'neutral' were common and considered to be bordering on praise. Very occasionally the panel heard 'fruity', 'complex', 'generous', 'mouth-filling', 'smooth', 'harmonious', 'delicious' and the like. In other words, these bare wines, *sans* powder and paint, were tough. However, the judges proved to be even tougher and would eventually complete the task, although at times several of their number had to retire from the field with battle fatigue. It usually took a day and several glasses of fine wine to nurse the palate back into something like a normal state.

Many of the grape varieties and clones, when stripped of their fancy clothes and held up against the harsh light of reality, proved to be unsuitable; many, but not all. There were several varieties that looked particularly promising for local conditions, such as riesling, chardonnay, sauvignon blanc, pinot gris and pinot noir. It was agreed that all of these warranted further investigation.

**'IT HAS A BRIGHT CRIMSON HUE** and a superb bouquet, reminiscent of raspberries, blackberries and black cherries, underpinned by hints of vanilla pod, chocolate and caramel. There is also an element suggestive of roast game, grilled meats and barbecued mushrooms. The wine is full-bodied and rich yet muscular and firm with a lingering velvety finish.'

Don was waxing lyrical while holding up a glass of red wine to the light. We were all sampling the same wine and were absolutely stunned by its sheer quality and power. It was truly an iron fist in a velvet glove, the classic description of red Burgundy, but this wine had another dimension that was found only in top Burgundies, namely a rich ripe fruitiness combined with savoury aromas and flavours. Like red Burgundy, it was made from pinot noir, but unlike red Burgundy it was made in the southern hemisphere and only about 15 kilometres from our own Mountain View Vineyard. It was the 1982 St Helena Pinot Noir made by Danny Schuster.

This was not the first pinot noir to be made in New Zealand and it was not the first to be awarded a gold medal, but it was the first wine from this country to really focus national and international attention on the potential for making world-class Kiwi wine from this grape variety. It was so clearly different from earlier examples, which tended to be just light red wines. This one had real personality, presence and quality. Many different wine regions around the world had tried to make good pinot noir wine and, with the exception of a handful, including Oregon in the US, they had failed miserably. Pinot noir was a grape variety that tended to sulk when taken from its home in France. It resembled the pouting beauty Musetta in Puccini's *La Bohème*. You could lavish it with special care and attention, fuss over it, put it on a pedestal and show it the high life, but the chances were that, like Musetta's sugar daddy, you would come away unrewarded and frustrated.

There was no trouble growing the vines or ripening the grapes, but the wines tended to be lacklustre and devoid of real character and excitement. For many winemakers around the world, the quest to make good pinot noir had become like a search for the Holy Grail. One Californian producer was to label it 'the heartbreak grape'. The variety clearly needed a very special soil and climate; it was a *terroir* freak. By contrast, black grape varieties from other classical European winemaking regions, such as Bordeaux's cabernets and merlots, had been used to make top-class wines in many different countries.

Rumour had it that when the 1982 St Helena Pinot Noir was judged at New Zealand's National Wine Competition the judges almost threw it out because it was considered to be so good that it might have been fraudulent. Wisely, they ended up giving it a gold medal, as they did to the 1984 version of the same wine. The wine and the winemaker became famous almost overnight, and in the following months and years a succession of wine writers, wine producers and wine merchants made the trip to the Holy Land to marvel at the miracle birth of such an immaculate pinot noir in a humble stable in a little-known village. One such wise man from the kingdom of wine was almost a god himself, Robert Mondavi, who at the time was the most prestigious winemaker in the Americas. It was said that he was considering investing in this new phenomenon of Kiwi pinot noir but eventually came to the conclusion that it would be too hard to control from his seat of power in California's Napa Valley. If so, he made no mention of it during the dinner he and his wife had at our home. He did, however, ask if he could try our humble Mountain View Vineyard Pinot Noir, which I reluctantly produced, knowing his reputation for honesty and forthright speech. Surprisingly, he was encouraging, but he warned against ageing it in barrel for any longer, to avoid smothering the wine's fruitiness by excessive oak character. I took his advice and removed the wine from barrel the very next day, and I have paid strict attention to this aspect of pinot noir winemaking ever since.

We did not realise it then, but those early experiments with pinot noir, which were orchestrated by David Jackson and Danny Schuster at Lincoln College, were starting to change the face of the country's wine industry. Up until that point, pride of place among New Zealand's reds had been taken by cabernet sauvignon, merlot or a mixture of the two, and they were largely grown from the middle of the North Island northwards. Pinot enthusiasts were thought to be nutters, wine geeks and wimps, who did not know how to appreciate a gutsy red wine. Over the following decades the emerging quality and unique character of New Zealand pinot noir would gain it such an international reputation and such respect that it would become this country's predominant red wine, and most of it would be grown in the South Island.

**I AM SURE YOU WILL HAVE NOTICED** that fate often works in strange, contradictory and even perverse ways. What seems impossible is sometimes achieved more easily than the apparently simple; not that developing medical neurosciences in Christchurch ever seemed simple. By comparison, however, starting the Mountain View Vineyard was a pushover. While I had not realised it when I made that fateful decision to return to Christchurch, all of the building blocks were there; they only needed people to put them into place. The shift to cooler-climate viticulture and the interest in the grape varieties that this involved were already developing. The first South Island planting of *Vitis vinifera* vines in modern times had already occurred in Marlborough.

On the other hand, there were no hopeful signs of the imminent delivery of modern clinical neuroscience services in Christchurch. In fact, the conception had not even taken place, meaning that the gestation was likely to be long and problematic. The city was known for being conservative, but in general the medical fraternity seemed to have a special brand of ultraconservative pessimism. Shortly after I took up my new combined position as senior lecturer at the medical school (which was part of the University of Otago Medical School) and consultant neurologist at Christchurch Hospital, I was asked to give a lecture to the medical staff on 'Recent Advances in the Clinical Neurosciences'. Part of this was devoted to the wondrous new advent of CT scanning, which I had been involved in first-hand at the National Hospital.

After my talk I was approached by several medical consultants who told me that there was no hope of obtaining such equipment in Christchurch, and that I would have to be content with the services that were already available. It was not that they were against progress; it was just that Christchurch had been the Cinderella of public hospital facilities in New Zealand, and the funding system, which was based on historic funding levels, ensured that it would remain this way. I was told that I had been lucky to gain additional monies to support my appointment and to be able to start a neurophysiology service (electromyography and electroencephalography — EMG and EEG). I was able to purchase equipment and to employ a technologist and a clinical neurophysiologist.

Dunedin, which was 365 kilometres by road to the south, had provided neurosurgery for Christchurch patients, and it was in no mood to discontinue this arrangement. Many clinicians in Christchurch felt they had been well served by Dunedin, and out of a sense of loyalty they did not wish to rock the boat. The fact that Christchurch had a much larger population, and that the majority of South Island neurosurgical patients were disadvantaged by having to travel a long distance, seemed of little importance. The injustice of this was readily apparent to those at the coalface.

'Gary, your headaches are caused by an increase in the pressure inside your head,' I explained to the worried-looking 29-year-old and his wife, who was cradling a six-month-old baby on her lap.

'This is due to a swelling that you have in the back of your brain, about here,' I said, indicating the midline, just a little above the spot where his neck joined his skull. 'This swelling is preventing the cerebrospinal fluid from flowing from the inside of your brain, where it is produced, down into your spinal canal, where it is absorbed.

'You have been put onto strong steroid tablets to try to decrease this swelling and to lessen the pressure inside your head. You will need an operation to find out what is causing the swelling and to relieve the pressure. This cannot be done in Christchurch and you will need to go to Dunedin to have it carried out. I have spoken to a neurosurgeon there and he will arrange everything. The operation needs to be done urgently, and we could fly you down to Dunedin in an air ambulance this afternoon.'

There followed a long discussion with my patient and his wife. Naturally, they had many questions and were very concerned, as well they should have been. It was a dangerous situation. The lump in the back of his brain, which was probably a tumour, had caused such a severe increase in intracranial pressure that the optic nerves at the back of his eyes had become grossly swollen. If the pressure was to rise any further, something that could occur unpredictably over the space of an hour or less, the vital centres at the base of Gary's brain could be crushed and he would die.

This being a Friday afternoon, the neurosurgeon wanted Gary in Dunedin as soon as possible. The small propeller-driven air ambulance (a Cessna), which could take Gary, a nurse and the pilot, was the only safe method of transport available and it would leave at 5 p.m. His wife and baby would have to travel separately by road. I wished them all the best.

I was doing my hospital ward round the following Monday morning when I was astounded to find the young father lying propped up on a pillow in the same bed where I had last seen him.

'Gary! What are you doing here?' I asked him. 'You're supposed to be in Dunedin!'

'I wish I was,' he said, 'but the plane could not land. The weather was too rough and the visibility too poor. When we arrived at Dunedin airport the pilot had to turn around and fly back to Christchurch.'

It transpired that a southerly storm had struck just before touchdown and the little plane had been forced to retreat, the pilot hoping to land at one of the other small airports scattered along its return flightpath. The storm, however, was sweeping northwards at such a rate that everywhere they tried to put down, including Christchurch, the weather had become too rough. Eventually they just managed to get to Wellington, about the same distance to the north as Dunedin was to the south, before the weather bomb hit and their fuel ran out. Because the sea was so rough all ferry services between the North and South islands were cancelled. Gary and the nurse had to wait in a motel until Sunday, when they were able to return to Christchurch by ferry and train. If only I had known I could have arranged for him to be admitted to the neurosurgical service in Wellington! Fortunately, the steroids had worked, his headache had gone and he looked decidedly better. Nonetheless, I was glad when later that day Gary again departed for Dunedin.

A few days later I learnt that Gary did indeed have a brain tumour, a medulloblastoma, which is uncommon in children and rare in adults. Happily, with surgery and radiotherapy it is completely curable. Although the outcome in Gary's case was fortunate, it might well have been fatal, and the experience of dealing with him and similar patients convinced me that we were in urgent need of neurosurgical services in Christchurch, even if we had an uphill battle on our hands with the powers that be.

But neurosurgery was also changing, and a CT brain scanner was becoming an essential tool for a neurosurgeon, especially a young one who had been trained in a large modern overseas unit where such equipment had become standard. We could not consider starting a neurosurgical service in Christchurch without a CT scanner. The first such machine in New Zealand was installed at Auckland Hospital in the late 1970s, ostensibly to evaluate its usefulness, although this had been well and truly established overseas. It was meant to provide brain scans for the whole country, but the service was rapidly overwhelmed by the volume of work and it soon became apparent that it was impractical to transport sick patients for long distances just to have a test.

On one occasion a colleague decided to act as a nurse and accompany a confused Dunedin Hospital inpatient, who had a suspected brain tumour, on the trip to Auckland for a CT brain scan. The patient had to be roused at 5 a.m. to get ready for the first leg of the journey, a flight to Christchurch at 7 a.m. They eventually got back to Dunedin Hospital at 9 p.m. In the meantime the patient had been in four ambulances, on four flights, travelled almost double the length of the country, and required to be taken to the toilet 20 times. The neurologist thought he was more exhausted than the patient, and he had new respect for the nursing profession!

As a result of multiple representations to the Christchurch Hospital authorities, the Ministry of Health and the Minister of Health, a CT scanner was installed in Christchurch Hospital in 1980 and Christchurch's first neurosurgeon, Martin McFarlane, started work not long after. With the appointment of two young neurologists, Philip Parkin and Stuart Avery, we had the nidus of a proper clinical neuroscience service for the city. In the end, my professional dream had been realised much sooner than I had thought it would be, but not without a huge amount of help and work by my colleagues in radiology, medicine, surgery and administration, who had all become enthusiastic supporters. When Chris, our four sons and I left on my first sabbatical leave, six years after I had taken up my post, I felt quietly confident about our future in Christchurch.

**YES, I DID SAY FOUR SONS.** Our family had mysteriously expanded over the years. First there was Matthew, who was born in 1970. Chris had briefly been a ward charge nurse before being offered a job as a tutor at the Christchurch school of nursing, where she fell seriously gravid. This was in the period before I had decided to go to Auckland for training and I had been offered an alternative job in Sydney. I had a trans-Tasman flight booked for a fortnight after her expected delivery date so that I could go and see what the position offered. Our calculations proved to be overly optimistic, however, as the day of our son's expected arrival disappeared into the past. In desperation Chris took to jogging, mowing the lawn with a push-mower and all other manner of unaccustomed physical activity, but it was to no avail. I wanted to cancel my trip, but she would not hear of it. We would lose the price of the ticket, and anyway, I would only be away for a day.

Perhaps it was the emotional stress of our fond farewell, or it may be that the fateful hour was always ordained. Whatever the reason, labour commenced as she was driving back to work from the airport. Yes, she was still working! It was a complicated affair that eventually required forceps and rotation in the middle of the night, but Chris's brother Brent sat in for me at the hospital bedside, keeping her 'amused' by rehearsing a medical presentation he was due to deliver the following day!

In 1973 Chris was also a fortnight overdue with our second son, Michael, when she felt labour commencing. I received a call from my mother-in-law,

Norma, who was babysitting Matthew, to tell me that I should make my way from the National Hospital to London's University College Hospital's delivery suite. My dear wife had decided that the quickest way to get there was by tube, in spite of having had a nasty experience on the underground a week or so earlier. She had been descending into the bowels of the earth at Holborn Station when the hem of her long dress became caught in the escalator. Frantically she tried to extract it with one hand while clutching Matthew with the other, but with no success. Gradually but surely her dress was being torn off her as it was swallowed by an invisible and menacing mechanism. It seemed that her feet might follow. She managed to hit an emergency stop button that seemed to rapidly flash by her heading in an upwards direction. She then calmly stepped out of the remains of her dress, which was frozen in the act of disappearing.

Norma also came to the UK two years later to help hold the fort when we were expecting our third child.

'Chris went into labour early this afternoon, and when she felt that it was well established she went off to University College Hospital,' my mother-in-law announced when I arrived home from the laboratory at Denmark Hill, where I was desperately trying to finish the experimental work I had been doing for my MD.

'I hope she hasn't done anything silly like trying to take the bus or a tube,' I said.

'No, she hasn't. She went off on the bicycle. She said she would leave it chained to a lamp-post outside the delivery suite entrance, and she especially asked me to instruct you to ride it home when you come back.'

'Good God!' I exclaimed as I turned tail and fled out the door. 'That must be all of about four or five kilometres. We agreed that she would take a taxi. Whatever will she get up to next?'

I found the bicycle exactly where Chris had said it would be, and it was a leisurely but very cold ride home as the dusk descended on central London that February evening.

'What is it?' Norma asked as soon as I let myself into the warmth of our small flat.

'More of the same — of course! Mother and Edward are both fit and well.'

It was a foregone conclusion that our fourth, Paul, would be a boy. Like the three others he was a fortnight overdue, but he still showed no sign of wanting to leave the comfort of the womb, so Chris had to be induced. On this occasion the mother behaved herself impeccably, if you overlook an emergency readmission to hospital in Christchurch. This was caused by fainting secondary to a postpartum haemorrhage that required an emergency blood transfusion.

## CHAPTER 6

# London Sabbatical

### 1983–1984

**'WELL, HAVE YOU DECIDED** what you would like to do with your sabbatical? Do you wish to renew your acquaintance with rats, do some other form of lab project, work in the hospital clinics or get involved in one of the clinical studies that we have going on?'

As I surveyed David Marsden through the haze of his cigarette smoke, which happily was being slowly drawn away from me and towards the open window behind him, I mused on how little he appeared to have changed. There may have been a few grey hairs starting to appear at his temples, but he still looked very much like a naughty schoolboy who could be told off at any moment for smoking. By comparison my wrinkles, receding hairline and salt-and-pepper hair colour would have fooled a stranger into thinking that I was his senior colleague.

David had lost none of his easy manner and charm. I needed to concentrate and not get seduced into a large project that would be difficult to complete. I wanted something simple; something that would not entail too much hard work and would be relatively easy to complete within the time available. It had taken a lot to chew the MD project that I had bitten off when I first met him. I did not regret it, but this time I wanted to enjoy London and all its extracurricular delights. Yes, we did have a year's sabbatical, but the time would fly by and there were shows to see, operas to attend, museums to visit, galleries to stroll through, buildings to marvel at, bargains to be found in markets, friends to look up and all of the thousand and one other things that beckoned in that great city. I did not want to get sucked into working day and night again.

I had earlier suggested to David that I might spend my sabbatical writing a book on movement disorders and I had asked him if he would like to be involved, otherwise I intended to do it myself. I had envisaged something of modest dimensions; something that would be easily completed within 12 months. Somewhat to my surprise he was quite positive, but felt it should be on a much grander scale.

'Have you thought any more about the book collaboration we discussed?' David now asked. 'There is no other comprehensive book on movement disorders. People have written books about Parkinson's disease, Huntington's disease and so on, but nobody has covered the entire movement disorder field. We could concentrate on the basement of the brain; the basal ganglia and their disorders, but these days the movement disorder field has expanded beyond that.'

I was very familiar with the term 'basement of the brain', which in 1925 had been coined by Kinnier Wilson. This famous neurologist had discovered a crippling and lethal disorder, which is now called Wilson's disease. He had been on the staff at the National Hospital, where he had made a particular study of the functions and disorders of the basal ganglia, the prominent clumps of grey matter that lie at the base of the cerebral hemispheres and connect them via the brain stem to the spinal cord. He had referred to them as the basement of the brain not only because of their position but because their purpose and mechanisms of action were surrounded by darkness and mystery. The precise functions and functioning of the basal ganglia had proved much more difficult to unravel than those of the cerebral cortex, and to this day many of the basement's secrets have never seen the light of day.

'It would be all the more significant in that the whole thing would be written by us,' David said, adding, as though as an afterthought, 'by the three of us.'

Perhaps I looked a little surprised, because David continued, 'Well, I think I would have to involve Stanley Fahn. I have discussed writing such a book with him as well. He is the recognised North American authority on the topic and, apart from being extremely knowledgeable, his participation would help the book sell in North America. That would be vital for its success in that marketplace.'

There was a reason why no one had written a comprehensive book on movement disorders, and that was because the subject had only recently emerged as a distinct entity. Most of the individual medical disorders that made up the topic had been known for a long time, and there were neurologists who had specialised in these and had written about them. Some of these conditions had been loosely grouped together, but the wider field of movement disorders was still developing and it was only just becoming recognised as a subspecialty of neurology.

As in the older subspecialty of epileptiology, the study of epilepsy, the clinical picture (i.e. the patient's symptoms and signs) was very varied and could be caused by a variety of different illnesses and pathologies that could be either inherited or acquired. The primary feature of a movement disorder was a disturbance of movement that was not just caused by weakness or loss of strength. These conditions particularly involved involuntary movements, with either the appearance of abnormal involuntary movements or the loss of normal involuntary movements. In Parkinson's disease, the best-known movement disorder, patients typically had both abnormal involuntary movements (tremor) and the loss or diminution of normal involuntary (i.e. automatic) movements (facial expression and arm swinging when walking). Both David Marsden and Stanley Fahn were very active and influential in defining and championing this emerging and vast subspecialty within neurology.

It sounded extremely tempting, but from the back of my head a pathetic little voice pleaded, 'Don't do it. It will be too much work.'

I should have listened to that voice instead of to my ambition and pride.

'Why don't we think about it over the weekend and meet again on Monday,' I said, procrastinating. But I knew all along that I was hooked. I wanted to discuss it with Chris, but I suspected that, as usual, she would agree to go along with my madcap scheme.

The following Monday morning I again caught my 'usual', the number 68 double-decker bus, from Russell Square to the small neurology department that was attached to the Maudsley Hospital and the Institute of Psychiatry at Denmark Hill in south London. Autumn's kiss was gently brushing the trees and the parks were carpeted with gold and russet leaves. An ornamental pond sparkled in the sunlight as model boats bobbed up and down, setting out on a long journey to nowhere. It was a propitious day to embark on an exciting project.

'I've thought it over, David, and if you are still keen, then I think we should do it. It will be a lot of work, but I think it's manageable.'

'Good. I will contact Stanley Fahn and see if he wants to be involved. We need to think who would be the best publishers. I think Oxford University Press would be good. Had you had any other thoughts? No? Why don't we start by organising a list of contents?'

A few days later, holding a long list of proposed chapters, divided into sections according to the different topics, I telephoned Oxford University Press (OUP). Yes, they could be interested in publishing the book, but did I really think that we could finish the job and deliver a completed manuscript? I was taken aback by the question. Why on earth should they have this doubt?

My co-author had not proved completely reliable in this regard in the past, came the reply. I assured them the manuscript would definitely be completed and delivered, but fortunately, I did not say when. It took several more telephone calls before it was finally agreed. OUP would publish the book.

On the basis of this verbal agreement I enthusiastically started to work, looking up published papers and dictating during the day, while Chris faithfully typed the text at night. We were living in a small apartment in William Goodenough House, a marvellous establishment for postgraduate students, where we had stayed for a time during our first visit to London. It was two blocks from the National Hospital and Institute of Neurology, where Chris would sit patiently typing, often until the small hours. This was 1983, and she had access to the one and only word processor in the whole place, courtesy of professors Roger Gilliatt and Ian McDonald. This spectacular new invention was regarded as one of the Seven Wonders of the World and was so special that it even had its own room. It was almost two metres high, a metre wide and a metre deep. It emitted deep growling noises, high-pitched hums and intermittent thumps; all very unnerving in a deserted building in the middle of the night. But, wonder of wonders, it allowed you to invisibly erase mistakes, add material and alter the text without having to type out the whole script again. Without it our difficult task would surely have been impossible. It was immediately apparent that this was the way of the future. I telephoned OUP excitedly and offered to deliver the manuscript on disk when it was completed. I received an unenthusiastic response. OUP's editors preferred to work from typed pages, and when these had been corrected the publisher would typeset the material. It was many years before OUP changed this policy!

**'I'M GOING TO CALL THE POLICE.'**

My concern had gradually become replaced by a rising sense of panic. Apart from going to the authorities and reporting that one of our sons was missing, I could think of nothing else that we could do. I had put our eldest, Matthew, on the bus that Monday morning, his first day at his new school. We had expected his excited face to appear in the doorway of our apartment at about 3.45 p.m. By 4.30 we were becoming disturbed and I had made my second visit to the bus stop where he should have alighted. By 5.30 we were agitated, and by 6.30 we were beside ourselves. Had he had an accident? Had he been abducted or attacked? A flood of ideas, most of them dark and unpleasant, was welling up within both Chris and me, ready to burst the floodbanks of our outward composure.

On the positive side, Matthew was a big, strong, quick-witted 13-year-old who would not take any nonsense from his peers. On the negative side, he was unused to being by himself in central London, and the only school that we had been able to enrol him in was North Westminster, which had the reputation of being rather rough, if not a blackboard jungle. Chris and I had taken him there for enrolment several days earlier and we had explained to him the route, the bus stops and the bus system. Euston Road was one of the busiest streets in London, and the journey to Paddington took about 25 minutes, passing Madame Tussaud's waxworks and other famous landmarks on the way. He did not, however, have to change buses. He simply had to get on and off at the correct stops.

What on earth could have happened to him? We were clearly the worst parents in the world and guilty of criminal negligence for not taking our little lamb to school each day for the first week. We were flagellating ourselves with the hard-knotted cords of grief.

It was 6.55 p.m. and I had just started heading off to the police station when a jaunty-looking Matthew, schoolbag over his shoulder, sauntered down the street towards me. It took me all my willpower not to burst into tears.

'Thank goodness you are all right, Matthew. Where on earth have you been? What has happened to you?'

'I'm fine, Dad. It's just that the bus coming home went a different way and I got hopelessly lost. I kept looking for my bus stop but it never came. Eventually we seemed to end up in the country. Then the conductor told me it was the end of the line and that I had to get off. I didn't like to argue as he was a very large dark man and he became annoyed when he saw my ticket. He said that I had paid only for a short ride and that I was cheating the system. I asked a man on the street which was the way home and he tried to explain it to me, then I started walking. After walking for a long time I asked another man, who was getting into his car, and I explained that I was lost. He gave me a ride to the end of the street.'

How had this happened? It seemed incredible. Why would the bus go a totally different route and not pass the end of our street with its friendly, familiar bus stop?

We did not have time to enquire then, because we actually had tickets to the opera at Covent Garden that evening, and the babysitter was already in our apartment. After tearful hugs we heartlessly rushed out. We had intended to walk to Covent Garden, a journey of about 30 minutes, but we were now desperately late. We owned only one bicycle so I ran while Chris cycled on ahead, then she would leave the machine propped against a lamp-post at the end of the block. She then ran while I cycled past and left the bicycle for her at the end of the next block … and so on. In this way we 'leapfrogged' our way to the opera house. We sweatily squeezed our way into our seats just as the maestro reached the pit.

Our unorthodox mode of transport had been so successful that from then on it became our regular way of going to the opera; and go to the opera we did. We kept a diary of all the operas we went to during that year's sabbatical. The grand tally was 56, and we never saw the same production twice! We had clearly become obsessed and were trying to set some sort of world record. But who would have thought that so many operas could be staged in one city?

The following day, however, we were determined to find out what had gone wrong with the buses, and to make certain it was not repeated. Chris accompanied Matthew to and from school. When they came to go home the mistake became apparent.

'This is the wrong bus stop, Mum. That's the one over there.'

Even though he was a teenager, Matthew had never travelled on buses before our sabbatical, and he had got off and on his buses at the same stop, instead of on opposite sides of the road! No wonder he had ended up in the suburbs. And no, he was not a slow learner. His slack parents were to blame. We thought it was ingenious of him to have negotiated his way back from the sticks so cleverly. He was clearly going to become a wily and resourceful character.

**I WAVED TO CHRIS, WHO WAS WAITING** patiently on the other side of Tottenham Court Road, looking for a break in the traffic. A few moments later she was crossing the street to where I was waiting for her outside the Dominion Theatre. I saw her stumble on the curb and there was a dull crack as the yellow plastic bag that she was carrying slipped from her hand. The corners of her mouth seemed to melt and flow downwards as her smile turned into an expression of frustration and anguish.

'Smell it! Just come and smell it because that's all you're going to get!' she cried out as I rushed forward in a vain attempt to reverse what had happened by offering her support that she now did not need.

We knelt there on the footpath, inhaling the heady aroma, which danced around us teasingly as it ascended heavenwards into the ether. The gods would enjoy their meal in paradise that night. We must have looked like a couple of old soaks, but we did not care. The wine trickled forlornly through a hole in the bag and hesitatingly made its way down the gutter to a nearby drain. Chris had just bought a bottle of Vega-Sicilia 'Unico', Spain's most prestigious and expensive red wine. It was produced in very small quantities and we had never tried it. There was a rumour in the wine trade that it had been requested to take pride of place at the wedding of Prince Charles and Princess Diana. Vega-Sicilia's owner was reported to have responded by offering them a dozen bottles. We were lucky to have found one in London, and because of the cost we were not going to be looking for another.

We entered the theatre and dispiritedly watched the musical *Blood Brothers.* It had been given spectacular reviews and had proved very popular with the public. But somehow it lacked lustre. We were in deep mourning.

Chris had bought the Vega-Sicilia at one of my favourite wine shops in London, Vintage Cellars in Old Compton Street, a curious little place in the middle of the red-light district of Soho. It incongruously rubbed shoulders with 'adult shops' and strip joints, whose touts tried to pull you inside but whose bouncers looked menacingly uninviting. Vintage Cellars was an enigma. It had a surprisingly good collection of wines and sometimes there were absolute gems. I found it hard to imagine the local clientele availing themselves of its services, particularly when there were other shops in the area with cheaper drinks. Perhaps I was underestimating the power and subtlety of Eros.

One Saturday afternoon, not long after the start of my sabbatical, I found myself sorting through some bottles at the dimly lit back of the shop when my eyes alighted on a line-up of 1977 vintage ports. They had only recently been released and the write-ups were excellent. 'Vintage of the century', some pundits had predicted. I was drawn to them, not only because they sounded exceptional but also because 1977 was our youngest, Paul's, birth year. Matthew had been born in that great claret year, 1970, but Michael and Edward were not so fortunate, arriving on the scene in 1973 and 1975, respectively. I had tried to get a few bottles of each of our sons' birth years to put down in my small cellar for special anniversaries or events. Here was the perfect opportunity, and the price was very reasonable. There was one small snag: our little central London apartment was bulging at the seams. We simply did not have room to store this wine, particularly since I had brought cases of New Zealand wine from home and these were crammed into every available nook and cranny. I explained the situation to the middle-aged shopkeeper.

'If I buy the wine now would you be good enough to store it for me until I am ready to go back to New Zealand in a year's time?'

'I would be delighted to do that for you, sir,' he replied helpfully, and so I happily tripped out of the shop weighed down by no more than my receipt.

I suspect that must have been a year of the Rabbit as it raced by like a bunny pursued by hounds. Not long before we were due to go home I received a letter from Kingsley Wood, a wine-merchant friend in Christchurch. He had managed to get a splendid supply of the marvellous 1977 vintage ports. Would I like him to put some aside for me? I was both pleased and annoyed to see that the prices were significantly less than I had paid for my little stash and I still had to get mine back to Christchurch without any breakages! It seemed too good an opportunity to turn down, but did I really need more port? This question assumed, of course, that Vintage Cellars still had my bottles. I decided it was time to find out.

'Yes, of course. We have them all ready and waiting for you, sir,' the helpful middle-aged gent confirmed.

I explained my position and enquired whether he might consider taking the port back and allowing me to spend the money on claret.

'That's fine, sir. We have a good selection of clarets and we can order in any others that you fancy. I will just work out what you have to spend.'

He went out to the back of the shop, returning a few moments later.

'Let me see now. You have quite a sum burning a hole in your pocket.'

I gasped. It was substantially more than I had spent on the port.

'But that is far more than I paid you,' I said rather reluctantly.

'I know that, sir,' he replied. 'But you bought them from me and I am now buying them back from you, and this is what they are currently worth. Quite frankly, I'm delighted to get them. Since you bought these bottles the world has discovered the 1977 vintage ports and it is clamouring for them. I can on-sell them at quite a comfortable profit.'

It had never occurred to me that I would get any more than I had paid for the wine, and I would have been happy even if he had deducted something for storage. I came away with a respectable number of reds from decent Bordeaux châteaux and a new respect for seedy old Soho and Vintage Cellars in particular.

The reason I had brought a range of top New Zealand wines to London with me was not that I felt I would be pining for a taste of home. No, these were wines from small producers who were turning out some of the country's finest, but the wines were not available in the UK. They represented the new wave of quality New Zealand wines made from classical *Vitis vinifera* varieties. Among them was the 1982 St Helena Pinot Noir. I wanted to show the movers and shakers of the wine industry just what my little country was capable of producing.

It had been my rather naïve intention to hold a tasting of these wines in London for top wine writers. I had procrastinated as it had seemed too hard to organise. Where would I hold it? In a restaurant? Who would I invite?

How would I contact them? What sort of food should I offer? Perhaps I should be done with the whole idea and we should just drink the wine. If that was to be the case, we had better start pretty soon as time was running out.

But there was another problem. I myself had started writing regular wine columns for newspapers two or three years earlier, and I had used my authority to lean on producers to give me examples of their very best bottles so that I could show them to the wider world. I could not let them down now. Then Chris, as was usual, had a bright idea.

'The New Zealand High Commission might be able to help you find the addresses of the people you want to invite. Why don't you ask them?' she suggested.

It was with some trepidation that I telephoned the High Commission, expecting to be fobbed off. The receptionist was surprisingly helpful, however, and before I knew it I was talking to the Trade Commissioner himself, Don Walker. I wondered momentarily whether he was bipolar and if he had stopped his lithium during a manic phase, but no, it turned out that he was a wine buff himself, a great enthusiast for and supporter of the Kiwi liquid product. When could I come down and meet him to discuss the details?

'Anytime it suits you,' had been my reply, and now here I was talking to him face-to-face. He was charming, urbane and extremely helpful.

'You can hold it here at New Zealand House,' he said. 'We have an ideal room, all the glassware and the other paraphernalia. We have the contacts of all the important wine people and we will send out invitations. All you will have to do is bring the wine here beforehand and turn up on the day.' And that is exactly what happened. I could not believe my luck.

Chris and I mingled among the guests, answering questions and talking about the wines. I was disappointed that my hero, Hugh Johnson, had cancelled at the last moment due to a bereavement. However, we met many other wine writers with whom we were familiar only through their articles. They genuinely seemed to enjoy the wines, and some proved to be very helpful in arranging contacts and visits for an upcoming tour of European wine regions that we were planning. One young lady in particular impressed us with her knowledge and flair. Jancis Robinson, who is now known to just about every wine lover, was then a relatively new but rapidly rising star in the vinous firmament. We were fascinated as her long silky locks covered her face when she leant forward towards the spittoon, but with a flick of her head the tresses parted and slid back towards her ears just as she scored a perfect bull's-eye. She never let go of her pen and paper or sullied a single hair. Great expectorations!

**THE END OF MY YEAR'S SABBATICAL** leave seemed to come and go like an express train passing through a suburban station. Throughout my time in London it had been a milestone rather than a goal. I had not been looking forward to the end of the year, but it represented a very important point in my journey. I had expected things to slacken off and slow down as we approached the station, but no, it was full speed ahead and on to the next leg.

I had been working hard on the book, or rather, Chris and I had been working hard. I had written what I estimated would be a third to a half of the final text. It was the part that dealt with hyperkinetic disorders; those with an excess of automatic or involuntary movements. I was keen that we should publish it then, before the material got out of date, and write the rest as a second stage. It would mean another volume but there was nothing to stop us immediately starting work on this with a fresh slate. I wanted to approach OUP and see if they would agree to it, but David Marsden was vehemently against this proposal.

'We can finish the rest over the next 12 to 18 months,' he assured me. 'I have a lot of material that I have already prepared. It only needs tidying up and to have minor changes made to it. We will make rapid progress. If it was published in two parts it would break the cohesiveness of the work. There are other books which deal with subsections of movement disorders. This book will be unique because it will be all-inclusive and comprehensive.'

Reluctantly I agreed to go along with his wishes. He undoubtedly knew the topic and the market better than I did, and he was so confident that we could complete it quickly that I felt optimistic about the outcome. The work would be delayed, but not by too much. I was to live to regret this decision.

**'DO YOU KNOW WHAT I HAVE ENJOYED** most about this sabbatical year?' I asked Chris as we cruised somewhere over the Atlantic on our way back home.

'No. Tell me.'

'Not doing the gardening.' I was being facetious but trying to make a point. 'Not just the gardening but all the other things that we do in our lives that are non-productive, or not very productive.'

'What are you trying to say?'

'Take Pleurisy Point, for example. I spend a huge amount of time making wine etc., but in the end all we get is a few bottles. It has been a great experience and I have really enjoyed it, but I think we either have to stop winemaking or we have to become completely professional about it. It's sucking away too much of our time for too little reward. It's a little like growing our own vegetables. It's fun and it's nice to have them, but realistically they are not worth the effort. Mountain View Vineyard has become my vegetable patch.

'All I am saying is that at the moment the game is not worth the candle. We need to become serious about vineyards and winemaking or get out of it entirely. Regretfully, whatever decision we come to, I'm going to have to tell the others that I'm going to leave the co-operative. To start our own vineyard and winery would take a huge amount of work and would be a considerable risk, but if we don't take the plunge sometime soon we will never do it. Then we might end our days wondering what it might have been like. Let's each have a really good think about it.'

At that moment the kids were being little angels; they were all fast asleep. Chris and I asked for a glass of dessert wine as a nightcap, then we settled down to join them.

## CHAPTER 7
# Just *the* Right Piece *of* Dirt
1984–1986

**A SCYTHE OF DAZZLING LIGHT** slashed a wide horizontal arc through the black night and I was momentarily blinded as I was cut by its beam. The car, which had roared around the tight corner, now came to a screeching halt. I heard doors slamming, voices and then a shout.

'Who's there? What are you doing? We know you're there. Are you all right? Do you need help?'

I lay spreadeagled in the long grass, gasping for breath. I had been winded by the fall and I had a severe throbbing in my right ankle. Silence: my embarrassment was as acute as my pain. I wanted to yell out in frustration and agony but I did not dare say a word. It would be too difficult to explain my actions and it might give my game away. I lay as still as a dead mouse.

'Is there anyone out there?' I could hear two or three people talking quietly among themselves. 'We know you're there because we all saw you. If you want to hide there in the wet grass and get cold then that's over to you. Have a happy life!'

Doors slammed, the unmistakable sound of a VW air-cooled motor roared into life and the Beetle sped away.

I lay quite still for five or 10 minutes to be sure they were not coming back, then I slowly and painfully levered myself into the upright position with the aid of my spade. My foot had caught in a rabbit hole while I was rapidly pacing and, just at the moment of my exposure, I had fallen heavily onto the ground. Using the spade as a walking stick I now hobbled back to the deep hole that I had dug and refilled it, carefully replacing the turf and treading it down with my good foot. Could I bear to finish pacing out the length of the field? I gritted my teeth and set out to do it, but this time I would switch on my torch or my headlamp; be buggered if I was going to risk tripping up in a rabbit burrow again!

Over the previous 18 months we had looked at every piece of land that had come up for sale within an hour's drive north of Christchurch. There was always a problem: it was too steep, the soil type was not suitable for a vineyard, it faced the wrong direction, it was not the right size, there was no water available, there was no site for a winery, the access was poor and so forth. We could not find anything that we felt would be entirely suitable for our purposes. Finally we came to the conclusion that we were going about it the wrong way. What we needed to do was find the piece of dirt that we thought was perfect, then convince the owner to sell it to us. But what was perfect? What did we really want? We needed to make a precise list of our requirements, and that we did.

The land needed to be within comfortable driving distance of the hospital in order to enable me to answer calls. The potential vineyard area would have to be large enough to allow us to generate sufficient income to employ other people, and it would need to have a site suitable for a winery and cellar door. Because of the types of grapes we wanted to grow, we felt that freely draining, stony soil would be optimum. We would require shelter from the fierce, hot northwesterly winds, which we called the 'Devil's breath', that were so typical of North Canterbury, and we needed a source of water. We also fancied the Waipara Valley area, where a line of hills, the Teviotdale Range, separate the Pacific Ocean and its cooling sea breezes from the valley floor. This gives the region more sunshine hours and warmth than most of Canterbury. We had earlier roamed the hills on both sides of the valley while collecting fossils, and we knew that this region had earlier been under the sea. Throughout the area there were copious deposits of limestone, which could be helpful for the cultivation of certain types of grape.

First we needed a topographical map and then we had to visit selected sites. We could see by looking from the road that many of these were unsuitable, but those that had potential would require further investigation, namely digging holes to assess the soil profile and to get soil samples. We did not want to go and ask a lot of different farmers whether we could check their pieces of dirt because we thought we might possibly like to buy their precious land for a vineyard. In North Canterbury sheep farmers reigned supreme. They drove, or rather had driven, the economy. Anyone wanting to do anything else with their land was clearly mad and to be discouraged or even thwarted. Perhaps the glint of gold might entice them to part with a pocket-handkerchief-sized part of their rural paradise, but they would doubtless prefer to pass it on intact for their sons to squabble over. If we weren't careful word would soon get around the district that there were loonies about, fools who might be prepared to pay a high price for poor farming land. Any stupid vineyard venture would be bound to fail, but then a shrewd operator might be able to repossess the handkerchief and make a handsome profit. We needed to be discreet and to be really certain which piece of dirt we wanted before we made our approach.

My preference was for moonlighting, but sometimes, as on this night, I had been forced to work by starlight alone, aided by my headlamp and torch. There had been a moon earlier, but its welcome sliver of a face had become obscured by the ragged clouds that had brought a brief light shower. As usual I had searched for banks, channels or pits in which I could see the soil profile, assessing the depth of topsoil and the underlying terrain. I had dug several holes and taken small samples. Since all this looked promising I would pace out the length and breadth of the fields to get an idea of the area involved. If the property warranted further investigation I would go to the Lands and Survey office where you could find out many things, including the total area of the property, but you could not find out the exact area of a fenced paddock. There were no Google maps in those days!

'What on earth happened to you?' Chris asked with concern as I finally hobbled inside dirty and wet.

'I was mauled by a savage rabbit and then chased off the property by an inquisitive Beetle … but I think I might be on to something at last!'

Our friends all thought we were mad when we mentioned that we were planning to develop a commercial vineyard. We assumed, without great regret, that this meant they did not want to be included in our seemingly hairbrained scheme. While a financial contribution would no doubt have come in handy, our experience at Pleurisy Point had taught us that we did not have the temperament for a co-operative; we were too bossy and obsessive. It was not that we were desperate to paddle our own canoe, but we were determined to be its captain and to steer its course.

The reason for our friends' lack of enthusiasm was that New Zealand was not only awash with its own wine but drowning in it. The wider world had not heard about the Kiwi product, which was why I had held my wine tasting in London. Wine exports were only a trickle, and excessive vine plantings had completely saturated the domestic wine market. The bargain bins in wine shops overflowed with $5 bottles of very good wine. It was being sold below cost because wine companies needed cashflow to pay their employees. Receivership and bankruptcy stalked the New Zealand wine industry. The situation was so desperate that the Labour government of the day paid vignerons to pull the vines out of the ground.

Pastoral farming was also having its own version of *The Grapes of Wrath*. After Britain joined the European Economic Community in 1973 it became progressively harder for British housewives to buy New Zealand food, especially butter and meat. The Labour government had reacted to the rapidly crippling monetary situation by introducing what became known as Rogernomics, a brand of far-right economic policies that eliminated farm subsidies and sent land prices into freefall. Being believers in the simple philosophy 'Plant potatoes during a potato glut' (because everyone else will pull theirs out), Chris and I felt it was the ideal time to launch our little venture. The only caveat was that we had to avoid debt because inflation and interest rates were skyrocketing.

**'DO WE HAVE TO DO ANY MORE, MUM?** We're sick of this now and we want to go and play,' a little voice pleaded.

'If you do another hundred each you can have an extra scoop of chips with your fish on the way home,' came the reply.

Although nutritionists would nowadays doubtless blame our epidemic of obesity on such wanton bribery, and unionists would accuse us of child slave labour, this tactic always worked. In doing so, it prevented the cracks that otherwise would have appeared in the supposedly smooth bond of parent-child relationships. The boys' faces brightened and they worked with new-found vigour at our task of making grapevine cuttings, using secateurs. It was a cold day towards the end of winter and we were sitting on boxes in a vineyard, muffled up with hats, coats, boots and gloves. Our cuttings, each of which was about 30 centimetres in length, were tied up in bundles of fifty. They would be put into wet sacks and stored in a cool place until they were ready to be planted out in a nursery during the spring. The boys had done this work uncomplainingly — well relatively uncomplainingly — for the previous three Saturdays, so it was perhaps not surprising that they were getting a little restive. This was not their idea of quality family time, in spite of what their parents told them.

Fortunately, we did not have to make all of the cuttings for our planned vineyard. Six months earlier Danny Schuster had asked if he could use our spare bedroom for a fortnight. He was still in residence, and we had leaned on him to use his contacts to get us cuttings of varieties and clones that were not locally available, such as sémillon. Although sauvignon blanc was grabbing the headlines as the rapidly rising star of the New Zealand wine scene, and the Kiwi version strongly resembled the Sancerre that had so much impressed me at the mess dinner at the National, our tastes had changed. We planned to tame down its strongly pungent aroma and flavour, add complexity and fill out its palate structure by blending it with sémillon, as is commonly done in France.

When the frigid breath of old Mr Winter had been chased away by the comforting body warmth of young Miss Spring, our family bent our backs and pushed our cuttings into the soft, moist earth. As yet, we had not found our special plot of dirt so Danny, who was doing the same work alongside us, allowed us to plant in the nursery that he was starting. He had formed a partnership with a local farmer and restaurateur, Russell Black, to develop their own vineyard. The plan was that a year later, in the following spring, Chris and I would lift our little vines. At that stage they would have roots, and we would then plant them into our own vineyard, assuming we had purchased land by then.

The unaccustomed stooping and crouching caused aching and stiffness in muscles and joints that we did not know we owned. It was hot, tiring work but we were all cheerful. We had started on our vineyard. What we did not know was that Danny planned to spend the New Zealand summer in Europe, which would leave us to tend both nurseries. We were about to become experts in the honourable art of weeding and lose what modest skills we had attained in the arts of holidaymaking!

**MR JONES HAD THE UNMISTAKABLE VISAGE** of a man of the land. There were the crow's feet wrinkles around the sides of his eyes and the forehead furrows between them, attesting to years of squinting into sunshine that was made piercingly bright by the unpolluted, low-humidity atmosphere of the North Canterbury countryside. His lower face, neck and hands were brick-red and showed the tell-tale hallmarks of skin that had been forced to rebel against chronic sun exposure. In contrast, he was unnaturally pale above his mid-face, the legacy of sensibly wearing a hat when outdoors. He was a generously constructed man, throwing into contrast his wife's more delicate physique. They were welcoming and helpful and, above all, keen to sell us a piece of what they regarded as their worst land: stony, unfertile and uneconomic, especially in the current agricultural climate. No, they explained, they did not have any sons; only a daughter who had left home, and they did not see a lot of her. Mr Jones wanted to wind down and would be pleased to have less land to farm.

It was a very dull late-winter's afternoon, and so dark that the invitingly warm fire caused the light in their lounge to waver and flicker. Over afternoon tea our real estate agent presented our proposal to them. I had drawn up a map that clearly outlined the fields that we wished to buy. The Joneses were being offered a sum for all the land within the enclosed area, regardless of how many hectares it contained. Neither they nor we knew the exact area as it had not been surveyed, but I was certain that we would need it all for future development. We would also have to establish a legal right to take water across a part of their land that we were not buying. As spring was just around the corner, we would also need access to one of the fields that we proposed to buy. This was so that we could plant out the young grapevines that we had grown from the cuttings we had planted the year before.

All was agreed and signed. It only remained for our lawyers to enact the necessary paperwork. The settlement date should not be too far off. We warmly shook the vendors' hands as we left. Both couples were looking forward to having such charming neighbours.

'What acreage should I put down on the contract?' my lawyer asked. I had received a message that he wanted to talk to me but I had waited until the end of my clinic before telephoning him.

'I don't know what the acreage is but the agreement clearly states that the price is for all of the land that is included within the fences that are outlined in colour on the accompanying map. Why do we have to include an acreage in the contract? The land has not been surveyed yet.'

'It is usual to put a rough estimate, with the wording "more or less" after the figure, so that it doesn't have to be precise.'

'Well, the vendor did have an old hand-drawn map on which he had written what he thought might be the approximate areas. It's the only indication I have had, and it is just that, a rough guess.'

'Let's use that. It will be near enough.'

**THE NORTHWEST BREEZE SEEMED** a good omen, further warming the sunny spring afternoon. Daniel Le Brun, the twelfth-generation scion of a respected Champagne-making family, sniffed the air and squinted into the bright light.

'Letz get to verk, men,' he commanded. He was a jovial but no-nonsense, bluff man who knew how to work and expected others to do the same. He had married a Kiwi and had started making Champagne-style wine in Marlborough. In a short time he had come to be well regarded and even something of a local legend. When we had told Daniel of our plans and asked for his advice he had generously volunteered to drive down from Marlborough with three of his men, to instruct us and help us with our planting. 'Us' in this case being Chris, because I, as usual, was busy bringing home the bacon by seeing patients. We would only have to pay Daniel's workers' wages.

That year we only had enough vines to plant out a fraction of our first paddock, but even this seemed an enormously daunting task. The men unloaded the truck and began to get to work, Chris toiling alongside them. By the end of the afternoon several rows of vines were happily soaking up the sunshine, with their dormant feet and tiny toes as yet unable to soak up the moisture from the earth in which they were embedded. It all looked very promising. Then it started to rain, rain, rain … and rain. The following morning it was still raining, and so it drearily continued for the next 24 hours. Men of the land hate being caged and idle. This crew was no exception.

'We goh back to my vinery. We 'ave bottling to do,' Daniel announced sadly. He was clearly disappointed and so was Chris.

'We 'ave shown you vot to do. Juzz caree on in zee same vay,' and so saying he piled his gear and his men into the truck, kissed Chris on both cheeks and drove off.

Chris described feeling as though she had been told she had won the lottery only to be informed later that it was all an unfortunate mistake. Our precious plants had been lifted out of the nursery and would soon dry out and die. The rain was not going to last forever. The clock was ticking so Chris had to act quickly to avoid a disaster. She set to work telephoning contacts, and by the end of the day she was confident that she could muster a small team of virgin vineyard workers, largely geriatric, to help her carry on with the planting. She, however, would have to measure and mark out exactly the positions of the rows and direct operations, as well as doing hard physical work herself. Ominously, this was setting the pattern of things to come in our matrimonial vineyard relationship. I would give a few impractical instructions and go AWOL, while she would be left to put them into practice. Thank goodness she is a practical lass, brimming with common sense, good at communicating and with more than a dollop of confidence. Without her our little vineyard and winery operation would never have got off the ground.

After three days the heavy rain had eased and the sun had reappeared. There was some minor flooding on the lower of the two north-facing terraces where they had been planting, and it was to be 20 years before the same thing occurred again. What exquisitely rotten timing for this inundation to have occurred just when we had had the expertise and manpower to get most of our planting done professionally. Chris did a stunning job, especially given that she has never claimed to be an expert in geometry, but her huge effort and sacrifice has not gone unrewarded. To this day there are a few lines of vines that are known as

'Chris's Rows'. Some swear that these are closer together at their north than at their south ends, and that at the north it can be difficult for a tractor to pass between the vines. Chris is certain that this is merely an optical illusion caused by parallax in psychologically suggestible individuals.

**'YOU HAVE PLANTED YOUR VINES** on my land!' an exceptionally florid-faced Mr Jones stated emphatically.

His neck veins were sticking out like the proverbial parts of a dog's anatomy and he was standing uncomfortably close to Chris, as judged by flecks of spittle that were impinging on her personal body space.

'You will have to pull them out of the ground or pay me more for the land.'

The farmer was extremely agitated, and making vigorous gestures with his upper limbs, as though he was directing an aircraft into its parking position. He was attempting to emphasise both the truth and the seriousness of his pronouncement.

'I think you are wrong, Mr Jones,' Chris replied, determined to hold her own but stepping back a little out of firing range. 'We have bought all the land that is contained within these fencelines.'

'No, you haven't,' he shouted. 'You only bought *X* hectares and the surveyor says that these fields contain more than that.'

'The figure of *X* hectares is the one that you said was contained in these fields. If there was a mistake it is because you provided the wrong number. There is no doubt about our agreement, which states quite clearly that we have bought and will pay a fixed amount for the land that is enclosed within the specified fencelines. At any rate, why have you decided that this so-called extra land is exactly the part on which we have planted? Why couldn't you claim some other area?'

'Because I don't wish to do so. I have chosen this area here and you have planted on my land! If you don't like it you will have to deal with my lawyer. Let me know what you want to do.'

When I arrived home that evening Chris told me all about the saga and we took out our copy of the agreement. We were in no doubt that the disputed land clearly belonged to us.

'Do you think he has tried to trap us by providing a false figure for the area?' Chris asked.

'I don't know, but if so he is not going to get away with it. There is no way we are going to rip those plants out of the ground and we are not going to pay him a cent more!'

The following day, after discussing the matter with our solicitor, Chris called at the farmhouse to give Farmer Jones the woeful tidings. We were sorry about the misunderstanding and we were happy to go over the document with him and his wife in order to sort things out, but we did not agree with his interpretation. Our lawyer agreed with us.

If Chris had thought he had been rather steamed up the day before, then clearly she was mistaken. By comparison, he had been in an almost agreeable mood. The chances that you will have annoyed an octopus are really quite slight, but should you happen to do this you will see it almost instantaneously change colour from an inconspicuous grey-blue to an intense, livid red. Farmer Jones's visage became that of an enraged octopus. Fortunately he also became almost apoplectic, allowing Chris to flee while he was still seething in an immobile and near-speechless state. She did not, however, escape with her reputation completely unsullied. His recovery was rapid. A parting broadside of colourful adjectives and vibrant expletives followed her flight.

The letter from Farmer Jones's solicitor duly arrived and there followed the expected costly legal game of ping-pong, with communications being batted from one side of the table to the other with monotonous regularity. The ball finally landed in our court; Chris and I were going to be taken to court for the additional sum of money that was claimed by the Joneses and, naturally, they would be seeking additional compensation and costs. We were told, however, not to hold our breaths. Due to delays in the court system it could be up to two years before the vine-pruning secateurs and the lamb-castrating knife met in the cold pale light of dawn. In the meantime we had a vineyard that was in serious need of attention or it would rapidly go to rack and ruin.

Was it the faintly earthy smell, the humidity, just the clouds or some other sensation that warned of impending rain? Chris had worked in the vineyard all day and was now making her way towards the gate that led to the road. She was keen to be on her way as the remnants of the afternoon had frayed rapidly and its previously bright fabric now threatened to be rent asunder by an early evening downpour. She reached down to unclip the catch that held the gate closed, then suddenly froze. A large chain encircled the gate and its adjacent post, and the chain's two ends were linked together by a closed padlock. She had been locked in the vineyard. It had started to rain when Matthew drove up several minutes later, and mother and son looked forlornly at their obstructed passage of escape.

'Perhaps we are here for the night, Matthew,' Chris said glumly. 'I could walk up the road to Mr Jones's house and ask him to open it for us. It must be he who has locked us in. I'll get soaked in the process but there really isn't another option.

'I wonder if he has done this on purpose. He knew we were working in the vineyard. I know we have worked longer than usual, but surely we are not limited in the hours we are allowed to work!'

'There is another way, Mum. Look there, on the left side of the gate. It's only resting on its hinges and we could easily lift it off.'

Having done this and passed through the gate, they then debated whether to put the gate back on its hinges or just leave it open. In the interests of peace and quiet they replaced the gate and sped on their way. They suspected that the next morning Mr Jones might be scratching his head, wondering how they had escaped his clutches.

Some weeks later Matthew telephoned the farm. 'Would you please tell Mr Jones that I would like to have access to the vineyard at nine o'clock tomorrow morning?' he said to Mrs Jones.

He heard a muffled conversation, then Mrs Jones returned. 'He will be busy at nine o'clock but he will meet you there at ten,' she said.

'Thank you very much, Mrs Jones,' our son replied, and hung up.

At 10.30 a.m. Mrs Jones opened the door of the farmhouse in response to Matthew's knock. He had been patiently waiting since 10 a.m. for Farmer Jones to appear.

'Is Mr Jones there? I would like to get into the vineyard.'

'Mr Jones has gone to town. He will unlock the gate for you when he gets back about midday,' Mrs Jones said, closing the door.

Matthew was quite a spirited teenager, sometimes rather too spirited for my liking, but on this occasion I thought he handled himself with magnificent restraint. Legal right of access had been written into the contract and we had used this in order to plant the vines. As we had found out at Pleurisy Point, however, planting the vines was the easy part; weed control, training the vines and the like were the real work. We needed almost daily access to our little plot of 'paradise' and it had become increasingly hard to gain entry. Farmer Jones normally only allowed us access via a tortuous, narrow, poorly formed and, in places, steep, dirt track. Not only was it nigh-on impossible to traverse this in a truck, but we had to enter it by way of the most remote farm gate, which he insisted on keeping locked 'for reasons of security'. It must have been the only locked farm gate in the district.

Occasionally we were told that the access route to our vineyard had changed and it was now across a poorly drained flat paddock. Curiously, this only seemed to occur when the field was flooded after heavy rain. At these times we were at risk of stalling our car in one of the many small ponds that had formed. We were forced to accelerate wildly in order to get sufficient speed to allow us to wallow our way through these mini-lakes as the car lurched violently from side to side. On one such occasion Matthew had slid into a barbed-wire fence and on another Chris had crashed into one of Farmer Jones's gates, almost demolishing it. We had begged for a key to the locked gate but were told this was not part of the agreement and that Mr or Mrs Jones would always be available to let us in. As on this occasion, farm time did not always have fixed relativity to Greenwich Mean Time, and it was becoming increasingly frequent for St Peter to be unavoidably delayed or to have lost the keys to the Pearly Gates.

Matthew had never previously been especially industrious in his school holidays but he now felt the urgent need to work. As mentioned, he was a high-spirited youth and he clearly thought one good practical joke deserved another. It had been riotously funny to have been kept waiting, so he decided to play a return trick on St Peter. Fortunately, the gate was made of wood and, happily, Matthew had an axe in the back of his car. It took but the twinkling of an eye to leave the Keeper of the Gates a decent pile of kindling, with which he could start a lovely blaze.

It turned out that the Holy Man did not have a great sense of humour, and rumbles of discontent were heard far and wide. I lightly chastised my wayward son but secretly thanked him, because thereafter our entrance to 'paradise' was significantly facilitated, although the Gates were certainly not opened wide.

It was shortly after this that we began to get strange mail deliveries. They were strange because the assortment of objects that arrived in our mailbox was distinctly unusual and because they always arrived during the night. Initially the deliveries were pieces of string, plastic bags, crumpled newspaper and a variety of other quite random but harmless objects. They then progressed to include dead animals, such as rabbits, mice and birds. We tried to ignore them and hoped that this unrequested service would just peter out but eventually it got the better of us.

'It all seems so childish and trivial that I don't want to make a fuss. What do you think we should do; just ignore it?' Chris asked our friendly local Mr Plod.

'Is there anyone you suspect: anyone who might hold a grudge against you and want to annoy you?'

'Well, we certainly don't suspect our local post lady. There is only one person in the district whom we seem to have fallen out with. I'll tell you about it.'

'Leave it to me,' Mr Plod said with a smile after he had heard a little more. 'I will pay him a friendly visit and ask if he has seen anything suspicious. I will let him know that we are going to be on the lookout and that the offender will find himself in serious trouble.'

Mysteriously, our deliveries ceased forthwith, so we did not have to resort to leaving a set rat-trap in our mailbox, as we had contemplated.

**'HAPPY CHRISTMAS, DEAR. I HOPE YOU LIKE IT.'**

'What is it, Ivan?' asked a bewildered-looking Chris, peering at the shiny red-and-black object that was sitting in the driveway of our house in Christchurch. It was about the same length and width as a trailer, but it sat much closer to the ground, being no more than 40 centimetres in height. The machine consisted of a series of murderous-looking sharp, broad arrowheads pointing downwards and forwards, each of which was on the end of a spiral of springy metal. At the back there was a large heavy roller, a bit like a giant version of Chris's very own kitchen rolling pin.

'It's a rotocrumbler, of course! It's just what you've always wanted. Every housewife needs one. I'm sorry I couldn't wrap it up, but don't you think the purple silk bow is a masterstroke?'

'I am not a housewife. I have never been married to a house, and the way you are behaving I am not going to have any time to spend in my own house. What am I supposed to do with the damned thing?'

'There, there, dear,' I said soothingly. 'That's not a very nice way to thank me for a lovely Christmas present. This little device is going to make your life a whole lot easier. Instead of weeding in those rows, you just have to attach this to the back of your lovely tractor and pull it along. The arrowheads dig into the earth and their vibration, on the end of those big curly springs, tills the earth. The roller behind crumbles up any clods and leaves the ground lovely and flat. In no time at all you will become passionately attached to it.'

'Why can't I get a diamond necklace and a fur coat for Christmas like any ordinary wife?'

'Because you're not ordinary, darling. You're amazing, and you know that you really wouldn't like those sorts of trinkets and five-minute wonders. This will give you many years of real pleasure.'

It was two months since we had planted our first vines and they were growing apace, but so were the weeds. We needed to do something about the latter before they sucked all of the valuable moisture out of the soil. The rotocrumbler was to be the solution to Chris's — I mean our — problem.

**A HUGE CLOUD OF GREY-BLACK** smoke swirled menacingly overhead and it was coming from the vineyard, just beyond the dense line of trees that formed a shelter-belt. It was stinking hot and several days of very warm northwest wind had turned the countryside into a tinderbox. I dropped the hammer I had been using to straighten the bumper bar and gunned the car into life. Chris was in the vineyard, and at any moment she could be surrounded by blazing shelter-belts and become trapped.

The vehicle lurched wildly over the rough track, fighting every rut and pothole like a heavyweight champion. Suddenly there was Chris immediately ahead of me, but it seemed it was her tractor that was on fire; or was it? There were no flames but she was enveloped in smoke. It was pouring out of the tractor while she was still driving it, apparently unconscious of the extreme risk she was running. The tractor might explode at any moment. What was she doing? Was she trying to drive it to a bare patch of earth where it could burn or explode without setting the whole field on fire?

Then it dawned on me. She was not being a heroine, she was merely testing out her Christmas present. The rotocrumbler was throwing up a huge dust storm from the parched earth, which the 'Devil's breath' was eagerly blowing up into the sky. She halted just in front of the car, covering it and me in a cloud of dust.

'It's working well but I'm going to stop now,' she said, jumping down from the tractor. 'The wind is too strong and it's just blowing away all our valuable topsoil. We have little enough of it as it is. What are you doing here? I thought you were supposed to be fixing the car.'

'I just thought I'd come over and see how you were getting on,' I replied sheepishly. 'I wondered if you were ready for a cool drink and thought you might like a lift back to our shady picnic spot.'

After the boss had surveyed her handiwork, she pronounced that her toy had done a wonderful job. The weeds had been ripped up and now lay wilting in the sunlight. But while the machine had solved the weed problem, closer inspection revealed that it had produced another. Tilling the ground had brought masses of stones to the surface; stones ranging from the size of a pea to that of a human head. We had unknowingly planted on a unique piece of dirt, which we later found out was the moraine of an ancient ice-age glacier.

'What are we going to do with all these stones?' Chris asked.

'Just leave them. They will be excellent, collecting the sun's heat and radiating it back on the vines.'

'But they'll create a very difficult surface to work on. They'll trip us up when we're walking and make it very rough for the tractor.'

As was so often the case, Chris's assessment of the situation was accurate. Over the ensuing months this stony landscape took its toll, not only on people's feet and ankles but also on our ancient tractor and other equipment. Before long I had sorted out a perfect birthday present for Chris, a huge metal roller made from ancient traction-engine wheels that could press the stones back into the earth. It was a compromise; we would have flat land between the rows but not within them. There would be a long layer of heat-absorbing stones immediately under the vines. Many years later we went one step further and added a sward of grass and wildflowers between the rows, but even then we still required the intermittent use of Chris's High Roller to deal with the odd errant boulder. What Chris said when she saw her birthday gift is unrepeatable!

**AT LAST A DATE WAS SET** for Farmer Jones's court case against the dastardly Donaldsons. It was set down to start at ten o'clock in the morning, almost two years to the day since we had signed the purchase agreement for the land. Chris and I had spent quite some time with our lawyer going over the evidence, but our case was a simple one. It was based entirely on the fact that the agreement said that all the land specified on the accompanying map was being purchased for a fixed sum and that an exact area had not been given.

While we felt confident, we were also anxious. We could not be entirely certain of the outcome. After a sleepless night I sat with my nervous wife and our lawyer in the corridor of the courthouse outside the hearing chamber. Not far away the Joneses and their legal representative looked equally unhappy. At 9.50 a.m. their lawyer approached ours and asked to have a private word. The two men disappeared into an adjacent empty room, accompanied by the Joneses.

'What do you suppose this is all about?' Chris whispered.

'I have no idea, but I guess we'll soon find out.'

It was only a few moments later that our lawyer gestured to us to enter the room.

'Mr and Mrs Jones want to withdraw their case if you will agree to it,' he told us. 'The judge is ready to hear the case, but they don't wish to proceed. Their only stipulation is that each party will be responsible for their own legal expenses. If the case is heard your expenses will clearly be more, but if the court finds in your favour you might be able to get your expenses covered. It would, however, be a gamble. What would you like to do?'

We were stunned and just stood there gaping. Eventually I stuttered, 'Do you mean to say that we will be able to proceed without delay to a settlement and transfer of title for the originally proposed sum?'

'Yes.'

The closest I had ever come to being a gambling addict was to buy a very occasional lottery ticket, and I had no intention of morphing into a big-time punter now. Our lawyer had substantially reduced his fees because we felt that we had been somewhat misguided into specifying even an approximate area of land.

'Yes! We agree to let them withdraw the case,' I almost shouted with joy.

Why had the vendors and their lawyer done this to us?

When our disagreement had become known in the district other farmers told us that the Joneses had a reputation for being litigious. If we had known this earlier we would never have approached them about buying the land. It seemed bizarre, not the least because of what it must have cost them. The settlement had been delayed for two years, and this was at a time when New Zealand was in the doldrums and inflation was running at a rampant 10 per cent per annum. It was matched by bank interest rates that were at about the same level. My rough estimate was that the delay had cost the Joneses about 40 per cent of the value they would have received if they had settled immediately and banked the money. As we had sold up assets to buy the property, we had had the money sitting in a bank earning interest over this time. However, we would have happily given this away to avoid the hassle to which we had been subjected. At last, however, the nightmare was over, and perhaps we could even mend the broken fences and become friends with our neighbours.

It was not long before this dream was shattered. 'There's no water!' cried Chris as the flow out of the tap quickly turned into a dribble, followed by a few spasmodic drips and then nothing.

There followed an obscene sucking sound as air found its way into the dark recesses of the pipeline. Chris was staring at the pile of dirty dishes in the kitchen sink of the humble little cottage that formed part of our new vineyard property.

'I'll go and see the Joneses,' I volunteered, not feeling at all enthusiastic.

It would be our first face-to-face meeting since the aborted court case. We had waved to them a few times when we had seen their car passing, but this had always coincided with their attentions being rigidly fixed on some fascinating object on the other side of the road.

The water to our cottage came from a bore that was on the Jones's farm, and our legal agreement and title clearly stated that they were responsible for supplying it to our house, garden and the adjacent property, but not the vineyard, which was situated some distance away.

It was with a heavy heart that I trudged up Farmer Jones's drive and knocked at their door. There was no response, although I could hear movement within. I rapped more firmly and after a considerable delay the door was opened a little.

'Well, what do you want?' demanded a belligerent-looking Farmer Jones.

'I'm sorry to disturb you but we don't seem to have any water. Perhaps the pump has stopped working.'

'No, it hasn't. The pump is working fine. I have turned your water off,' replied Farmer Jones, allowing himself a faint flicker of a self-satisfied smile. 'You have planted grapevines around your house and I am not going to supply you with water for those. Pull them all out and then I will turn the water back on again.'

'It is only a small garden nursery of valuable vine cuttings that I am trying to establish so that I can plant them out in the vineyard next spring. They will die without water so I would be grateful if it could be turned back on straight away.'

'Get lost. It is not going to be turned back on,' Jones spat out with a snarl, firmly closing the door.

There was clearly a tap somewhere that controlled the flow of water to our cottage without affecting his house. If I knew where it was I could perhaps secretly turn it back on, but I had no idea where it might be. We had no option but to consult our lawyer again and we would need to act quickly because the weather was dry, and our cuttings, which were already shooting leaves, would not survive for very long without water. As our little garden could not be seen from afar it was clear that our neighbour had been poking around our little house. The thought of this made me feel quite uncomfortable. What else might he get up to?

We did not have a choice, our lawyer informed us. We would have to get an urgent court injunction if we were to have any hope of saving our cuttings, not to mention having the extravagant luxuries of flushing our lavatory and cleaning our teeth. This time we would be taking legal action against the Joneses, and there would be no dragging things out for two years and then withdrawing at the last moment! Within days a judge found that our water had been illegally discontinued and ordered its immediate reinstatement.

'I don't think there's any hope of getting back on friendly terms with our neighbours,' Chris lamented.

'Quite frankly, I couldn't give a toss about that now,' I replied vehemently. 'What we have to do now is spend all our time and energy getting the vineyard fully established and producing. It has proved beyond doubt the existence of black holes — up until now it has just been a huge black hole in the earth that has sucked in and devoured money!'

If we had had an inkling that it would take another nine years for our daily income from our little venture to equal our daily outgoings, without any consideration of recouping capital or making a profit on our investment, I suspect we would have given up then and there. In retrospect, I am glad I do not believe in fortune-telling.

CHAPTER 8

# *The* Trials *and* Tribulations *of a* Grape Grower

## 1986 and Beyond — Not a Drop to Drink

**'LOOK AT ALL THOSE BLACKBIRDS** fluttering about … or are they jumping up and down? There's an immense flock of them. What on earth are they doing there? Are they trying to peck something out of the ground? But they all seem to be in lines. Perhaps they are trying to peck up something that you have planted,' hypothesised my intrigued visitor.

I squinted in the bright sunlight. It was a hot, cloudless but windy day, one of very many that we had had recently. I was equally perplexed but much more concerned than my visitor, Bruce Collard. This Auckland winemaker's chardonnay was recognised as being as good as it got in Kiwi white wine and, call it vanity, but I was keen that my vineyard should make a good impression on him. As we approached the line of restless birds my emotions evolved from concern to anxiety and then to agitation. I began to run, stumbling over the rutted, stone-covered earth.

'They're not birds,' said Bruce. 'I think they're flags. What are they, Ivan?'

My black shoes and trousers were thickly covered in dust by the time I was close enough to realise the unpleasant solution to the enigma.

'They're neither birds nor flags, they're pieces of plastic. The black polythene that the vines were planted through has disintegrated and left thousands of little fragments. One end is embedded in the earth while the other is merrily flapping in the breeze!'

It was February 1988, and the previous October Chris had carefully planted out this block with our small, precious pinot noir plants, making sure to get the rows straight and, on this occasion, absolutely parallel. That had been the second spring during which we had access to the vineyard property and, as yet, we still did not have title to it. Because we did not officially own it we were unable to apply for a right to irrigate our young vines and Farmer Jones was certainly not going to put in the application on our behalf.

Deep down, however, we felt that we would not need to water them. After all, we had visited vineyards in Portugal, Spain, France, Italy and beyond and we smugly felt we knew it all. Many of these vineyards were in hotter and drier areas than the Waipara Valley and they had no sign of irrigation. We knew that once our vines got their roots down then we would not need to give them water. We believed that it was good to make vines struggle: after all, 'Spare the rod and spoil the child' was a maxim that should surely be applied to vines as well as children.

We had been advised that, if we were to go down this path, it would be as well to put down long, wide strips of black polythene, the edges of which would be buried in the earth. The vines would be planted through holes poked in the centre of the plastic. The polythene would help retain the moisture in the earth, encourage growth by warming the roots of the vines, and prevent weeds from competing with them. We had used this technique during the first spring and the results had been excellent. It was now apparent that we had a catastrophe on our hands. Our sad-looking plastic, which had a guaranteed life of 10 years, had simply disintegrated into a useless mess in less than six months. Our vines, all of which had developed small shoots and leaves, now looked like lines of miniature soldiers that were straggling home defeated after a failed campaign. On some the leaves were wilting, and on others they had turned brown. Quite a number of plants appeared to be dead.

Three weeks earlier Chris, the boys and I had left for Auckland so that I could attend the Second International Cool Climate Symposium on Grape-growing and Winemaking. The vines had all seemed in good health when we left. We had chosen to drive to and from Auckland, stopping to visit a number of vineyards along the way, unaware of the tear-jerking surprise that would be awaiting us on our return.

'I'm terribly sorry, sir,' the young man said unctuously. 'By mistake, a stabiliser was left out of the mixture during the manufacture of that batch of polythene. This means that it rapidly perishes in the sunlight. We have had other customers report the same problem. But don't worry, we will give you your money back or replace it free of charge.'

He looked anything other than terribly sorry, with a customer-friendly grin that spread from ear to ear. It appeared as though he might burst into chuckles at any moment. I was tempted to throttle him, but 'Don't shoot the messenger' charitably came to mind.

'But what about my vines? The cost of the plastic is nothing compared to their worth, and I'm sure I couldn't fit new polythene over them. Those that are alive now have fragile shoots and leaves that would be knocked off in the process.'

'I'm sorry, sir, but we can't accept any additional liability. Our guarantee solely relates to the cost of the product.'

The young man had clearly been given instructions from further up the money chain on how to deal with the fallout from this piece of industrial incompetence. I was uncertain about the finer legal points of the matter, but I felt it was not worth arguing. Money would not compensate us for the disappointment and emotional turmoil that we felt.

The heatwave and drought continued relentlessly, and despite our attempts to mount a rescue mission our now withered little soldiers fell by the wayside in battalions rather than squads, their skeletal upper limbs still clutching on to their dried-leaf banners. Farmer Jones would not allow us to take water from the little stream that flowed through his property. We thus had to cart it from afar, and this was possible only in small amounts because of the narrow, steep access track. By the time we had got a little water to all of the vines those that had drunk first were already parched again. Cheerful verdant flashes, signifying life, were to be seen only here and there. In spite of the depressing and mounting losses we continued the battle until autumn petered out and the first frost of winter frizzled up the few remaining green leaves.

Spring is a time of renewal and hope and we were full of optimism when we finally got title and took full possession of our property in the dying days of winter. Our main task in the spring of 1988 would be to replace the vines that had died during the preceding drought-stricken summer. We decided to abandon the idea of new polythene and to plant directly into each spot where there was a dead vine. After all, we now owned the place and we could apply to the authorities for a permit to take water so that we could quench our vines' thirsts in the unlikely event of having another dry summer.

'What do you mean when you say that it is necessary for us to have a hearing?' I asked the heavily made-up but cute little blonde behind the information desk of the local catchment and drainage board.

'When you apply for a permit to take water we have to notify your immediate neighbours. Unless they all agree then we have to notify the public of your application by way of advertisements in the newspapers. People then have to be given a month in which to submit in favour of, or in opposition to, your application. Once the responses of all interested parties have been collated the matter will have to go to a tribunal, at which you and these other people, the submitters, will be asked to present your cases. Then the tribunal will consider the matter and eventually give a written judgment.' She adjusted her trendy glasses before continuing, 'Unfortunately, one of your neighbours, a Mr Jones, has objected to your application so it will now have to be notified publicly and go to a hearing. Otherwise, we would have issued you with a permit straight away.'

'What is the timeframe for all that to happen?'

'It is likely to take several months, and it won't be this side of the Christmas and New Year holidays. As you know, New Zealand effectively goes on holiday during January so that the hearing will be some time after that.'

I let out a groan. We had decided to replant our vines directly into the ground before being issued with a permit to take water, otherwise our planting programme would have been put back by a year. Our agreement with Farmer Jones was that we could bring water across his land in an existing underground pipeline and that he would give up his disused water right so that we could apply to take this over. It had never occurred to us that he would be so bloody-minded as to then object to our application. What naïve fools we were!

'But what about all my new grapevines? Ninety per cent of them died last summer and I just can't afford to let the same thing happen this season! Isn't there any alternative way that I can get water to them?'

'Other than carting water from some authorised off-site source, the answer is no,' the blonde replied, fluttering her dark-blue eyelids and adding in an official bureaucratic tone, 'We have to follow due process.' She then started to type, signalling that my interview was at an end.

As the weeks dragged themselves into months there unfolded one of the hottest and driest summers on record, and as 1988 ground itself into 1989 it was clear that these two back-to-back drought years were going to punish the farming community, not to mention aspiring vignerons. First, all the remaining grass in the fields turned brown and became tinder-dry. By this time those farmers who had animal fodder were feeding it out, but they were few in number since the previous drought-plagued summer had meant most had had difficulty making hay and silage. Next, the fields became devoid of any sign of feed; they were simply fenced areas of hard, bare brown earth. It was not long before bloated, black, fly-infested, rotting sheep's carcasses covered the land. Finally, the farmers who had the energy and sympathy dug large trenches and slit the throats of their animals before throwing them in. Although it was theoretically illegal to leave dead animals lying in paddocks the authorities were forced to turn a blind eye.

All the while Chris and I valiantly tried to cart water to our newly planted vines, but it was largely in vain. As in the previous season, they had all started to grow, their buds bursting and sending out cheerful little leaves, only for them to wilt and become desiccated before being blown off by the chuckling 'Devil's breath'. In spite of all our efforts, we lost 90 per cent of our replanted vines. When the dead ones were removed there were so many blank patches in the vineyard plot that the following spring we decided to transplant all the survivors into the few gaps that had appeared in our successful first season's planting, which had been carried out three years earlier. As we gently lifted these plants out of the ground we found that their roots did not seem to have grown at all. We rued our theory that making the vines struggle, by not using irrigation, would make them stronger and better, forcing them to drive their roots deep into the earth in search of water.

**'WHY HAS THE IRRIGATOR STOPPED** near the start of the row? It can't have been irrigating since this morning, when we set it going. I wonder if it's run out of water.' Chris sounded concerned, as well she might, since we could not afford to lose a day's watering.

'Let's go and see if we can fix the problem, whatever it is,' I said.

As we approached the large mobile irrigator we looked up at the gun, which was in effect the barrel of a big cannon that was supposed to gradually rotate horizontally in full circles while jetting out pulses of water that covered the width of 11 rows. The cannon was mounted on large wheels, and as the water passed through the machine it caused the irrigator to move along the length of the row it was in. It took a whole day to travel this distance, so we could water a maximum of 11 rows in 24 hours.

Looking up at the gun we could see something very odd. Pink polystyrene was gradually oozing from its mouth.

'How on earth could that polystyrene have got inside the cannon? Perhaps it's a part of the machine that's broken loose and been forced into the barrel. I'll climb up and have a look.'

There was a good view from on top of the cannon but I did not stop to admire it. I was fascinated by the pink polystyrene, which seemed to have discoloured the small amount of water that was managing to ooze past it. Suddenly I realised the pink colour in the water was blood!

'It's flesh! There's a piece of meat stuck in the mouth of the cannon, and there's also part of a broken bone protruding out. It looks quite ghoulish! Do you want to come up and have a look?'

'No thanks! I'll take your word for it, Ivan.'

It was not a simple job to disassemble the irrigator and extract the poor offending creature, which turned out to be a rabbit.

When we had finally admitted that we needed irrigation to establish our vines we decided that we would use an overhead sprinkler, and the water cannon had seemed the best option. We felt that when the vines became established we would no longer need water and the irrigator could be sold. Others had suggested that we should put in drip irrigation so that an individual dripper would water each plant but we thought we knew best. We soon found that, although the mobile irrigator kept the grapes alive, the weeds grew faster than the vines and soon covered the vineyard in a waist-high jungle. This smothered our little treasures and stole their precious water.

It was also a very labour-intensive business, as each day the irrigator had to be moved by a tractor. Then a whole series of long aluminium pipes, which were about the diameter of a sumo wrestler's arm, had to be taken apart, shifted and then fitted together again in order to bring the water to where the lumbering beast was working. All of this, involving two to three hours of hard physical work, needed to be done every day, including weekends and public holidays. We now had no days off, but we had learnt two things that would make our lives easier. The first was that before assembling our irrigation line it was best to peer down each aluminium pipe, to make certain there were no animals taking refuge inside them. The second was that we should listen to advice and put in drip irrigation. But we found that drip irrigation was also good for growing weeds, or rather, one weed in particular.

We had hired two young men, teenagers really, to help us establish the vineyard and they seemed to be good workers. Chris and I had to go overseas for some weeks and we agreed on a vineyard work programme with them. They felt it was perfectly achievable and it was in line with what they had been doing over the preceding few months. All was agreed and Chris and I felt comfortable about leaving them to work alone. When we returned we were in for a nasty surprise.

'I can't understand it. They hardly seem to have done any work at all while we've been away,' Chris reported over dinner one night soon after our return. She had been to the vineyard while I had been working at the hospital.

'Let's look at it together and compare it with the proposed work programme,' I suggested.

Sure enough, as we moved along the rows and inspected the vines it was clear that Chris was correct. It seemed as though our two workers had also been on holiday.

'Look!' Chris cried out. 'They must have taken to market gardening. Look at all those pots with tomato plants growing in them.'

'Those aren't pots,' I replied. 'Those are pot.'

What incensed us most was not just the lack of work but that these two young men lived on family farms themselves, with plenty of room to grow cannabis if they'd wanted to. Why had they chosen to grow their dope on our vineyard and put us and our business at risk? If Farmer Jones had seen it, he would doubtless have reported us to the police.

We had a serious talk with them, and our property rapidly became weed-free. It was not long before they chose to depart for greener pastures, and shortly after that we employed a middle-aged ex-farmer, who proved capable of doing the work of two, and doing it willingly.

**PERHAPS YOU HAVE TRAVELLED AROUND** some of the more ancient and venerable wine regions of the world and seen gnarled old grapevines that are grown simply as small bushes, without any supporting trellis. From their roots several short trunks are trained upwards and outwards, like arms reaching skyward, and it is from their bulbous upper portions, or 'hands', that short finger-like spurs give rise to the new season's pendulous growth. It is as though many upper limbs are stretching towards the sunlight; sunlight that is so bright and hot that the foliage has to hang downwards to provide shade and prevent the berries from being burnt and wizened. These so-called 'bush vines' stand about waist-height. As mentioned earlier, they are known as *gobelet* by the French because the general outline resembles that of a goblet.

This primitive form of training is almost universally restricted to very hot climates. In cooler, more quality-focused areas, such as France's Bordeaux and Burgundy, vines are usually grown on a long straight trellis, a bit like an elevated wire fence. The lower wire supports the fruiting part of the vine, which is between knee- and hip-height, while the foliage is held straight up in the air to avoid excessive shading of the grape berries. As our new vineyard was situated in a cool-climate viticultural region we opted for the latter system, which is standard throughout New Zealand.

But when to install such a trellis? Young vines are like children and need to be trained to grow into straight, upright citizens. Left to their own devices they can become twisted and deformed individuals. Their formative years are all-important. For the first year or two they can be trained up stakes, but sooner or later they need to be pulled up straight and restrained on a trellis. I am referring to vines here, not children, although if you have brought up a family of four boys you will doubtless know that there are moments when you might wish to do the same to them! The paediatric gurus of today are inclined to take a dim view of such straightforward and logical action, preferring a more devious psychological route to obedience. We decided not to temporise too long before disciplining our children and our vines, but, just for the record, let me make it clear that the methods we adopted were quite different. We started to erect our vine trellis in 1987, the year after we had planted our first vines. We had not, however, anticipated the problems ahead of us.

If you cast an experienced eye over a trellised European vineyard and compare it to a New Zealand one you will notice an immediate difference. Europeans use relatively flimsy material compared with Kiwis. In fact, the New Zealand vineyard trellises are surely the strongest in the world, and they are generally constructed of long, thick posts which are driven well into the earth. Why is that? It is because New Zealand, consisting of two long thin islands surrounded by the largest ocean on the planet, is an extremely windy place. It never ceases to amaze me that the wind speeds reported during continental hurricanes are frequently little greater than those experienced on a regular basis in a Kiwi vineyard. Such blasts can cause damage, and we have had rows of mature vines blown over and their supporting posts snapped in high winds. Fortunately, this is infrequent.

We knew we would need to use very solid posts for our trellising, and that they would have to be brought to us on heavy trucks.

'Farmer Jones says that we cannot truck the posts along his track and into the vineyard. He told me we will have to carry them along the track by hand,' reported a worried-looking Chris.

'Why?' I asked, with a rising sense of frustration and anger.

'Because he says it will damage his track and that his ewes are lambing. He doesn't want the truck to frighten them.'

'But that's ridiculous. His rotten old track is so potholed and rough that it couldn't be made any worse, and he drives his truck through that sheep paddock each day to check on the lambing.'

'Don't get worked up,' my dear wife said consolingly. 'Let's ask our neighbours on the other side if we can bring the posts by truck through their farm. We would have to cut some fences to get the truck into our property but we could pay to have them repaired. I know we haven't met them yet, but I've heard that they are helpful.'

It turned out that our neighbours were happy to help but, not unreasonably, appeared to think we were unhinged. They were intrigued and wanted to know why we were planting our vineyard on some of the boniest and meanest land in the district.

'Why don't you plant on the airstrip?' they asked, referring to part of our property that had earlier been used as the district's runway for light planes. 'It's good land there. You could even grow potatoes on it.'

'That's the very reason we do not want to plant our vines there,' I said. 'The soil is too heavy, fertile and water-retentive. It's no good for growing quality winemaking grapes.'

'But most of our farm consists of exactly the same type of soil that you have chosen for your vineyard.'

I thought that even then I could see the implication of what had been said gradually dawning on them, but it was well after we were selling our wine that they sold part of their farm to a Californian investor who planned to start a vineyard. They later took the plunge themselves and planted grapes.

We heard that Farmer Jones was incensed when he learnt that we had bypassed his kind offer to allow us to carry our posts over his track, but by then our contractor had started driving them into the ground.

'What do you mean, Joe, that you think you can't do the job?' I was staring incredulously at the contractor, my mouth hanging open. He was a practical man with many years of farming experience, including post-driving and fencing on the roughest terrain. Joe Richards was not big, but he had been toughened and weathered by years of working outdoors. He was as strong and wiry as a roll of number 8 fencing wire and he would not give way under any normal pressure. He looked very unhappy, and it was clear that he was under enormous stress. He was a simple man of action and he felt uncomfortable talking, especially if it involved negotiating.

'It's too hard. There are far too many stones and the earth is just like concrete.' Joe, a man of the earth, shuffled awkwardly from one foot to the other while staring at the ground; the dirt that was normally his friend had now become his enemy and was in the process of defeating him.

'If we were to carry on, me and m' mate, I would need to double the price or just drive the posts half the agreed distance into the ground. But I would prefer just to quit.'

'But you can't do that, Joe. You gave Chris and me a quote to do the work and it was on the basis of this that we have paid for the posts, the wires and their delivery. You can't just walk away now. There is no way we can afford to pay you double. And driving them only half the distance into the ground would mean that the trellis would be too rickety and it would probably blow over in the first decent wind. When a trellis has a full canopy of grape leaves it catches the wind, just like a sail. The pressure on it is enormous. It's not like a normal wire fence.'

'If you wait until winter, when the ground will be wet, I could return and do the job for the original price, but it's just too hard at present,' Joe conceded reluctantly.

'It would be too late then, Joe. We need the trellising put up now so that we can begin to train our vines on it this season.'

That evening Chris and I were discussing our latest problem over dinner. We did not know what to do. Suddenly a voice piped up from the other end of the table.

'I'll drive those posts for you,' said Matthew. 'I'll do it in my school holidays, they're starting soon. I could get my friend Shaun to help me. You could just pay us by the hour. I'm sure we could do it.'

'If Joe Richards, with all his many years of experience, is unable to do it, then it will be quite beyond you, Matthew,' I replied rather deprecatingly.

'It isn't that he can't do it. It's just that he can't do it and make a lot of money. That wouldn't be a problem with us because you wouldn't be paying us as much, and we have six weeks' holiday in which to do the job.'

During his spring holidays a few months earlier Matthew had worked for two or three weeks with Danny Schuster, helping in his winery and vineyard. Matthew had done some post-driving there. When he returned home Matthew had announced that he was going to become a winemaker. We had tried to talk him out of it, arguing that he would be better to do a more general degree, perhaps in biochemistry or microbiology, rather than specifically committing himself to a life of winemaking. After all, we argued, our vineyard might turn out to be a total flop or it might be many years before we produced any wine, let alone had a profitable venture. It was too risky. But he persisted, and we were glad that at least this gave him an ambition, as before that his career path had not exactly been focused. At 17 he was a biggish lad, muscular and strong. He also had a will of his own and knew how to get his own way by wearing down his poor parents. He was keen to work, not least because he wanted to buy a car.

'What do you think about Matthew's suggestion?' Chris asked me later as we were lying in bed.

'Right at the moment I don't have a better one, and at least it would keep him off the streets! We would have to hire or buy a post-driver, though.'

And that was how Matthew and Shaun came to spend their school vacation living on the vineyard in the little old caravan that we had purchased to use as a workstation. We did not care to enquire what hijinks they got up to and how they amused themselves in that remote spot, but we suddenly noticed how quiet it was with only the three younger boys at home.

The post-driver that we had bought second-hand was a fairly basic homemade affair. It consisted of a massive block of concrete, the monkey, which the tractor lifted to a great height on a steel pole. When a lever was depressed the block hurtled downwards and crashed against the top of a post, driving it a small distance into the ground. It took very many such dramatic thumps and much ear-splitting noise to get even one post to a satisfactory depth. We found it was necessary to spike each hole, otherwise too many posts would shatter. Thus, Matthew had to drive a large metal spike, resembling an elongated torpedo, to the required depth before withdrawing it and then driving a post into the pre-formed hole.

'Come quickly, Dad! Matthew has been badly hurt. He's lying on the ground groaning. I think he might be unconscious.'

Fortunately, I was in the vineyard and not far away. I felt physically sick as I looked down at my son, who was lying on his side moaning unintelligibly.

'What happened, Shaun?' I demanded of his friend, a sallow, sandy-haired, lanky youth who was supporting himself against the post-driver, looking as though he might faint.

'One of the posts snapped in half when the monkey slammed onto it. The upper part was blown out of the machine and it hit Matthew on the thigh. I think he must have broken his leg.'

It was a relief to know that Matthew had not been hit on the head. If he had been unconscious, then he must have fainted. His moaning had settled with my arrival and he was now able to talk coherently. I took out a knife and cut his jeans lengthways, from the hip to the ankle, in order to have a good look at his leg. The back of his thigh had started to swell and it was clear he had suffered a severe blow but I was fairly certain he had not broken his femur. We managed to get him into the back of our estate car and drove him quietly home, where a neighbouring orthopaedic surgeon confirmed our hopes.

'He will make a good recovery, but he will be off work for a week or two.'

In spite of this setback Matthew and Shaun were able to finish the post-driving during their vacation. This was not all of the post-driving that needed to be done on that block, but it was all that Joe and his sidekick had been going to do. It allowed us to train up all of the vines that were in urgent need of support. We congratulated the boys on their magnificent effort and the result looked marvellous. Not infrequently, however, a large subterranean boulder had obstructed the downward progress of a post, requiring it to be moved to a different spot. And here and there stones might have made a post slew to one side so that it was no longer completely vertical. These little hassles meant that the posts that were driven that summer lacked the boring exactitude that typifies most vineyards, in which perfectly placed rows of straight trellis march into the distance with mathematical precision. Our vineyard now had a devilishly rakish and individual appearance. If this was to signal things to come, then we were clearly in the grips of an artist rather than a tradesman.

**'IT'S AN ABSOLUTE DISASTER, IVAN!** All of our leaves have disappeared,' wailed a distraught Chris.

'What do you mean when you say that they have "disappeared"?' I responded. 'Is there absolutely no sign of them? Perhaps sheep have got into the vineyard and eaten them.'

'No, it can't be that because you can still see the veins of the leaves. They just form the skeletal outline of the leaves, but otherwise there is nothing left of them. It must be some small bird or insect. What should we do?'

'First of all we have to find out what has caused it and then deal with that. Have a good look around and see if you can get any clues.'

I put the phone down and returned to my outpatient clinic, but my mind was elsewhere. Chris had never before disturbed me while I was seeing patients. The situation had to be grave. It was a beautiful sunny spring day and she had gone to the vineyard to train young vines on the trellis. If the vines had no leaves then perhaps she could not train them, and even if she could, was there any point in it?

That evening over our meal and the inevitable dinner glass of wine, we discussed the situation further.

'I wonder if it is night beetles,' Chris hypothesised. 'There seemed to be lots of them hanging in spider webs around the vineyard. But if it was beetles then there must have been thousands of them, because they have destroyed virtually all the leaves on the vines. What should we do?'

'I think we'll just have to wait and see what happens. I don't want to start spraying pesticides around the vineyard.'

And that is what we did, absolutely nothing. Over the ensuing weeks we were thrilled to see delicate little new leaves magically unfurl and we held our breaths, waiting for them to be molested in their turn. But no, their virginity remained inviolate. After a month or two it was hard to appreciate that there had been a problem. No doubt the vines had been set back by the loss of their energy-producing leaves and the growth that year would be less than it might have been, but it was not a complete disaster.

Chris's detective work had solved the case. The mischief had indeed been caused by night beetles, sometimes called bronze beetles, which are the adult form of what Kiwi gardeners know as grass grubs. These little nasties live as translucent whitish grubs, 20–25 millimetres long, under the ground, gorging themselves on the roots of grass, tussocks and other plants. On a warm evening in late spring the now bronze-coloured beetles come to the surface and take flight, devouring whatever tasty greenery they can find, no doubt to compensate themselves for their miserable childhood diet. They live another two to four weeks if they do not earlier end up as a spider's or a bird's dinner. They are uniquely Kiwi, in that they are both native to and restricted to New Zealand. Unfortunately, they love grapevines.

Over the ensuing years the amount of damage caused by night beetles gradually diminished and became relatively minor, although it tended to fluctuate from year to year. The improvement was possibly because of the relative reduction in the amount of pasture as we expanded the planting of our vines. Nonetheless, occasionally they could descend like the proverbial plague of locusts. The only good thing about the first incident was that we made a firm decision not to use pesticides, a policy to which we have held fast ever since.

For the first few years we saw no sign of the various disorders that can affect *Vitis vinifera*, then slowly they began to appear. We did not realise then that this is not an uncommon pattern. The main problem for us turned out to be powdery mildew, or oidium, which causes a powdery grey film to develop on the leaves and fruit, delaying growth and ripening, and causing the berries to split. Fortunately, this is easily controlled by spraying a harmless solution of sulphur.

**IT WAS A DESPERATE FIGHT.** My assailant was bigger and stronger than me. I was pinned down on the ground while he held a knife at my throat. I could smell his overpoweringly foul breath, and his disgustingly matted locks were dangling in my face. I had disturbed him in my wine cellar after I had responded to the sound of the burglar alarm — the alarm that kept on ringing and seemed to be getting louder. Why did he not become frightened and flee? With a desperate wrench I managed to free my right arm and silence the alarm. The burglar had gone. I lay there sweating, but it was a cold sweat. In fact, the room was cold, freezing cold. I shook my head vigorously and leapt out of bed, only half-awake. It was 1 a.m. I had been fighting for my life, but now I had to pull myself together and fight for the vineyard's life.

I flung my dressing gown over my naked form, put on my slippers and went downstairs with a torch. In the garden the mercury had plummeted to 8°C. I had to get moving quickly. I slipped on some warm clothes before climbing into the car and heading north. It would be three-quarters of an hour before I reached the vineyard, even though the road was deserted. I had calculated that it would be about 7°C in our Christchurch garden by the time I turned into the side road that led to the vineyard gate, but it might be only 3°C or 4°C among the vines. Because we had chosen a very sheltered spot for the vineyard it became much hotter than Christchurch in the summer, but the downside was that still air favours a frost. This meant that our spring and autumn nights were not infrequently disturbed by frost warnings and we were always on tenterhooks at those times of the year.

As the headlights cut a small tunnel of light through the moonless night and myriads of stars twinkled above I mused on the irony of it all. Soon after graduation I had decided that obstetrics were not for me; too much night work. Neurology was relatively good in that regard. Now I frequently had disturbed nights, but they were to look after my own baby, which eased the pain. But we shared the night beat, Chris and I. If I had to be at the hospital in the morning she would drive out, but at other times I would do it. If there was a very high risk of frost one of us would sleep in the cottage on the vineyard property.

When we purchased the vineyard we really did not spare a thought for frosts. I had been involved with the Pleurisy Point vineyard for just on a decade and we had never seen hide nor hair of frost damage. It was in the spring of 1993 that we first found out just how spiteful Jack Frost could be. He was a thief who could steal a whole year's work. I was judging at the Air New Zealand Wine Awards competition in Auckland in November when I heard other winemaker-judges talking about a serious frost risk that night. I telephoned Chris to inform rather than warn her, as we did not really have a frost-management plan. We had simply thought it was not necessary. Marlborough, immediately to our north, had never been frosted. Nonetheless, I half-heartedly suggested that she phone around and see if she could get a helicopter if we needed one. When I phoned home the next day it was a subdued Chris who answered.

'We did have a frost,' she said.

'How bad is it?'

'It's too early to say. The full extent of the damage won't show up for several days, but it looks quite nasty.' Time proved her to be correct. 'I stayed at the vineyard last night and I conferred with Matthew at about 11. At that stage it still seemed quite warm outside although we didn't measure the temperature. We were sure it wouldn't freeze.'

After that we quickly developed a frost-management plan and we made certain we believed the mercury rather than our own subjective impressions.

Tonight we had a helicopter on standby. From the time of that disastrous night in 1993 we had contracted the services of a helicopter and pilot to be at our sole disposal during periods of risk. It is the leaves, shoots and flowers of grapevines that are sensitive to frost. If a vine gets frosted during the spring it can kill off those parts and you will lose some or all of that season's crop. New buds will give rise to more shoots and leaves so the vine will survive and may crop again the following season. If a frost occurs in the autumn it does not harm the fruit as the berries contain so much sugar that they do not freeze. The leaves, however, can be killed and that stops further ripening. Should you get a rogue frost in early autumn you might be left with a crop of green or underripe fruit. It was now autumn, and although our grapes were fairly good we still wanted to get a bit more energy out of the leaves to give our wine that special oomph that comes from optimal ripeness.

I started to walk about, torch in one hand, thermometer in the other. As is common, the temperatures varied wildly from one place to another within the vineyard. The anatomy of a frost is never simple. I would have to make my call on the temperatures in the coolest areas. The mercury kept heading south, and eventually I felt it had gone far enough. In my calculations I had to anticipate the time needed for the pilot to get to his helicopter and for the helicopter to fly to the vineyard. I also needed to allow myself time to light the drums of fuel that marked out the corners of the vineyard, in order to show the pilot the area he needed to protect. Finally, the temperature had dropped to a level that made it imperative to act. I drove back to the cottage to make my urgent telephone call. My hands were trembling as I dialled the number, but I told myself that this was due to the cold, not stress. The ringing seemed to go on interminably and then there was a click.

'We are sorry that Helicopter Professionals cannot take your call at the moment. If you would be kind enough to leave your name and telephone number, we will respond to your call as soon as we are able.'

I was stunned. We had usually telephoned the pilot in the early evening if a frost was predicted. But only a week earlier he had said, 'You don't need to call me to let me know about a possible frost. I'm contracted to you and I will always be available. You only need to call me at the time I am required to fly.'

I redialled the number several times but always with the same result. I started to curse and swear and pounded my fist against the wall but it was pointless. I was panicking and needed to pull myself together and try to find a way out of this disastrous situation. I suddenly remembered that the pilot had an unusual double-banger surname so perhaps I could locate a relative who would be able to go and wake him. My hands continued to tremble as I thumbed through the dog-eared telephone book. There were only three entries under that surname and one was the pilot himself. I dialled the number immediately under his. The ringing seemed to go on forever and

I prayed that an answering machine would not kick in. Finally, the voice of a confused-sounding, sleepy elderly man came on the line.

'Is that Mr Highgate-Brown?'

'Yes. What is it?'

'Is Bruce Highgate-Brown of Helicopter Professionals related to you?'

'Yes. He is my son. He hasn't had an accident, has he?'

'No, but I need to contact him urgently. He is contracted to frost-protect my vineyard and I need him to fly now. I can't raise him. All I get is his answerphone.'

'I am sorry but he has flown down to Wanaka for the weekend to watch the air show. You know — Warbirds Over Wanaka? The aerobatic show of old warplanes.'

I was stunned and momentarily speechless.

Then I heard myself saying, 'No, it is I who am sorry for your son. He is contracted to be available to fly his helicopter for me any night that I need it and I need it now! If you know of anybody else who can bring a helicopter to my property within the next hour then I'm sure he will be forever grateful to you. Otherwise I will sue him for at least $1 million for loss of crop.'

I was probably exaggerating, but I was desperate.

'I will see what I can do.'

'I will be waiting in the vineyard and I will light the markers that show the corners of the property.' I gave him directions to pass on to the pilot.

The wait in the dark seemed interminable and extremely cold as I watched the temperature drop below freezing point. Eventually I heard the welcome thub-thub sound of a helicopter approach, and then it started to circle the vineyard.

Within a couple of days we could see that some but not all of the leaves had been frosted. The helicopter had arrived rather too late to be fully effective. Whether it had really done any good could only be determined by the gods. This experience, however, did Chris and me some good. It taught us that helicopter pilots are cowboys or, at the very least, adolescents in adult bodies. They are risk-takers and inherently unreliable. From that time on we decided to curb such wayward behaviour. We gave our helicopter contract to another pilot and insisted that if there was a serious frost risk he would fly onto our property before sundown. There he would sleep in our cottage, where we intended to keep him imprisoned until he and his egg beater were needed.

'Wake up, Jim! We're ready for you to start flying over the vineyard now.'

It was 2.10 a.m. The tousle-haired bear of a man stirred, and after being shaken several more times he was sufficiently awake to throw on his clothes and groggily make his way to the helicopter. We prayed that he was sufficiently alert to be able to fly it. Gurr, gurr, gurr, gurr … gurr, gurr, gurr, gurr … gurr, gurr, gurr, gurr … the sickening noise went on until finally it began to slow. It was clear that the damned machine would not start and the pilot was simply flattening his batteries.

'I'm sorry, but I can't get it to start,' he said at last, after fiddling around with the motor for quite a while. 'It just won't work. Perhaps I should have put a heater in it. It's a cold night. I think I might as well go back to bed — there's nothing more that I can do.'

'Of course it's a cold night,' Chris snapped. 'That's why we have got you here.' Then she added more gently, 'It's springtime, and if we get frosted tonight we stand to lose the entire season's crop. It could cost us millions. We accept that you have done your best, and it is certainly not your fault that you can't start the helicopter.' Then, pleadingly, she continued, 'You are such an excellent pilot and so helpful to others that surely you must know another pilot who owes you a favour. Perhaps you could telephone one of your colleagues and persuade him to bring his machine here.'

Jim looked pleased with this recognition of his fruitless but valiant attempts and his inestimable worth. He thought for a moment then pulled a grubby notebook from his pocket.

'Where's the telephone?' he asked.

Before long we heard the cheerful sound of another helicopter arriving and it was this that saved our bacon, or rather, our crop.

Although we had successfully used helicopters on a number of nights, this second unfortunate episode made us determined to control our own destiny and free ourselves from our dependence on these Magnificent Overgrown Boys in Their Flying Machines. Although it would cost us considerably more money upfront, we needed something less nerve-racking and more reliable.

There are different types of frost, but in our vineyard they had always been inversion frosts. This means that they are due to a very cold layer of air which covers the ground and that as you go upwards the air becomes warmer. This is the *inverse* of the normal, non-frosty situation in which the air becomes colder as you ascend. There is a common misconception that the so-called *inversion layer*, which is found during such an inversion frost, is the warm air above, whereas it is really the cold layer blanketing the ground. Helicopters can protect vineyards because they bring this warmer air from above down to ground level and this disperses the frost-forming inversion layer. The same thing can be done by wind machines (frost fans), which have high installation costs but are cheaper to run than helicopters. Wind machines consist of a vertical tower with a large motor at the bottom and helicopter-like rotors above. The precise statistics depend on the make, but generally the tower is

10 metres high and the device can bring warm air down from about 30–40 metres in the air. Each machine can cover four to six hectares. We initially decided that we would install four wind machines.

The ringing of the telephone awakened me from a deep sleep. I reached groggily for the handpiece.

'Hello. Hello. Hello …' I got no response. I had received a number of such anonymous nocturnal calls over the years. Sometimes they were accompanied by the sound of heavy breathing on the other end of the line, and inevitably they were terminated by a click as the anonymous caller hung up. We had complained to the telephone company and asked for their assistance in tracing these calls, but they had assured us they could not do this. Although we did not believe them, our inertia prevented us from taking the matter further. These nocturnal pranks were childish and annoying but not worth getting steamed up about. We suspected our friendly neighbour. Tonight's call, however, was subtly different; there was no heavy breathing and the caller did not hang up.

'What is it?' Chris asked groggily.

'The temperature at the winery must have dropped to 2°C. It's only 1 a.m. so I'll have to go out and see what's happening.' With a clear sky the temperature drops by about 1°C per hour, so it could start to freeze by 3 a.m.

In the garden adjacent to our distant winery we had installed a frost alarm system that was connected to our office computer there. It would ring our home telephone number when the temperature dropped to a predetermined level. Although it was almost half a kilometre from the nearest of our grapevines, we could generally rely on this garden temperature to be a little lower than that in the vineyard. This anonymous night-caller now demanded instant action. This might be the first time our newly installed wind machines were tested in anger.

After roaming around the vineyard measuring temperatures for an hour or two, I decided it was time to crank up the new wind machines. To some extent wind machines resemble helicopters, and although I have never started the latter, it seemed to me that the processes were probably very similar and equally complicated. There were various switches and levers to operate and dials to read before I finally kicked it into life with an impressive large red button that was enigmatically called the 'Murphy switch'. I prayed that Murphy's Law of Disasters would not also swing into gear.

The diesel motor started with a roar. It had to be left idling for 10 minutes before the clutch was slowly engaged to start the rotors turning. Then I had to gradually wind up the throttle as far as it would go. The noise became deafening and the blades whirring above me seemed malignant and menacing. I was glad to get out from underneath the devilish machine. The whole process had taken at least 20 minutes. It was quite clear that I could not spend this amount of time starting each machine at the same time as monitoring the vineyard temperatures in order to know which machine to kick into life next. I would have to warm up all the motors and only engage the blades on each machine as it was required.

If a wind machine resembles a helicopter then our vineyard had become nothing short of a war zone. It brought to mind that unfortunate skirmish which the Americans conveniently call the Vietnam War and the Vietnamese inconveniently term the American War. I hoped that my little fleet of lookalike helicopters would prove to be more effective in winning my personal war. The temperatures around the vineyard were certainly improving, but this did not mean that I could put my head back on the pillow, however tempting that might be. Perversely, these enormous fans can be damaged if they operate in a breeze, thus I would have to watch that a zephyr did not spring up unawares. Then, once they were no longer needed I would have to shut each one down, which involved the same rigmarole as starting them, except in reverse. There would be no more sleep for me that night, but I felt happy that at last we had taken control of our own destiny.

The rapid and slow advances in technology and our finances, respectively, eventually allowed us to get our wind machines upgraded so that they were automatic. This meant that if the temperature dropped to a preset level they would automatically start, warm up, engage the rotors and then wind up to the required speed, then automatically shut down when the temperature rose sufficiently to place the vineyard out of danger. However, we were still required to go to the vineyard to make certain that all the wind machines had started when they were needed and that they were not operating in a breeze. Then we got anemometers retrofitted. The gentlest zephyr would set their busy little cups spinning, measuring the wind speed and preventing the machines from operating if the wind was too strong.

One day I saw an article in the newspaper about a little device that could turn switches off and on by using a portable telephone, and it gave me an idea. Maybe we could use such a thing to turn our wind machines off and on. Yes, father and son, Jeff and Jay Furness, thought that this was definitely possible and could be combined with our new monitoring system. We would just have to work with them to develop it. Nowadays, we are sent a warning text whenever the temperatures at various places in the vineyard drop to preset levels, and we can view these on a map on a smartphone. Although the wind machines will still work automatically, we can override this function and control them from our phones. We can see whether each one has started or stopped and what effect they have had on the vineyard temperatures. We now spend more time making certain our wind machines do not start unnecessarily than we ever do starting them, making frost protection more environmentally friendly and economic.

But there was a persisting problem: wind machines protect large circles, but nobody plants their vineyards in this configuration. There were places in our vineyard that the wind machines could not protect, so for these we turned to using water sprinklers. It sounds counterintuitive, does it not: pouring cold water on plants to stop them getting damaged by frost. As the sun peeps its face over the eastern hills and starts to chase away the cold fingers of Jack Frost, it is likely to see row upon row of bejewelled grapevines sparkling in the light of the new day. Tender young buds, sensitive shoots and new leaves are frozen in a clear casing of ice that hangs in looping pendants, stalactites and icicles, more glorious than the most expensive chandelier. Trapped inside all this jewellery the vines' new season's potential rests safe and sound. It really is a spectacular and beautiful sight, and it works like this: when water freezes it releases a small amount of energy, or warmth, that protects the plant. As long as you keep sprinkling on water it will provide enough heat to keep the plant at 0°C, and it is only temperatures below this that are damaging. This system can also be monitored and controlled from our smartphones.

Technology has become so advanced that we have almost forgotten the many years of circling the vineyard at night with a hand-held thermometer. We are at risk of becoming self-satisfied, overconfident couch potatoes; but not quite. There is one frost situation in spring that brings us up with a jolt and requires the immediate, hands-on participation of the family team. That is when the inversion layer becomes so deep that wind machines, or even a helicopter, cannot pull down enough warm air. Should this happen, then it is usually in the hour or two just before dawn. At these times we all 'scramble' and light heaters ('frost pots') that are spread in a circle around the wind machines. The wind machines entrain the rising warm air and spread it out around the vineyard. Crawling in the dark on frozen ground underneath the trellis wires, in order to get from one row to the next, is not my idea of absolute bliss but it beats the pants off losing the crop. It is just one of the things one has to suffer in order to get a glass of wine. So much for the romance of the wine biz!

**IT USED TO BE THE GOSSIPS** who created the news, spread tales of village happenings and predicted the dire consequences of things to come.

These days it is the media. No doubt you have totally forgotten about the Y2K disaster that was predicted to paralyse the world at the start of the new millennium. We were all advised to make certain we had supplies of non-perishable foods, water, flashlights and radios. I guessed, however, that the authorities could not be very serious when they omitted to mention really important matters, such as checking that our cellars were adequately stocked with decent wine. This Book of Revelations turned out to be a damp squib when New Year's Day 2000 dawned quite peacefully, although many of us may not have felt entirely happy, having toasted the arrival of the new millennium with a few of our best bottles.

Having got it wrong, however, there were those who argued that our ancient forebears could not have celebrated the end of the first year AD until it was over. Ergo, we could not celebrate the end of the second millennium and the start of the third until the end of the year 2000. Thus, they claimed, it was on the next New Year's Eve that we could expect a real disaster. After the events of that night I am grudgingly inclined to believe that these soothsayers of misery and doom knew something that I did not.

On that fateful evening Chris and I were sitting with a group of friends on the terrace of our holiday house at Akaroa, drinking a toast to the dying old 2000 and celebrating the birth of his baby 2001. The old man had been good to us and we had the makings of a splendid vintage hanging on our vines. We had escaped any frost damage, and mild weather over flowering had ensured a good set, so we had the potential for a plentiful crop of grapes on our vines. We had no inkling that this child would be so spiteful.

It had become something of a tradition for us to have our friends to dinner on New Year's Eve. From our hillside terrace we had a splendid view over Akaroa Harbour, which fills the crater of an extinct volcano. We were looking in the direction of Pegasus Bay and our vineyard, although they were obscured by the hills that form the crater's rim. The night was warm and balmy as there was a slight breeze from the northwest, and on this occasion it was definitely the 'Devil's breath' at work. Gradually, however, we became aware that the sky to the south was becoming obscured, which could only mean one thing, that there were clouds billowing in from that direction.

Suddenly we were blinded by an eye-searing flash of light, which was soon followed by a deafening clap of thunder. We sat in stunned silence as a pyrotechnic display unfolded itself over Pegasus Bay. It was surreal because Akaroa Harbour is open to the sea at its south end and usually any storm coming from that direction blasts the little township of Akaroa with freezing air before reaching Pegasus Bay. Yet here we were still sitting comfortably in our shirtsleeves while observing irrefutable evidence of a savage battle between the winds of the south and those of the northwest that was going on directly in front of us. For 10 or 15 minutes they threw their lightning bolts and head-butted each other with peals of thunder, while our guests celebrated the spectacular display with wine glasses held high. Chris and I were less enthusiastic and sat quietly pensive, there being nothing else we could do.

Being born in Australia, the 'Devil's breath' is hot and dry, while the Antarctic is the pure white cradle of the south wind and its child carries all of that continent's frigidity and fury. When they choose Canterbury to be their battleground, the southerly often wrestles the northwest wind downwards, while the latter throws its opponent high into the sky. This can cause the southerly's moisture-laden clouds to freeze and, under the influence of lightning, hail may form. Chris and I were hoping that the lightning bolts might strike Pegasus Bay itself and thus be over the Pacific Ocean, rather than our patch of dirt.

Suddenly, the jangling sound that we had been dreading shook the pair of us from our lugubrious musings. Although the storm had now stopped, the freezing wind had eventually reached our little party and driven us indoors. I had to force myself to get up to answer the telephone.

'Hello, Dad, I thought I should let you know that we've just had a heavy hailstorm at the restaurant.'

Edward was at a New Year's Eve celebration at the winery restaurant. He sounded worried.

'How bad was it, Edward? Do you think it hit the vineyard?'

'I suspect that it did, but I can't be certain. There's a lot of hail piled up around the restaurant and the hailstones are enormous, about the size of big marbles.'

Chris and I spent a restless night worrying about the possible consequences of the storm. In the light of the following day Matthew visited the vineyard, where he found a scene of devastation.

'It's really bad,' he reported. 'The leaves have been shredded, many grapes and bunches have been knocked off, and those that are left on the vines are bruised and split … but it's patchy and some areas look okay. The hailstones dented the roof of Edward's car. It looks as though somebody has tried to panelbeat it with a hammer!'

It was not the first time that we had been hit by hail, but the few other events had been mild in comparison. In the space of less than 15 minutes we had lost about a third of our crop, and where the hail had struck, the vines had been largely stripped of leaves. Even though these would grow back it would very significantly delay the ripening of those grapes, making harvest extremely difficult. The damaged fruit would be liable to infection and mould. It would take a huge amount of remedial work to save the remaining crop and to nurse the fruit to optimal condition, but we had no option. We had to do it if we wanted to make half-decent wine. When hail hits it often comes in well-defined bands or patches. Some grapes may be virtually annihilated, while those a few rows away can be completely unscathed. The affected areas may differ from one hailstorm to another, as may the direction from which the hail comes. Such are the vagaries of nature.

As it turned out, the rest of the growing and ripening season was excellent. We had to leave the remaining fruit on the damaged plants until very late in the autumn in order to get similar ripeness to that in the grapes from the undamaged vines. This made harvest prolonged and difficult, but in the end it was all worthwhile. By and large the quality of the resulting wines was up there, making it one of the better vintages that we had experienced!

**THE MAN ON THE MOTORBIKE** was hunched low and bundled up against the cold. The peak of his cap was pulled down to shield his eyes from the wind. The approaching dusk and the occasional leafy branch straying across his path made it difficult to see the narrow way ahead. He was riding full tilt, or rather, going as fast as the wet, rough surface would allow him. Now he was happy to see the clearing ahead, indicating the end of the seemingly interminable tunnel of shade through which he had been passing.

Suddenly a deafening explosion and a blinding flash of light assailed him from the right, causing him to swerve inadvertently and almost lose balance. He was dog tired. It had been a long day, riding almost continuously from daybreak, with only a short break to snatch a snack and knock back a drink. There had been other unexpected and frightening noises. At times he had heard what sounded like someone or something crying for help. On other occasions it had seemed as though someone was being strangled. Occasionally, menacing black shapes had passed overhead, hovering, as though searching the landscape for sign of their enemy. Inquisitive eyes had stared at him as he passed by and guards had stood stiffly to attention. But what could you expect? After all, it was war, although he had not been expecting gunfire so close at hand. He had been told where the cannons were stationed and had spent the day weaving in and out so that he was never close to them. Never, that was, until that moment!

'Good God!' he exclaimed under his breath. 'That's not friendly fire. I'll silence that guy!'

When he reached the clearing he dismounted and circled back, coming up from behind to reach the spot where he guessed the blast had originated. Parting the foliage, he peered through and saw his target directly in front of him. With a satisfied smirk he reached forward and firmly grasped its neck, screwing tightly as he did so.

'We are not going to hear any more from him,' the rider thought to himself as he backed away and then turned to make a hurried exit towards his motorbike. He had had enough. He needed to get away from all this.

'How was your day?' Chris asked cheerfully as I entered the warm kitchen and started to peel off my layers of clothing. It was already dark and sombre outside, but the smell of dinner cooking and the thought of a glass of wine were already reviving me.

'Okay, but only just. I'm half deaf. I mistook my row and rode down one that was next to a gas cannon. It almost blew my head off! Its timing mechanism must be faulty, as it should have stopped firing before dusk. I had to circle back and turn it off at the cylinder. It was so wet and slippery that I had to hold it by its half-freezing neck. Stupidly, I lost my gloves somewhere during the day, so my hands are really cold. How people can ride around like that every day for six to eight weeks is quite beyond me. One day is my limit.'

'You poor dear,' said Chris with a tinge of sarcasm in her voice. 'I'll do Sunday morning and you can cover the afternoon. The vineyard staff will do the rest of the week.'

'Thanks,' I said gratefully. 'It's an absolute war zone out there! You have to circulate continually in order to keep the birds away.'

One of the things that always strikes us as strange in Europe is the relative lack of birds. Vineyards, orchards and even lone fruit trees show no sign of bird damage. Ripe figs, which send New Zealand birds into an absolute feeding frenzy, remain deliciously plump and unsullied in Europe. Some say that this is because for centuries, if not millennia, even small birds have been part of the traditional European diet. In bygone days the culinary needs of the peasants severely depleted bird numbers, and there is many a delicious-sounding old recipe for blackbirds, thrushes, starlings and the like. European friends tell us that even sparrows are not immune. You may turn up your nose but, after all, were not four and twenty blackbirds fit even for a king? A quick flick through any French hunting magazine will show that shooting and eating these small birds is still *de rigueur* among self-respecting sporting types.

Whether or not this is the total explanation for the current dearth of our feathered friends seems to me uncertain, and loss of habitat may also play a part. On the other hand, it could be our side of the world that is the abnormal one. Before a human foot left the first imprint of humanity on some sandy beach on one of our islands, New Zealand was devoid of terrestrial mammals, with the exception of a small bat. Birds occupied every normal mammalian ecological niche, from that of mice to those of gigantic grazing herbivores and enormous rapacious carnivores. Birds were everywhere and in great numbers.

But our natives cannot be blamed for vineyard damage, as none of them eat grapes. The birds that wreak havoc amongst the vines, such as the starling, blackbird and thrush, are not indigenous to New Zealand. They are all interlopers, including a cheeky little Australian scoundrel, the waxeye (silvereye), which just goes from one grape berry to another, pecking holes and never really seeming to satisfy its appetite. Perhaps these foreigners have just found fertile ground in New Zealand and their relative numbers have ballooned compared with those found on the other side of the world.

Whatever the explanation, vineyards and birds are not a happy combination, at least not from the viticulturalist's point of view. This liaison is most fraught in the South Island, possibly due to the proximity of the high mountains. Waxeyes live in the alpine forests over summer and migrate east into vineyard territory when the first autumn snow appears on the mountains. There they assist the resident starlings, blackbirds and thrushes in their attempts to destroy the fruit of the labours of the poor vigneron.

Gina and her husband had planted a six-hectare vineyard several years earlier, and after many trials and tribulations they were expecting their first crop. It was not going to be large but they were hoping to get a few tonnes of grapes, quite enough to make a respectable number of barrels of pinot noir and chardonnay.

'How are you going to protect your crop against the birds?' I asked Gina one day. Like Chris and me, she and her husband were idealists and romantics at heart, but even so, her reply surprised me.

'George and I believe that you have to live in harmony with nature. The birds need food to live so it's only natural that they will eat some of our grapes. They will take some and leave the rest for us. There is a natural balance in all things.'

'But don't you think you should do something to scare the birds away,' I cautioned. 'After all, they can be very destructive, and even if they don't eat your entire crop they may damage most of it so that the grapes go mouldy. Once the skin of a berry has been broken by a bird peck any subsequent rot can spread to the whole bunch.'

'George has had a lot of experience in vineyards overseas and he is confident that we will be all right.'

About two months later I met Gina in the street in the same little village of Amberley.

‘How was the vintage?’ I enquired.

‘Terrible!’ she replied, looking crestfallen. ‘We went away for a few days and when we got back the birds had been at work. We only managed to harvest two buckets of grapes off the entire property. The birds here don’t seem to understand the principle of sharing!’

We had started protecting our crop from avian predators by resorting to the good old-fashioned scarecrow, which we still used from time to time. Our enemies were not entirely bird-brained, however, and after a few days we found them sitting on the scarecrow’s menacing outstretched arms and soiling its old jacket with their grubby little calling cards. Moving the amiable old boy to different places every day was minimally more effective, but it was soon eminently clear that our adversaries were brighter than crows. We next resorted to the gas cannon, a type of imitation gun that is run by a cylinder of butane and intermittently lets off loud explosions. A number of such devices are usually needed to protect a vineyard, so it really does sound like a war zone. After a week or so, however, the birds become used to all the kerfuffle and, like Pavlov’s dogs, they come to regard it as a signal to get ready for dinner. The music of the gas cannon is as enticing to birds as the sound of the dinner bell to hungry boys at boarding school. There is, however, an even greater frustration with gas cannons than their lack of efficacy. Their manufacturers are not like the artisan gunsmiths of yesteryear. They are, in fact, decidedly second-rate and their produce is shonky, particularly with regard to the all-important timing mechanism or clock. It is this that decides the hours of operation of the cannon and its exact pattern of firing.

‘I am sorry to disturb you, Mr Donaldson. It’s the police here; we have had a complaint from one of your neighbours to say that one of your gas cannons is still going off.’

‘Thank you for your call, officer,’ I responded. ‘It’s pitch-black outside, and as owls are strictly carnivorous they don’t eat grapes. I don’t need any of my guns going off at present and I checked them only half an hour ago. They are all turned off, so it must be somebody else’s cannon.’

I hung up with a nasty self-satisfied smile. I knew the officer, who was a thoroughly decent chap, and I was well aware that he was only doing his duty. Irritatingly, a few weeks earlier one of our guns had played up and had kept on firing after dark. Even more frustratingly, this had happened on two or three occasions over the preceding months. We just could not seem to get the timing mechanism functioning correctly. On each occasion one of our neighbours had telephoned the police to complain, rather than simply calling us. This time I had heard the errant cannon booming out and had gone to our vineyard, only to discover that the unfriendly fire was coming from another property. I was not going to complain but I was delighted to receive the officer's telephone call. He had had enough of his valuable time wasted with such trivia.

After an hour the telephone rang once more. 'I just thought I'd let you know that you will have a peaceful night, Mr Donaldson. We have found the culprit, and much to their embarrassment it was the complainants' own gas cannon. We have given them a warning.'

'Thank you, officer. Should you get any further complaints about our guns please just ask the caller to phone us directly. We are always very happy to respond and to fix the problem.'

It was the last time the police were called on to adjudicate in the vineyard wars.

At an earlier stage we had decided to be sporting and to shoot our enemies, although, unlike our European counterparts, we never planned to eat them. I had always fancied myself as a bit of a sharpshooter, but sadly reality proved this to be mere fantasy. I am not sure that I once hit my target. When I added up the number and price of the shotgun cartridges that had aimlessly filled the sky with lead, this was clearly not a cost-effective bird-frightening exercise. I was further discouraged when a lad scaring birds in a local vineyard lost part of his hand. The breach of his shotgun exploded, fortunately sparing the side of his face.

Noises other than explosions can also scare birds. We knew that high-tensile tapes would produce a nasty whistling sound in the wind, and with great difficulty I stretched these high in the air above our vineyard, from one shelter-belt of trees to another, a distance of about 350 metres. They certainly produced quite an unpleasant noise and they seemed to be a deterrent, but they were useless if the weather was calm. Unfortunately, one of the shelter-belts was on Farmer Jones's property, and although we were careful only to use branches that were overhanging our own vineyard, he scaled the high trees and selectively cut these off. We had to admit grudgingly that it was a splendid feat for a man of his advanced age and generous girth.

But human ingenuity has no limits and there are a variety of other noise-emitting devices that are claimed to scare our feathered friends, including sounds that mimic their loved ones being maltreated and pulses of ultrasound that we humans cannot hear. Acquaintances, however, claim to have discovered the silver bullet for the poor vigneron's bird flu; the noise that signals avian Armageddon and will send birds flying helter-skelter. They assure us it never fails, but on principle we refuse to try it. They strategically place large stereo speakers throughout the vineyard and turn the volume knob fully clockwise before playing OPERA! *Sacré bleu!* They assure us that sopranos such as Maria Callas, Joan Sutherland and even our own Kiri Te Kanawa going full tilt make the ultimate weapon. As opera-lovers we refuse to try or countenance such barbaric behaviour.

Unexpected movement also signals danger, and it can frighten birds. For many vineyards this forms the basis of their bird-scaring programme, as it did ours at one stage. Thus, one or more motorbikes, preferably with their mufflers removed, are continually on the move throughout the day. Teenage boys and young men go glassy-eyed and start to salivate when they are offered such a job. Several days later, however, the excitement begins to wane, and after a week motorbike monotony sets in. Given a fortnight, all but the most hardened of the leather-jacket set are dying to quit, particularly after a period of cold, wet weather.

There are many other ingenious bird-scaring devices, including mirrors that rotate with the wind and flash in the sunlight, helium-filled balloons with huge googly eyes that sway in the breeze, and self-launching kites shaped like huge birds. There is a maxim that states that if there is a long list of treatments for a medical disorder you can be certain that none of them is very effective. The same applies when it comes to methods for scaring birds away from delicious ripe grapes. Because of this, many years ago, Chris and I decided that we would try a novel way of protecting our crop by fighting fire with fire.

'Pull over, Chris! There are a couple of beauties back there.'

Our ancient car skidded to a halt and I sprinted back down the verge before making a dash out onto the tarseal. I had to weave between a couple of oncoming vehicles in order to retrieve my prize, and I was panting as I slung them in the back and climbed aboard.

'What did you score?' asked Chris.

'A couple of relatively fresh road scabs. Not too minced-up or rotten. In fact, not too bad for road kill.'

'Yes, but what are they?'

'A rabbit and a possum. I could also have got a hedgehog but he looked a bit far gone; too dried out to be of interest.'

We left the main highway and after a short distance pulled onto the dirt track that led to the vineyard.

'If you drive right into the rows I'll climb up on the car and put them on the platforms,' I volunteered.

I firmly nailed the carcasses onto the two well-separated wooden platforms that we had erected above the vines.

'Let's hide behind the trees and see what happens,' Chris suggested.

We had started feeding the local hawks some weeks earlier, and they had quickly learned where they could get a regular bite, or rather peck, to eat. We had decided to nail down their snacks so that they could not just fly off with the meat or knock it to the ground, where it might get lost under the vines. We crouched behind an adjacent shelter-belt and peered out from behind the leaves.

It didn't take long before Chris whispered, 'One's coming … no, there are two. Perhaps they are male and female.'

The silhouettes hovered majestically against the bright-blue sky, slowly moving in diminishing circles before diving downwards, one towards each platform. They hit their targets almost simultaneously and began to tear at the flesh. They seemed to gorge themselves for an age, but perhaps it was not more than 10 or 15 minutes before the larger of the two lazily flapped its wings and rose slowly and majestically into the air. The other followed soon after. They circled the vineyard and appeared to be about to depart towards the summit of the nearby hills when Chris called out in surprise, 'Look at that! Look at that mob of starlings!'

From the trees of an adjacent shelter-belt a large flock of starlings rose up towards the sky, wheeling in unison, as though they were an aerobatic squadron of jet fighters, piloted by true professionals. They did not circle the vineyard but made for the smaller and slower of the two hawks, diving down on it from above in arrowhead-like formation. Their target slid sideways in the air and then, wings flapping wildly, it ascended up into the ether, madly pursued by the pack that were apparently intent on blood. We had witnessed the raw power of the mob, and we were to see it not infrequently during the weeks to come. It unravelled our plan to fight birds with birds. This rapacious king of the sky, which could easily dismember the much weaker and smaller starling, gobble it as an entrée and then look around for the main course, could be scared off by its opponents en masse. True, hawks will fight back and may also dive-bomb a flock of starlings, seeking out the weakest member of the troop, but they do not have it all their way. Too often the underlings chase off their masters, then the supposed underdogs waste no time in tasting the sweet rewards of their success.

**'HOW DID IT GO?' ASKED CHRIS** as she welcomed me home with a wide smile and a big kiss.

I had been away with Matthew for several days at one of the early annual workshops that, over 20 years later, are still a must for any serious Kiwi pinot noir producer. It was a show-and-tell type of meeting at which the participants sat down together to blind-taste and frankly evaluate each other's pinot noir wines, warts and all. Each of the wines tasted had to be accompanied by a data sheet outlining all the viticultural and winemaking details. The group then gave advice on how the wines might be improved. The aim of this little band of 'Pinot Pioneers' was to improve the overall standard of New Zealand pinot noirs so that Kiwi pinots could develop into an internationally known entity of the highest standard. Everyone knew that in order to attain this goal we had to lift the game of all players. We had to sacrifice self-interest for the greater good and openly share information with competitors.

'Okay,' I replied.

'Only okay?'

'Good and not so good, I guess. I made quite a fool of myself by savagely criticising one of the wines, then later on, when the line-up was revealed, it turned out to be one of our own. I felt such a fool.'

'Did everyone agree with you?'

'No, the others thought it was reasonably good, although not exceptional. We got some good suggestions about how we might do better next year.

'These meetings are great for getting all types of information and solving practical problems, too,' I continued. 'I think I might have the solution to our bird problem, although it is going to be expensive.'

'What is it and how much will it cost?' asked the holder of the purse strings with a look of mock concern. 'Nothing could be more expensive than losing a fair proportion of our fruit, not to mention our sleep,' she added.

'Nets; nets that will go over four or possibly five rows at a time. Herman Seifried from Nelson was there. He kindly took me to his vineyard and demonstrated the machine he uses for putting the nets over the vines. He made it himself. It's like a big cotton reel that contains all of the net wrapped around it. It's raised high in the air by the forklift on the front of his tractor. The net unrolls and can be pulled into place over the rows as the tractor moves down between them. I'm going to get the engineers in Amberley to make a similar machine for me.'

We had earlier tried nets that fitted over single rows but the birds could perch on the outsides and reach in to peck the fruit. By having nets that spanned multiple rows only the outer edge of the outermost row could be damaged in this way. Although simple, this concept proved very effective, and the following autumn our entire vineyard looked as though it was covered in a giant white spider web. No longer would the birds pressure us into picking before our grapes were deliciously ripe and well coloured. In addition, a truce had been signed between us and our feathered friends. The guns fell silent and all the other ugly vestiges of war were cleared away. From now on vintage would be a time of peace and harmony.

Yet something else niggled; something was not quite right. Yes, I was happy, but not ecstatic. It was the pollution, the visual pollution. Like all proud parents we considered that our baby looked beautiful, yet we had dressed it in ugly clothes. Our vineyard, which was the first in the Waipara Valley to be entirely netted, now stood out like a sore thumb, or rather a bandaged sore thumb. Soon other vineyards began to follow suit so it looked like the district was full of DIYers who were incompetent with hammers. What could we do about it? We had been told that it was essential to use white nets. White appears as it does because it reflects all visible light. Black, on the other hand, absorbs all of the light and leaves nothing for us to see. Thus, white nets do not absorb the light and they enable the grapes to ripen at a normal rate, whereas black nets steal some of the light and slow down ripening. Or do they?

That was certainly the hype of the net vendors, but we decided to set up a trial. We found that the rate of ripening was identical with both colours. Black nets, however, are virtually invisible from a distance of about 10 metres and the vines can be seen clearly through them. We thus started a programme of replacing worn-out white nets with black, and our autumnal eyesore started to disappear. There was also another advantage, which is perhaps best explained by way of an analogy. The more observant of you will have noticed that a ladder or hole in black net stockings seems to irresistibly draw your eye if the leg is pale, more so than with nets of another colour. It is all a matter of contrast. Thus, birds find it harder to discover holes in black nets because the background is dark. You will doubtless understand their frustration at not being able to easily penetrate the paradise that they see behind the alluring veil.

All the time we had been developing our vineyard in the Waipara Valley I had continued making the wine for our little co-operative at Pleurisy Point, thus ensuring that I kept my finger on the pulse of winemakeing or oenology, to give the gentle art its proper title. Finally, having coped with the innumerable problems and frustrations of setting up a vineyard and growing grapes, we were now in a position to reap the rewards of our toil and to focus on harvest and winemaking. It was in the year that we had expected our first harvest at Waipara Valley, 1990, that I had left the Mountain View co-operative with feelings of both sadness and excitement.

## CHAPTER 9

# *The* Man *with the* Three Balls

1975–2006

**I HAVE NEVER CLAIMED** to have great physical prowess, agility or athletic ability, but from the time I was a junior medical officer I did become quite adept at juggling. My skill was not outstanding, and in fact by some people's standards it would be classed as modest. It was of a type that anyone can pick up with a bit of practice. In fact, I have to come clean and admit that I never succeeded in juggling more than three balls at a time. No one taught me, and it was by chance that I stumbled upon the juggler's secret, which I will share with you. This is that you have to keep your eye on the ball in the air, the one that you do not have in your hands. Everything depends on that.

The balls that you hold in your fingers are safe and you can move them about almost automatically. However, the one in space, the one that is for the moment 'active', needs all of your attention. If you let it fall then the whole show will be a flop. I do not know why I found it necessary to have three balls. Perhaps it was because there is a type of reliability in three, rather like a three-legged stool. This provides stability on uneven terrain, while those with fewer or more legs can become wobbly when the going gets rough.

As far as I could tell, most of my colleagues only had two balls and they seemed quite happy with this arrangement. Perhaps they really had an extra one that they kept out of sight. Although three balls should have been simple stuff, I found my juggling difficult because each ball was incohesive and multifaceted. Bits stuck out at odd angles and were liable to fall off or, worse still, a whole ball might disintegrate. The balls that I had to keep twirling were my family, medicine and wine.

**WHEN I RETURNED TO** Christchurch Hospital in the mid-1970s, after my study in London, my medical work had a number of different aspects. As time went on others became attached to these. It was a bit like a rolling snowball that increases in size and weight. Although I was officially employed by Otago University to do research and teaching at the Christchurch School of Medicine, 50 per cent of my time was paid for by the public hospital, where I was to work as a clinical neurologist. Prior to my arrival, clinical neurology had been in the hands of a general physician who over the preceding few years had restricted himself to neurology. John (Jake) Cunningham was a lean, hard-working, sober man with a marvellous economy of speech. He did not waste words needlessly, and with the exception of um …, er … and ah …, and a tendency to repeat certain words or short phrases, every one of his verbal soldiers had a precise job to do. Seen against today's background of media talkfests, gossip and general tittle-tattle, it was an admirable quality and one that he had honed to perfection. I have often regretted that some of his expertise in this domain did not rub off on me.

Jake had never mastered the art of talking into one of those newfangled dictating machines and he always had his correspondence transcribed by his shorthand typist, an elderly and charming expert in the now lamentably lost art of stenography. She did not have to accompany him on his clinical duties, except when a neurosurgeon from Dunedin made one of his fortnightly visits. On these occasions Jake and the stenographer paid the surgeon the courtesy of trailing in his footsteps for the entire visit. Even in those days it seemed rather quaint. To the slick-typing, computer-raised junior medical staff of today, however, it would appear positively archaic; but it worked.

Jake had a sense of loyalty to the Dunedin neurosurgical unit. He felt that Christchurch had been well served by it and he had no desire to see that changed. He was a very private person and every inch a gentleman. A respiratory physician, Bill Smith, shared private consulting rooms with Jake and they split all the running expenses. Bill told me once that quite by chance he had remembered that nine months earlier the pair had agreed to give their shared private secretary a salary increase but that they had not subsequently discussed the matter. Bill had forgotten to increase the amount of the monthly cheque which covered his share of the costs.

'Jake, I've just remembered that we agreed to give the secretary a rise but we have done nothing about it,' he told his colleague.

'I did raise her salary, Bill, just after we talked about it.'

'In that case I must pay you my arrears. We should sit down and work out how much it amounts to.'

'It is $567.57,' came the instant reply.

Jake had been too polite or shy to raise the matter with Bill, although he had clearly followed the mounting debt in precise detail. Indeed, Jake was shy, but behind a somewhat austere exterior was a thoughtful, kindly, reliable, self-effacing colleague.

I was somewhat surprised when a year or so after I had taken up my appointment Jake asked me if we could have a private chat. I was uncertain what he had on his mind but he came straight to the point.

'I would like you to become head of the neurology department, Ivan.'

I was quite taken aback. I did not know how long he had to go before retirement, but I had not expected anything as sudden as this. In fact, there was no real department, only the pair of us, the secretaries, the junior medical staff and the nursing staff. Jake knew, however, that I had plans for enlarging the department and for establishing neurosurgery in Christchurch. This was his way of saying that he approved, and giving me the green light. Because of his feelings of loyalty to Dunedin he preferred not to drive the changes himself, however. Even as I accepted his offer I knew that the extra work would put pressure on the university's share of my time, which was already under attack from the large public hospital caseload.

The clinical work consisted of organising and running a ward of 25 neurology inpatient beds, which accepted all types of acute neurology admissions through the emergency department as well as taking arranged neurology admissions, doing neurology outpatient clinics, performing neurological consultations for other services and wards in Christchurch Hospital and surrounding hospitals, and providing a neurophysiological service (electromyography [EMG] and electroencephalography [EEG]). As there was no neurosurgical unit in Christchurch, the pre-operative and post-operative management of patients with neurosurgical conditions was also done by neurology, while these patients were transferred to Dunedin for the actual surgery. Thus, patients with suspected subarachnoid haemorrhage, brain tumour and the like were admitted, investigated and managed by the neurologists. There was no intensive-care unit, so patients with life-threatening neurological disorders that required intensive management were looked after by the neurologists in a type of modified post-operative recovery room.

Then there was the teaching and assessment of junior medical staff and medical students. There were 10 or more fifth-year medical students attached to neurology, and every five weeks these groups moved on to another discipline, only to be replaced by a fresh batch of enthusiastic new faces. I would not wish to suggest that my situation was particularly unusual, for I had many medical colleagues who were in the same boat. We all had to man the pumps and row hard in order to keep our crafts afloat and make any headway. The amount of clinical work in public hospitals was overwhelming, and it frequently demanded immediate attention. Those doctors who worked in larger departments were generally more fortunate, as they could roster their time so that one of their number would handle the acute calls, allowing the others on the service free time for study or research. Doctors employed by hospitals were not obliged to do research, although many of them did and were excellent at it. University employees, like myself, were expected to do research, but it was often difficult to find the time, especially when your office was immediately adjacent to your ward.

After some time it dawned on me that I was spending at least 75 per cent of my nominally 50/50 university/hospital job doing hospital work, but if you can turn your back on acute calls and the immediate needs of your patients then you should not be in clinical medicine. I really enjoyed what I was doing and decided to box on, making the most of the limited time I had available for research.

It was about this time that Jake asked to have another talk with me.

'I would like to go away for several months, Ivan. I have long-service leave from the hospital that is owing to me and I have decided to visit a number of overseas neurological centres. Would that be all right?'

'Of course it would, Jake. I would be delighted to help you out. After all, it will be no more work than you did before I arrived.'

'I think it will be,' Jake said. 'The amount of work seems to have built up very considerably since you came. It must be your ready availability. After all, I am always in my private consulting rooms in the afternoons, while you are here all of the time.'

If I thought that I was busy before Jake went away then I was dreaming. I did not realise that I had been living on easy street. Being the only person on call for neurological and neurosurgical patients in Christchurch, in fact in the provinces of Canterbury and the West Coast, proved to be rather daunting.

After what seemed like an indecently short period, in reality about six years after taking up my neurological job at Christchurch, I was made president of the New Zealand Neurological Association. This was the official, but very low-key, organisation that was responsible for the educational/research meetings and the political/advisory functions of the country's neurologists and neurosurgeons. It was clear that they were scraping the bottom of the barrel in order to get somebody to do the job, but I could not refuse without seeming to be impolite and shirking my duty. It did, however, have some compensations, as I found out when I went overseas. Suddenly, neurologists, neurosurgeons and their respective national bodies seemed somewhat in awe of this young upstart from the colonies, inviting me to comment at their meetings and inviting Chris and me to their prestigious dinners. It was all good fun.

Somewhat later, I was invited to join the scientific advisory committee of the Neurological Research Foundation of New Zealand, which turned out to be much more serious stuff. It involved reading lots of applications for research funds, along with the associated background literature and the referees' reports from overseas and local experts. I enjoyed the work, but my heart bled for all those researchers who had submitted really good applications and who deserved to be funded but had to be culled out for lack of sufficient money. It is the bane of all medical and scientific research in New Zealand, this severely prostatic flow of funding that makes it extremely difficult to get even high-quality clinical-relevant studies done. It reduces to only a few per cent the number of successful applicants to most major funding bodies and proves to be the rock on which the hopes of many a bright young researcher founder.

Not long after I returned from sabbatical leave in London in 1984 an ophthalmologist friend of mine, Rod Suckling, told me excitedly that he had found a way of getting botulinum toxin. By chance, he had met a man from the British Embassy in Wellington and, after Rod had made a dramatic plea, the diplomat had arranged for some of the toxin to be flown out from England. It was said to have originally been manufactured as a weapon of selective or mass destruction at Britain's germ-warfare establishment, Porton Down.

Botulinum kills by causing severe muscular paralysis, but in 1980 an American ophthalmologist reported that tiny injections into the extra-ocular muscles, those tiny muscles that move our eyeballs, could be used to treat squint. It worked by weakening the overactive muscle that was causing the problem. Botulinum was subsequently used overseas to treat other involuntary muscular hyperactivity and spasms, particularly those caused by movement disorders, such as dystonia. It was thus that via this backdoor route I came to start New Zealand's first botulinum toxin clinic, which was an adjunct to my regular EMG clinic. Several years later botulinum was to become available through commercial suppliers (Dysport from the UK, Botox from the US), but it still all originated from the dark recesses of germ-warfare establishments.

I began by treating involuntary spasms and twitches on the face or torticollis (neck spasms), but soon moved on to a miscellaneous variety of other disabling neurological conditions. Botulinum only works by causing temporary muscular weakness and patients always return for further injections if treatment is successful. I rapidly found that I had made a rod for my own back as word got around that this new therapy was available. It just added to the weight of the medical ball that needed to be juggled. Fortunately, I escaped the later wave of wrinkle-free and expressionless faces that were to become the cosmetic fashion.

'**GOOD MORNING, DR SMITH.** This is Dr Peterson, and I am Dr Donaldson. Please come this way.'

The young man in the freshly laundered and scrupulously pressed white coat gave a flicker of a watery smile and extended his hand.

'This one is definitely on a beta-blocker,' Jack Peterson whispered to me as we followed Dr Smith into the examination room.

We were used to the moist, cold hands of fear, but this one was more like a pack of frozen fish fingers than a wet fish. Candidates sometimes took beta-blockers to control their nerves and to mask any anxiety-related tremor. A side-effect of these medications is that they constrict peripheral blood vessels, cooling the hands and feet.

Some years earlier, the Royal Australasian College of Physicians had asked me to join its examination committee. Many people appear confused about the nature of physicians, whereas they are quite clear about the function of surgeons. As mentioned earlier, New Zealand follows the British system in which the basic qualification in clinical medicine is two bachelor degrees, one in medicine and the other in surgery. After this one may train to become a general practitioner/family doctor, a psychiatrist, a surgeon, or a medical specialist (physician). I rather naïvely felt that being invited to join the examination committee was some type of honour, only to find out later that it came with a high price, the currency for which was time and hard work. Not only did it involve many hours of unpaid labour, examining aspiring physicians who wanted to become specialists in every imaginable branch of medicine, but it also meant a lot of organisation and committee work. It was a major operational exercise for the locals when the travelling circus of the examination committee came to town, and for me in particular when the show rolled into Christchurch. Fortunately, over the years I had grown and then sharpened my deputising skills.

After years of hospital medical practice and study the hopefuls had to sit multiple examination papers and those that passed went on to sit the clinical exams. There was a lot at stake. If they passed these examinations in general medicine then they could go on to do further training, over a minimum of three years, in the subspecialty of their choice, e.g. cardiology, neurology, gastroenterology, renal medicine and so forth. This was supervised by the relevant specialist advisory committee. Successful completion of this phase would allow them to become Fellows of the Royal Australasian College of Physicians (FRACP), which was a basic requirement to become registered as a specialist physician. I had much earlier served a stint on the Specialist Advisory Committee for Neurology, but I was now on the college committee charged with conducting the clinical examinations in general medicine. After eight years on the committee I had rather foolishly allowed myself to be elected its chairman.

'We would like you to examine Mr Fletcher's abdomen and report your findings to us,' Jack Peterson now said to the candidate.

Dr Smith had a good examination technique, exposing the patient's abdomen after asking his permission and then observing it carefully before reaching out to palpate it. The hand was just about to descend onto the unsuspecting flesh when Jack said, 'Perhaps you had better warn Mr Fletcher about your cold hand, and perhaps try to warm it before palpating.'

The candidate's hand remained frozen in mid-air, in more senses than one, before being quickly withdrawn, rubbed vigorously, and then, without further warning or mucking about, placed purposefully on the target. Even after being warned, Mr Fletcher jumped, let out an expletive and tightened his abdominal muscles, making it impossible to feel anything.

'I'm sure Mr Fletcher would appreciate it if you warmed your hands under the hot-water tap over the bedside basin,' Jack suggested helpfully.

'Damned beta-blockers,' he said to me later when we were alone. 'I wish candidates for this examination would not take them.'

'Yes,' I agreed, 'but we really should have given the poor chap and the patient more warning. Otherwise his examination technique was up to scratch, he identified the major abnormalities and his discussion on the liver function and kidney test results was reasonable. He scores a pass on that patient's case in my books. It will be interesting to see how he fares with the other short-case examiners.'

'Please take a seat, Dr Scott, and tell us about your long case, Mr Greenwood,' my co-examiner, the congenial Jim Short, said to the young man, indicating the hot seat with a wide flourish of his arm.

The Australasian system of long and short cases was similar to that used in the UK, as described in Chapter 3.

'Were there any particular problems that prevented you from getting a good history or interfered with your ability to carry out a satisfactory examination?' I asked.

Although all patients were volunteers and generously and willingly gave their time, there were occasional disasters, including reluctance to discuss their symptoms or sudden and persistent diarrhoea striking the patient, the candidate, but hopefully not both, during that one crucial hour.

'W…, W…, W…, Well, in fact, y…, y…, y…, y…, yes,' replied the young Doctor Scott, blushing. 'M…, M…, My patient had a st…, st…, st…, st…, st…, stutter. It sl…, sl…, sl…, sl…, sl…, slowed up m…, m…, m…, my hi…, hi…, hi…, hi…, hi…, hi…, history ta…, ta…, ta…, ta…, ta…, taking dreadfully. I di…, di…, di…, didn't manage to fi…, fi…, finish in ti…, ti…, ti…, time.'

It did not take a clairvoyant to see that we had a major problem on our hands. While any physician might be expected to be able to cope with a stutterer, it was clearly unfair to have one in an examination in which the candidates were under a major time constraint. Somehow this problem had not come to the attention of the examination organisers and the patient had slipped through the net. But here we had a double whammy; two severe stutterers had been thrown together by sheer malicious chance. I cringed when I thought of them both trying to do their best under severe pressure.

'Thank you for bringing it to our attention, Dr Scott. We will certainly take this into consideration when assessing your performance. Why don't you just relax, take your time and tell us about your patient's history and examination findings before we ask you how you might go on to manage his problems,' said Jim with a reassuring smile.

'Well, what did you make of that?' I said to him after Dr Scott had left. 'Even if you make allowances for difficulty in eliciting the patient's history and symptoms, Dr Scott misinterpreted some of the physical findings and his plan of management seemed only just adequate, possibly as a result of his incorrect findings.'

'That's true, Ivan, but perhaps he became flustered by the patient's stutter and panicked.'

It seemed curious that neither Jim nor I had noticed a severe stutter when we had interviewed and examined the patient earlier that morning before the candidate arrived. We would clearly need to re-evaluate the situation, and that we did. Back at the bedside it was clear that the patient did have a mild speech impediment but it in no way prevented us from obtaining a clear history in a relatively short time. It seemed as though it was the candidate's own speech problem that had slowed him. How much allowance would we have to make for that? We pondered the problem and added up all the parts that he had got correct, weighing them carefully against the things that he had got wrong and making some allowance for his own speech difficulty.

Eventually, we decided that he had passed his long case, but only just. There was no fat to spare and he would have to gain a pass in both his short cases to be successful.

At our end-of-day committee meeting, when all the examiners got together and discussed the aspirants' performances, tallying up their results, it transpired that Dr Scott had failed both his short cases, in which he did not have to discuss the patient's symptoms or history. The two different pairs of examiners who had observed his short cases had independently found the same problem. His examination technique was inadequate, leading him to misinterpret the physical findings. While this meant he would not pass the examination on that occasion, it did raise an interesting point. What allowance, if any, should be made for candidates who had disabilities that might slow but not otherwise impair their performance during examinations? Being a good physician is not the same as being a virtuoso concert pianist; speed is not everything. Doctors often deal with and have to be advocates for disabled patients. We should be sympathetic to disability in our colleagues, so long as it does not affect the quality of their work.

Being chairman of the examination committee also carried with it the responsibility of being chairman of the board of censors, a triumvirate that was responsible for adjudicating on the misdemeanours of our fellow Fellows and for assessing the qualifications and standing of overseas-trained physicians who wanted to practise in New Zealand or become Fellows. Decisions relating to the latter could often be made quite simply if the applicant came from a country with similar qualifications and standards to New Zealand and it was easy to check on their character and good standing. Problems arose where this was not the case, and such applicants had to be examined in order to protect the unsuspecting public.

Dr X was one such case. This charming middle-aged gentleman purported to be a diabetes specialist. He had lost the documents related to his training and qualifications when he was in a refugee camp, and there was absolutely no way of getting information about them from the university and hospitals where he claimed to have trained. He had to be examined. Having presented the history and physical findings of his long case with a show of great confidence, he was about to proceed to tell us how he would manage the patient's problems.

'Thank you very much, Dr X. Before you proceed, we just want to make certain that we understand you correctly. Would you be kind enough to tell us once again your findings related to the patient's eyes,' I asked.

'Ophthalmoscopic exam showed zat patient's retina have diabetic change, mod'rate. Show microaneurysms.'

'And had this affected his vision?'

Dr X looked slightly taken aback and after a moment's pause said, 'No, acuity normal, both eye.'

'Were his eye movements normal?'

'Fine, without problem.'

'Was there any sign of a diabetic peripheral neuropathy?'

'Perhaps little numb on feet to pin.'

'So all of his reflexes were present in both legs?' my co-examiner, Stan Watson, asked in a surprised tone.

'Fine, no problem.'

'Would you be good enough to demonstrate these findings to us?' Stan requested.

At the bedside the candidate looked perturbed when he found that the patient appeared to have become blind in the left eye during the preceding half-hour, and then it slowly dawned on Dr X that it was a glass eye. He looked positively aghast when he drew back the blankets fully and saw that the patient had a below-knee amputation on the right. He had even missed the clue of the prosthetic lower leg and shoe propped up against the patient's locker. He had been cutting corners and just making things up. His plan of management for the patient was hopeless. He had clearly picked up a smattering of medical knowledge somewhere; as a nurse or a medical orderly? We would never know, but we were certain of one thing: he was not going to be let loose on trusting patients!

**BUT THERE WAS ONE OTHER** little pastime that added to the pressure of my medical life, and that was private practice.

'Sh…, sh…! Michael, turn the television down. If you kids can't stop squabbling then turn the television off, go out into the backyard and play quietly. Matthew, stop pushing Edward's head down onto that chair, you might dirty the fabric!'

'He started it, Dad. He pulled my shirt and he's ripped it. Mum'll be furious.'

'Ow! Stop pulling my hair!'

'If I have to tell you off again you will have to go and do your homework. Go and tell Paul to stop kicking that ball against the house. You're making far too much noise. I can hardly hear myself think.'

I slammed shut the sliding panel between the kitchen/living room and the formal dining room of the house, fortunately remembering to withdraw my head before I did so. The panel had been made to look like part of the woodwork and it concealed the opening through which platters of steaming food could be passed, thus avoiding the need to trek between the two areas of the house. I now used the dining room as a consulting office, and an adjacent converted sunporch served as an examination room. A downstairs lounge doubled as a waiting room when there were patients to be seen. Unfortunately, the patients had to come through the main front door of the house because a second, smaller front door was kept tightly locked. This latter door opened directly into the examination room and I reasoned that it might upset the odd sensitive soul if we were suddenly joined by a pack of strangers in the middle of their examination. The setup was not perfect but it worked reasonably well: reasonably well, that is, provided the boys did not yell, fight, turn up the volume of the TV, etc. In other words, it was okay so long as they did not behave like normal boys but sat as quiet as four little mice.

After a pause, which I estimated would be long enough for the patient to partially disrobe, I gave a knock and entered the examination room. Jason Daniels was a robust, sandy-haired 28-year-old who had previously been in good health, apart from an unexplained transient episode of left facial numbness 18 months earlier. He was now troubled with tingling in his right foot and lower leg, which had been present for 10 days. I suspected multiple sclerosis but there were other possible explanations, including blockage of blood vessels causing small strokes. After performing a neurological examination I launched into a general medical one. I was in the process of auscultating his heart when I heard a very squeaky noise. Was it coming from his heart, lungs, pleura, ribcage or elsewhere? It was very brief but quite definite and, wait, there it went again. It was not quite the same as the first time but definitely similar. Yes, it was repeating intermittently but quite irregularly. What could it be?

The penny dropped just as the squeaks elongated and started flowing into a continuous but varying sound. It had been Michael tuning his violin, and now he was starting to play, somewhat tentatively. Fortunately, the rest of the examination did not involve using the stethoscope.

While Jason was dressing I nipped up to the 'music room', a large upstairs lounge that overlooked the garden. Michael stopped playing abruptly and looked up as I entered.

'I thought you were seeing patients, Dad. Have you finished already?'

'No, Michael, but I need you to stop playing now. This room is directly above my consulting office and the examination room. The music is too loud down there. I want to talk to the patient about a very serious matter and I can hardly hear myself think.'

'But my music teacher will be cross if I don't do my practice, Dad, and by the way, you said that before.'

'Said what?'

'Said that you couldn't think. Do you really think you should be seeing patients if you can't think?'

'Don't worry about it, Michael. I'll explain it later.'

'I think Matthew's coming upstairs to practise his drums.'

'Go downstairs and tell him that under NO circumstances is he to play his drums until all of the patients have gone!'

When Matthew practised his drums it sounded as though Armageddon had arrived. The whole house reverberated with a noise that seemed to insinuate itself between the skull and the brain, levering off the former to squeeze the latter into a painful little ball. I could not evade it even when I escaped to the outside garage. It was impossible for anyone to actually like this cacophony, and I was convinced that Matthew used it as a kind of punishment for his siblings and blackmail on his parents. I muttered unspeakable oaths as I descended in a hypertensive crisis.

'Nice to hear a budding musician, isn't it?' Jason said cheerily as I entered the consulting room.

'Yes, I love to hear him play,' I replied with a guilty smile. 'I don't know why, but he never seems to do it for very long. Just like that, he starts, plays for a little bit and then stops. No stickability, I guess.'

The physical layout of our house worked well for seeing private patients, and it would have been a great setup if it had not been for the kids. On the other hand, the boys would have been fine, even if I could not say well-behaved, if it had not been for the patients. Our home was where two of the three balls that I had to juggle came into contact, sometimes with the risk that one would disastrously disturb the equilibrium of the other. The problem arose because my full-time university/hospital appointment allowed me to do some private practice but I was determined that I would restrict this to outside normal working hours. Thus, I only saw private patients during the evenings or at weekends, which were just the times that the boys were at home. This meant that some interaction between the professional and domestic sides of my life was inevitable. While this could cause problems it did have potential benefits by educating my boys and me. On occasions when Chris was out, the boys had to let the patients into the house, leading them to the waiting room through the entrance hall that was scattered with splendid examples of the taxidermist's art. My sons became adept at making their own spot diagnoses.

Remarks such as 'I let Mr Ranfurly into the waiting room, Dad. He's got

Parkinson's disease', or 'I think your next patient has had a stroke', were run-of-the-mill.

I am sure if I had paid more attention to my boys they could have improved my clinical accuracy.

Occasionally, just to enliven proceedings, one of them would add something like, '… and he looks more stuffed than the badger'.

Nonetheless, I always had a sense of tension and I felt that I was excessively strict with the boys when patients were in the house. I was suppressing their naturally boisterous behaviour. Another disadvantage was that this private work meant I had less time to devote to my family, but fortunately the ever-resourceful and cheerful Chris stepped in to help plug the gap. As well as filling in for me as a surrogate father, she handled calls from the referring doctors, made the appointments, welcomed the patients, acted as a chaperone, made the doctor cups of tea and typed the reports and letters. Normally, I did not sit down to dinner until 8 p.m., an hour at which unfed boys tend to become particularly truculent, so I missed out on their dinnertime. Chris and I were forced to have our evening meal alone in peace and quiet, listening to background music. While such enforced segregation has its little compensations, I am sure that most young parents would feel woefully distressed at such an arrangement.

'Don't give up your day job or, for that matter, your night job. We need them both to feed that money-eating monster of a vineyard,' was Chris's frequently expressed sentiment.

'Who has been cutting their fingernails in our bedroom?' I demanded, poking my head into the living room, where the boys were wolfing down breakfast before they headed off to school.

'What's the trouble, dear?' asked Chris sympathetically, looking up from the waffle-maker. She had decided to give the boys a special breakfast treat.

'I have just eaten part of a fingernail!'

'That's a strange thing to do, Ivan. It might irritate you but don't worry, it will eventually pass. You must have been particularly hungry.'

'No,' I thundered. 'It was sitting on the folded-down sheet in front of me and I thought it was a flake of desiccated coconut! It has to be one of you lot. Own up, who was it?'

Receiving nothing but blank stares and head shakes I stormed back upstairs to finish my bowl of fruit and muesli. Breakfast in bed had become something of a routine for me since starting private practice. Chris had insisted on it and I weakly acquiesced. Initially I had a sense of guilt, but I soon found that this was easily put down. I had to admit it was not too bad, given the alternative.

'It's the only time in the day you have to read and correct the letters that

I've typed,' Chris had argued persuasively, 'because you always dictate them after we have finished dinner. You never seem to come to bed before 10 or 11 p.m., especially if you have to write one of your newspaper wine columns.'

**BUT IF I ABROGATED MANY** of my paternal duties during most of the year, I tried to make up for it during the boys' school holidays, when I endeavoured to devote my time exclusively to our family. These vacations were mainly spent in the countryside of Banks Peninsula. The peninsula was formed by the remains of two ancient volcanoes that thrust themselves out into the sea adjacent to Christchurch, like a pair of clenched fists pressed tightly together with the thumbs held upwards. Over millions of years the craters or palms at the centres of the fists have become large, twin safe harbours, and their existence is the reason the early English settlers chose to site their city there.

The peninsula has many wild and beautiful smaller harbours and ocean beaches, some with lagoons. We usually holidayed adjacent to one of these. We swam in the sea, dried ourselves on the warm sand, caught fish, hiked in the hills, barbecued our meals and played games. Sometimes we broke out the canvas and camped under the stars, while at other times we hired remote old houses. For many years we rented a dilapidated old farmhouse that sported a billiard room and came complete with a resident beehive contained within its walls. The dwelling had a stream flowing alongside its green lawn, on which we played badminton and bowls. We ate the eels that the boys caught in the creek, and made rollmops out of the herrings that swam up it to our front door on the incoming tide. In the evenings we all played the board games that, like the old magazines, furniture, ornaments, kitchenware and albums full of faded family photographs, had been left in a time-warp. They were exactly as they had been left when the owners' parents had died many years earlier. It was a very rustic paradise, made all the more exciting by a locked shed-cum-sleepout in the garden which carried a crooked sign saying 'Fantasy Hut'. We peered through the grimy, cobweb-covered windows, but apart from the hint provided by a faded old calendar picture featuring a pinup, what had passed in this fantasyland was left to our fertile imaginations.

One night I took the boys 'exploring'. We carried torches but they were hardly needed as the sky was clear and a full moon sailed on high. We made our way through the lush grass, following the lazy stream that gurgled and shimmered enchantingly. Suddenly we came across something amazing that I have never again observed. There, basking in the moonlight, were dozens of eels lying quite motionless in the riffles, those shallow patches in a streambed where the water just trickles over the stones. These shyest of creatures, who normally lurk in deep holes or under a hollowed-out creek bank, concealing themselves and inhabiting the darkness, were lying fully exposed, moon-bathing. They were like a crowd of happy holidaymakers perfecting their suntans on the beach. The eels seemed to be entranced, and whereas normally they would have darted away at our approach, this sinuous school moved only languorously at our touch. It was as though the moon had enticed them from their lairs, only to bewitch and tame them. Although we had been fishing for eels earlier in the day, the spectacle was so amazing that we ourselves must have been entranced as we left them to rest in watery peace.

But leisure is the thief of time, and on every occasion that the sun slipped down behind the gradually darkening crater rim, setting the sky on fire with spectacular shades of red, orange and mauve, the boys were a day older. Without us being fully aware that they were losing their innocence they were gradually stalking each other through adolescence towards maturity. Edward was knocking on the teenage door that Matthew and Michael seemed to have bolted through. Even Paul looked set to forsake childhood. An impending testosterone storm led the older ones to hanker for more action than our isolated Arcadia could provide, so we started spending our summer vacations in Akaroa, the picturesque little harbourside village that had once been the haunt of tattooed Maori warriors, whalers and European colonists. In bygone years its narrow streets had echoed with the romantic lilt of French, being the chosen site, in the mid-1800s, of France's only attempt to establish a New Zealand colony. But the boys were not driven by the dusty pages of history books; they sought the company of their peers of both sexes and shops where they could fritter away their meagre pocket money.

'I think we'll have to say something to the boys,' I said to Chris one night after they had gone to bed, 'because I don't think we can keep up all this smelly work. It's spoiling our holiday.'

'You can't do that, Ivan. They are having so much fun that you would only disappoint them. After all, we have only got another week to put up with it.'

'But we have already had a week of it,' I whinged. 'I can't get the smell off my hands and the house is starting to stink.'

Chris looked at me over the pile of cod that we were filleting and tossed another skeleton, complete with head and tail, into the rubbish tin.

'Buck up! I know that we have had 30 cod and upwards to fillet most days and that we have had fish for breakfast, lunch and dinner every day since we got here, but the kids love catching them. These fish that I'm freezing will last us over the next month or two. They could not be fresher.'

And that is how we left it, and why we kept smiling every time we heard them coming up the path with yet another load of cod, all caught off the end of the Akaroa wharf.

**'WE'VE ONLY GOT THE SHERRIES, PORTS** and the sauternes-style wines to go and then we've finished!' Don shouted encouragingly, his face unusually flushed with perhaps more than just the prospect of imminent success.

'Well, I'm damned if we're going to do them,' Brian said forcefully. 'They'll all be crap.'

'Hear, hear,' added Alan, while the rest of us shouted 'Yes' almost simultaneously.

'It won't take us long,' pleaded Don. 'We'll probably knock them off within the next hour. I'm under a time constraint and I have to get everything finished by the end of the month.'

'We are going home, and we are going home now, Don. We have had enough and can't concentrate any more. It's 11 p.m., we are tired and our palates are shot,' I said definitively. 'It will have to wait for another day.'

'What about next Monday night? If we start at 6 p.m., as we did tonight, we would probably be finished by eight. I will put on a good meal for you, which we could have before, during or after the tasting. We'll finish up with a few very special bottles from my own cellar,' Don added by way of a bribe, concluding before anyone could object, 'Well, that's settled then.'

Earlier that evening, the eight or so people in Don's lounge had all tasted, scored, written tasting notes and then discussed about a hundred wines, which had been divided into flights of six. While we were all wine enthusiasts and not simply tasting virgins, or should I say virgins at the noble art of wine tasting, we had never been subjected to such a palate-shattering experience. Our tongues and teeth were stained a vivid purple, our gums felt both raw and numb at the same time, and our mouths rebelled against even the thought of wine glasses advancing towards our lips. We had had enough and felt totally unenthusiastic about a repeat performance a few nights later. Because we had all been spitting the wine, however, our central nervous systems had stood up to the assault rather well. We were reasonably confident that any slurring of speech resulted from the physical damage to our oral apparati, since our coordination, balance and gait attested to the fact that at least the lower parts of our brains were functioning acceptably. On the other hand, our meek acquiescence to the command of a further tasting suggested that the higher centres controlling judgement and wisdom might have been impaired.

'Don, please call us taxis, and these special wines you're promising on Monday night had better be bloody good! Go to the top shelf and be sure to make your special steak and kidney pie,' Brian said emphatically.

And so it came to pass that one Monday evening in 1977 we finished, in relatively leisurely and painless style, the rest of the tasting that formed the basis for Don Beaven's book *Wines for Dining*, a practical guide to buying, cellaring and serving New Zealand wines. In addition, the book contained a scored evaluation of all the New Zealand wines that were currently on the market. They ranged from a retail price of $1.50 to a staggering $4.25 for a cheeky little state-of-the-art 1974 Nobilo Cabernet Sauvignon, with most wines being between $2 and $3. This was one of the first, if not the first, buyer's guides to New Zealand wines: not a bad effort from a busy professor of medicine.

It was a decade later that I teamed up with Don Beaven and Graham Watson to write a more comprehensive book on wine; a much broader volume that did not look at individual wines but covered history, wine styles, wine appreciation, physiology, wine and health, social aspects of drinking, and so forth. We were on a crusade against binge-drinking, boozing and excessive alcohol consumption, with all the health-related and social problems that these bring. Our aim was to promote the consumption of small to moderate amounts of wine with food and to emphasise the civilising effects of wine, which is the perfect accompaniment to food, unlike other forms of alcoholic drinks that are better suited to the role of beverages. *Wine: A New Zealand Perspective* ended up being distributed to all medical practitioners in the country, and Don became a member of what was to become known as the Alcohol Advisory Council of New Zealand (ALAC). His powers of persuasion were such that he even managed to persuade the ALAC board, an organisation with a reputation of sombre sobriety and fervent crusades against the Demon Drink, to partake of a little wine at their occasional shared dinners.

The drinking culture in New Zealand in the 1970s and 1980s was only just emerging from the effects of the 'six o'clock swill', which was invoked by the law that all bars and taverns had to close at 6 p.m. This resulted in patrons drinking as many jugs of beer as possible between the end of their work day and the appointed hour. Then they would be unceremoniously thrown out in an inebriated state so that they could happily drive or weave their way home to share their evening meal and bonhomie with their lucky spouses and kids. The law was an unfortunate experiment aimed at curbing drunkenness and promoting the happy family unit, but it did just the opposite. Apart from the occasional glass of spirits, beer was the only drink readily available in pubs and it was guzzled down without food. Only snobs drank wine, and beer was the staff of life for the macho Kiwi bloke. Sharing a glass of wine with your beloved over the evening meal at home was not enticing, because one or both halves of the equation was likely to be well topped up already. The limited number of cafés and restaurants that existed were prohibited from serving drinks with their food, and only in a hotel dining room was it possible to order wine with your meal. Not surprisingly, the New Zealand market for wine was minute, and the size of the New Zealand wine industry reflected this.

Fortunately we have become much more sophisticated in our drinking habits, but our dreams of limiting drunkenness in the young have been frustrated by misguided legislation that has targeted all forms of drinks and punished all classes of drinker, rather than focusing on those that are causing the problem. Having a meaningful legal minimum price for every unit of alcohol would go a long way to improving the situation as the large majority of drinks of abuse are cheap. But allow me to dismount from my hobby horse as I have become all too serious, and permit me to lead you down some other meandering and overgrown vinous paths.

Among those that I wandered down was that of the teacher, which I suppose was only natural, given that another part of my life was devoted to teaching medical students. At first I taught intermittently in the viticulture and winemaking diploma course run by the local technical institute, and later I lectured in the diploma and degree courses at the former Lincoln College, which had morphed into Lincoln University.

Another track I followed was that of the wine writer. Next time you are having your dog shampooed, visiting your podiatrist or nervously waiting to have your teeth drilled, just pick up one of the many magazines that festoon such classy offices of attendance. Casually flick through the pages and the chances are that you will come across a wine column. Every self-respecting magazine or newspaper has one, or so it seems. Naturally, I am excluding specialist publications like *Hunting and Fishing*, *The Vatican Daily* and certain sorts of pornographic literature, which tend to deal with moral and personal issues, often padding out their extra space with glossy photographs rather than informative articles on wine.

It was in the early 1980s that Don Beaven, Graham Watson and I joined forces to write what must have been one of the first regular wine columns in New Zealand. Our only qualifications were that we were all seriously interested in wine, had poured quite a bit of local and international product down our throats, and were self-opinionated and 'ballsy' enough to think that our opinions counted for something. We each produced a column every third week, working as a trio because we felt that our other commitments would not allow a more frequent contribution. At that time the *Christchurch Star* was the city's daily evening newspaper. Having put our toes into the water, or rather the wine, Don and I found that we had enough time, energy and material to write a weekly column as well for the Wellington-based *Dominion Sunday Times*, which later merged with the *Sunday Star* and became the *Sunday Star-Times*.

'The editor of *The Press* wants to see you,' Chris casually dropped into the conversation one evening when we were sharing paella, washed down with a glass of deliciously tangy, lime-flavoured riesling. *The Press* was Christchurch's morning paper and had a larger circulation than the *Christchurch Star*.

'Why? What have I done?' I asked, feeling mystified.

'I had to meet one of the subeditors on opera-related business. The paper has offered to help with Canterbury Opera's next production and I was chosen to sort out the details,' said Chris, who was now a member of the opera company's board. 'It looks as though they are going to come on board in a big way and sponsor the publicity and advertising.'

'What's that got to do with me?'

'Our vineyard and wine-related interests came up in the conversation. When I told him that you were a national and international wine judge his ears pricked up. They have evidently been looking for a wine writer with experience to back up his opinions. I recommended you,' Chris said cheerily. 'You had better make sure you make a good impression. Don't be too modest,' she advised with a wink.

'It would probably mean I would have to write a column every week. That's quite a big ask. I don't know if I would have the time. On the other hand, the stipend would prevent me having to mortgage my mother-in-law every time I wanted to buy a decent bottle for the cellar. That would definitely make it all worthwhile.'

So it came to pass that not only were my evenings occupied by dictating patients' letters but also in writing wine columns, and both of these had to be corrected over my breakfast fruit and muesli. While time and motion studies have never been strengths of mine, I feel proud to have discovered a major efficiency, without which I could not have coped. I found that it was not only possible to do research for my wine columns while dictating my letters, but that a glass of wine also improved the speed and quality of my medical opinions. It was a win-win situation!

I am sure that there are those amongst you who think that being a wine writer is a cushy job and one for which you would happily volunteer if you were so asked to sacrifice yourselves. I will admit that there are times when it rises above the tolerable, but it also calls for a good deal of self-control to avoid letting oneself be seduced by junkets and freebies. Wine companies are inclined to offer you lunches, dinners and trips in order to show off their wares, which you have to judge impartially. Then there are what I call 'mushrooms', those tempting little things that appear out of nowhere, often in clusters. When you open the front door in the morning you may do yourself a serious injury by tripping over a heap of unsolicited packages that couriers have left. A few of these mushrooms will be magic, while most are modest and a few mediocre. You always hope that there are none that are really toadstools. Each package contains one or more bottles.

It is hard to be a wine writer without accepting wine samples because you are much more likely to strain yourself lifting up one of the mushrooms than you are by picking up your pay packet. You would need a serious private income if you were to buy all the wines you need to try to keep up to date. However, should you truly aspire to the doubtfully noble profession of wine writing then there are two things that you must remember before all else: firstly, you are writing for the reader and not the wine producer, and secondly, the truth lies in the glass. Because of the latter I never actually picked up the mushrooms, but rather grandiosely left this to Chris. I thus remained blind to what the harvest had brought.

In wine writing, just as in viticulture and winemaking, I had gone my own way, but I still worked closely with Graham Watson and Don Beaven, who cultivated their own little mushroom patches. On Sunday nights our heaps of fungi would be put together and one of our wives would arrange the wines in flights of like varieties, then serve them blind for evaluation. Since the bottles were masked, not even she knew exactly which wine was in each flight. Every wine was personally scored by each of us and our friends Bruce and Marie Todd, and then discussed before its identity was revealed. All wines were thus evaluated by eight experienced tasters and given the same stage on which to strut its stuff. Our only clue to what we had tasted lay in our glasses. We found this gave each wine the fairest chance to shine, enabling us to tell our readers the truth, at least as we saw it. Naturally, I never showed our own wines or commented on them in my columns.

Although wine writing proved to be a lot of work, I never found it hard because I enjoyed it thoroughly, not only the liquid research but the actual writing. It made a pleasant change from that of the medical fraternity — the staid, cautious language of consultation reports and the dry, dusty words of scientific articles and books. I revelled in the change of writing style between the worlds of medicine and wine, between the factual movement disorder book that I was working on and the throwaway newspaper articles on what to drink. Wine writing opened doors, and none were more important to me than those of wineries. Because of my connections it was now possible to visit almost any national or international winery and find out what made it tick, how the grapes were grown, how the wines were made and, more importantly, it allowed me to taste the wines and to understand them. It was inspirational stuff to an aspiring grape grower and winemaker, and I tried to interpret it into the vernacular of my own situation; to find the best direction for Chris and me to paddle our own little vinous canoe, which was at risk of losing its way without clear navigation and destinations.

Occasionally, people wanted to fête us, and although the purists among you would doubtless have turned down such offers, we felt it would be churlish not to allow ourselves to be pampered once in a while, like the time we were guests of the Champagne House of Moët & Chandon at its Château de Seran. Multiple silver-service dishes were presented by white-gloved waiters, and naturally there was a special Champagne to accompany each course. We rubbed shoulders with the rich and famous and slept in Moët and Chandon's wedding beds (yes, that's right, they were two single beds), complete with those abominable French pillows or *polochons* that look and feel like large logs. Perhaps, however, the happy honeymoon couple were not intent on sleeping. Unlike the other guests, who chugged off the following morning in their Lamborghinis, Porsches and the like, Chris and I had to be taken to the local railway station by the chauffeur. He looked decidedly downcast when we insisted on carrying our own luggage and scuttled off down the platform to find our second-class carriage for the trip back to Paris.

Champagne is a curiosity, in that it is almost the only wine area in the world where the high ground has been seized by the big players. In virtually every other region the small to medium-sized wineries and the boutiques are regarded as the most prestigious producers. In Champagne it is the other way around, and any budding marketing guru ignores this anomaly at his or her peril, for that is what it is based on: marketing. It is not that the big houses or *Grandes Marques* produce rubbish. They do not, but their wines are no better than those of many an *artisan producteur* or small Champagne house, and in some cases they are not as good. The *Grandes Marques*, however, have one of the most sophisticated marketing systems in the world for selling luxury goods at high prices. There is an unwritten rule that they promote the region as a whole and that one *champenois* does not criticise others or say that his or her own product is superior. That would be far to crass.

A wine-merchant friend of mine organised a large tasting of Champagnes and, surprise, surprise, the *Grande Marque* that he represented came out on top. Naturally he advertised its success in the local newspaper, but within a week he had been contacted by the producers of the fine product. He was told that if he did not cease to promote their wine in this way they would withdraw his right to represent them. Of course, *champenois* compete, but they do not cut each other's throats. If they forced their neighbour to his knees he might sell his product cheaply. What would that do to the image of the world's priciest party-maker, which on the side launches thousands of ships? Who would gain? The marketing of Champagne is much more subtle, and while hard times have forced direct advertising on some of the houses, most of their substantial promotional budget goes on supporting associations with prestigious events or other luxury goods, and on high-flying PR. They promote themselves by the company they keep.

Some years after our little sortie to Château de Seran, we paid a visit to one of our favourite *artisans producteurs*, Huré Frères. It was a beautiful sunny afternoon and we were sitting with the Huré family on their lawn about to start lunch when François, a delightful young scion of the tribe, who had worked two vintages at our own winery in Waipara Valley, held up his glass in a welcoming gesture and in a thick French accent proudly proposed, 'Up your bum!'

His family beamed approvingly while the Watson's, Chris and I sat stunned, our glasses frozen in the raised position. Then we broke into laughter. It is well known in the medical profession that Gallic doctors have a strange penchant for prescribing their treatment by suppository or pessary, but I had never heard of wine, let alone Champagne, being administered by this route. It seemed a strange custom and I wondered if it made the mousse more titillating or easier to appreciate. Then it dawned on me. After all, the French themselves have a similar toast, *cul sec*, the literal translation of which is 'dry bum'.

'Don't let us hold you back, but we will decline this one. I think that the expression you probably want, François, is "Bottoms up". It has quite a different meaning from the one you have just used,' I corrected him as tactfully as I could.

'Oh, I am sorry,' a flustered-looking François replied, reddening. 'When I worked at your winery Bridget told me it was the right thing to say.'

'Well, she must have been trying to play a trick on you because it is really a bit rude. At any rate, "Bottoms up" really means to drain your glass in a single gulp and I don't think you want us to do that to your very delicious Champagne. We want to take our time to savour it. Perhaps it's best just to say "Good health".'

I laughed inwardly when I thought of the rascally Bridget leading François astray. She had worked for us at the same time as he had, and she would have loved to have seen the result of her mischief. Luckily François enjoyed the joke and had a good laugh at his own expense.

**I HAD BEEN WINE WRITING** for almost 20 years when the first columns on beer appreciation began to appear in newspapers and magazines. They extolled the enticements of this ale over that and the niceties of one lager versus another. They talked about the big producers and the microbreweries. This was fair enough and it was all good stuff, but beer had been produced in the motherland and its colonies for eons and nobody had paid it much attention in print. Everyone had their preferences, but they knew what they were and they ordered them. The brews remained faithful and consistent from year to year because they were made from a recipe. You didn't have to read about them. If a brewery started a new line or wanted to promote itself then it reached the public by direct advertising. It did not need some fancy column to promote it. If the wine industry was David, then the breweries were Goliath; they were where the real money was.

At some point a bright beer-company accountant had noticed that something strange was beginning to happen. The figures on the bottom line did not look as rosy as they had in the past. They were still black but they were gradually becoming smaller. The accountant puzzled over this for a long time: it could not be, it was against all natural laws. The brewing industry's profit had not become so small that he needed to put on his glasses but he did that at any rate. In looking up to the shelf where he had left them he found the cause of the problem. And in doing so, he found the cause of the problem. The figures on the top line had shrunk and this had trickled through to the bottom. Yes, from the 1970s through to the 1990s, while wine was becoming more popular and its sales had been increasing, those of beer had been heading south. In spite of the heroic advertising budgets, the giant billboards and the attempts to piggyback on football, rugby and other macho sports, blokes were drinking less beer. To make matters worse, amalgamation of distribution had produced fierce competition in the marketplace so that selling breweries' fine products on promotion had become the norm. All this was causing the worrying loss of fat around the profit line's middle; although at no stage did it threaten to become anorexic.

News of the accountant's discovery was gradually passed up the line until it reached the boardroom, where it threatened to upset the digestion of the directors' agreeable lunch. The CEO was directed to hire consultants and to report back ASAP.

After extensive and expensive consultations the CEO had a 'Eureka!' moment. 'If you can't beat 'em, join 'em — or rather, buy 'em!'

So plump men in suits, flashing toothy smiles and fat cheque books, appeared between the rows of vines and popped out from behind barrels, making offers that only the brain-dead would refuse. Now everybody would be happy, and so they were, at least for a while.

Slowly, it dawned on the new owners that wine is not like beer, and vineyards and wineries are not like breweries. Wine is not like Coca-Cola that can be made from a recipe, as needed, in any amount required, from reasonably cheap ingredients, in a cost-effective factory in which the plant and equipment are in continuous use and with a profit margin that is readily calculated. No, wine is a product of raw nature, with all its unpredictable foibles, including frosts, reduced crop levels, hail, birds, fungal diseases and the like. It is capital-intensive and ties up a lot of plant and equipment that is only used for several weeks of the year. You do not have a consistent product from one year to another; each vintage is different. The worst revelation, however, was yet to come: wineries are not as profitable as breweries!

Thus, brewers lost their enthusiasm for buying into the wine industry and decided to stick to their knitting but they needed to increase their sales. To make this work they had to lure back previous 'beer-totallers' and bring on board new drinkers. And what better way to do this than by using the experience they had gained from dabbling in the wine industry? Why not encourage the media, which benefited from the brewers' advertising budgets, to promote interest in different types of beer? Would not beer columns do just that?

The phenomenon of brewers, and even soft-drink-makers, buying into the wine industry and then becoming disillusioned with their purchases was international, not just a local aberration. In the end most of these corporate high-rollers on sold their purchases.

Almost 20 years after I had first put pen to paper to help fill newspaper space, I received a letter from the editor of a circulation for which I was writing, informing me that my services were no longer required. Not long before, the publication had started to publish an erudite column on beer, and the author had written an article saying what simple stuff wine was compared with beer. All you had to do to make wine was to ferment the grape juice. In effect, wine made itself, and the winemaker's task was simple. The brewer's art, however, required much greater skill because beer and related beverages had to be constructed, according to a recipe or formula, from multiple ingredients, many of which had to be treated in a special way before being incorporated into the final brew. Beer was thus a much more complex and interesting drink than wine.

I have never claimed to be a phlegmatic individual and so I rose to the bait, thinking it would all be a bit of fun. I wrote a tongue-in-cheek article, explaining what a pure and natural product wine was: in essence, liquid sunshine stitched together with the finest poetry. You did not even have to add yeast. The winemaker only had to gently guide the process to make certain it did not go astray. By comparison, beer was a concocted drink and needed to be manufactured according to specific formulae, often secret, and the brewer was more like a chemist. These two articles were published within a week or so of each other, and it was just a few weeks later that I received my letter of dismissal from the editor. Not satisfied, I asked to see him. The brief interview was tense. Although it was not explicitly stated, I came away with the distinct impression that beer barons, who contributed very significantly to the publication's advertising budget, had senses of humour inversely proportional to their purchasing power.

It was irritating, but what the heck? I had had a good run and I had benefited enormously from the experience of tasting and critically analysing so many different types of wine from so many wine regions of the world over such a long period. This experience had been vital in helping me to decide what types of wine I wanted to make myself.

**WELL, IF THE PRICE OF WRITING** all those columns and articles seems too high to pay for the privilege of sipping the odd glass of free wine, then how about having a crack at wine judging? It may sound like a cushy number but, having judged wine competitions both nationally and internationally for over 20 years let me assure you, it is not.

My formal induction into the gentle art had come a few years after I started wine writing and probably because of it. I am not really certain, because I just received a letter out of the blue inviting me to be an associate judge at the Air New Zealand Wine Awards, the wine industry's main annual competition. I guessed that my babblings must have come to the attention of somebody high up. In those days there were few who were silly or egotistical enough to put their vinous opinions in print, so that I must have stood out like a sore thumb. The fledgling wine industry had kept a tight rein on this show and its predecessor, the New Zealand National Wine Competition. Most of the judges were professional winemakers. As an associate, I was like a paralysed arm, an ineffective fourth member attached to three strong ones, and that is how it should have been, for I was there to learn and to be judged myself.

I went through the motions of judging and, in spite of my scores being recorded and my opinion politely listened to, they played no part in the ultimate decisions of the powerful triumvirate of senior judges. Although I often felt foolish showering praise on wines that the real winemakers dismissed as seriously faulty, or marking down those that they judged worthy of gold medals, I guess I must have slowly learned because after three or four years I was promoted to being a real judge.

If you want to become seriously involved you have to be prepared to give up quite a lot of your time, and for me this meant chewing into my holiday allowance. A small regional competition may take only a few hours but a national show may run into several days, while an international one may tie you up for a week or more, including the travel. The format is also quite variable. At competitions sanctioned by the OIV — the Office International de la Vigne et du Vin, an intergovernmental body based in Paris — communication between judges is *interdit*. Thus, every one of the five judges on each of the panels sits in a separate booth, proudly sporting their national flag. They all receive the same wine at the same time and they score its many attributes on a pre-printed page, according to a highly structured system. The pages are then pounced upon by the minions of the number-crunchers and the next wine is ceremoniously delivered up to the slaughtermen. A wine's performance is based on its averaged total score, which is very fair and democratic but, as in elections, the winner may be a candidate that nobody thinks is the best; merely a mediocre performer that nobody hates. In one such competition in which I judged, to everybody's surprise the champion red wine turned out to be Japanese.

'This is a very generous, full-bodied red wine,' I commented as I sipped the wine and congratulated the proud Japanese judge standing beside me at the awards ceremony. It seemed like an Australian Shiraz puffed up with a fair dollop of American oak. 'I didn't know you made this sort of wine in Japan.'

'Yiz, velly good. Law in Japan zay only need 5 per cent Japan vine to call Japanese.'

This was quite a number of years ago and I suspect the scrupulously strict Nipponese may well have tightened up their regulations.

As mentioned, the five judges on each OIV panel are forbidden to discuss the wines while judging and thus do not work as a team. This is probably just as well, because by regulation they all come from different countries, and frequently they do not speak a common language. I certainly found that my Turkish, Bulgarian and Croatian language skills, to mention only a few, were a bit rusty. The official language of communication is usually French. Like many of my époque, I did three years of French at high school before dropping it like a hot potato (which I now much regret). I thus had a rudimentary grasp of the language, but still I found that the judges' briefing sessions were a little hard to follow.

During one such competition there was an extraordinary meeting of all judges one morning to discuss a catastrophe that had occurred the day before. The organisers were clearly very embarrassed, more so, I suspect, by my presence than by the actual matter at hand. Had I been more wicked than usual? Why were they so upset? It took me some time to work out what was happening. *Quelle horreur!* Something terrible had come to pass. A cheeky little New Zealand wine had won the fortified sweet wine section, beating all of the grand Spanish sherries and Portuguese ports. However, *Dieu merci*, a solution was at hand. This dastardly little new-world pretender had been arrogant enough to label itself as 'port' and, after the OIV regulations had been consulted, it was discovered that such insolence had been outlawed by the European Union. The fact that the wine may have been bottled and labelled before the law came into effect was of no matter. It was unceremoniously discarded, in spite of my protests regarding the process. Surely, I argued, it should have been eliminated from the competition before the judging, which would have avoided embarrassment and saved the entrant some money.

In these OIV competitions you never seem to taste more than about 12 wines without a half-hour gap for a cuppa, or judge more than about 50 wines over a day in case you might abuse your palate. The pace is so leisurely that an army of judges is required and the event can be expected to run for several days. Generally half of each day is spent judging and the rest is sightseeing. Because there are so many judges, whose expenses need to be covered, the fees for entering these competitions can be eye-watering for small producers.

**IT WAS DARK BUT WARM INSIDE** the small, rustic inn-cum-restaurant, and there was a comforting log fire in the hearth that was throwing shafts of light dancing over the rough-sawn wooden walls. A delicious gamey smell wafted in from the kitchen, enticing our salivary glands into free-flowing action. We were a smallish band who had ventured deep into the Slovenian countryside, as many in the judging circus had crashed on their beds back in Ljubljana, exhausted by the hard morning's work. I had asked for the menu, but the interpreter told me that such a thing did not exist. The restaurant served the same meal to all the guests, changing this from day to day as befitted their whim and the available produce. Judging by the tempting aroma that wafted from the kitchen they knew what they were doing, so I relaxed back and sipped a little of the house red, which came in a carafe and suited the unpretentious atmosphere of the establishment.

'Goodness gracious me!' exclaimed Chris after our generously laden plates had arrived. 'This meat is fantastic, so savoury and rich.'

'Yes,' I agreed, 'both the meat and the gravy are so dark and tasty. It's almost as though they have been caramelised without any sugar, if that makes any sense.'

'It's a bit chewy. I guess that's because the fibres are so big. Surprisingly, this rough red wine suits it, perhaps because they are both a bit coarse. The roast vegetables are equally delicious.'

We had finished the main course by the time the waiter reappeared and our interpreter could ask the question that had been on everybody's lips.

'What is this beautiful meat that we are eating?'

After an earnest discussion, which seemed to go on for an age, the embarrassed translator turned to us and confessed, 'That meat be bear, Slovenian brown bear from forest.'

We were aghast at the thought, and started to protest. I was not exactly a gastronomic pussycat and in my time had savoured such delightful morsels as raw Australian witchetty grubs, Japanese sea worms, Peruvian guinea pigs, turtle steaks and similar exotica. I had never quite understood why Anglo-Saxons consider ungulates with a single hoof as sacrosanct while those with two are fair game. While the thought of eating horse can invoke hysteria we happily sink our fangs into the gentle brown cow that devotedly provides us with milk, cream, butter and cheese. What have these latter creatures done to deserve the ignominy of being ground up and served to teenagers in McDonald's, while beasts of burden get off scot free? Having been served both horse and foal and having considered them to be delicious, I cannot see what the fuss is about.

This, however, was different. What a sacrilege! We had mental images of a cuddly, furry, gentle giant of the forest being sacrificed for our eating pleasure, and it was enough to raise our ire.

As we started to protest the interpreter added, 'Him child molester. He come out of forest and attack children in school yard. Take him back to forest several time but he come back always to school so police shoot him. Pity to waste, no?'

A wave of contentment and self-righteousness flowed over us as we settled back in our chairs and greedily wiped the remaining gravy from our plates with pieces of crusty bread. Our translator went on to explain that these brown bears had once been common in mountain ranges throughout Europe, including the Pyrénées, where they had since died out. Because of this they had recently been reintroduced into the Pyrénées but he had heard that the bears had caused problems and were regarded as a danger to humans. I suspected that the wily locals were more likely to be a danger to the bears. It would be hard to ignore such a delicious protein source that had suddenly arrived in their midst.

If OIV-style wine competitions do not sound like palate-breaking work the same cannot be said for the average wine competition in the English-speaking world, including Australia and New Zealand. How would you fancy being confronted with a flight of 30 or 40 glasses of sauvignon blanc, chardonnay, riesling or similar to help you wash off your toothpaste at 8.30 in the morning? But that would only be the start. You would then be expected to continue in a similar fashion throughout the day, eventually finishing at about 5 or 6 p.m., by which time you may have evaluated between 150 and 200 wines. In order to survive the day you have to repeat to yourself the rule of the six S's (Swirl, Sniff, Slurp, Spit, Synthesise and Score) before you leave the trenches and go over the top.

You cannot afford to let your concentration slip or your mind wander. Not only will you have to score each wine for colour, bouquet, taste, body, balance, mouth feel and the like, but you will also need to write notes. This is because at the end of the bracket all the judges who have been working on the same flight (three plus one or two associates) will sit down and compare their scores and impressions in order to come up with a final mark for each wine. If there is any significant difference between the individual judges' scores on particular wines, these may be retasted by the panel until a consensus is reached.

This is real teamwork and not just averaging numbers. It also has the advantage of enabling direct comparisons between different wines in the same class, something that the OIV system does not allow. Any judge can argue the case for or against any particular wine. Potential disadvantages are that a self-proclaimed prophet can dominate a panel and that unstoppable forces may meet immovable objects. In the event of a likely gladiatorial fight to the death, the panel leader takes the case to appeal. The competition's chief judge adjudicates before mopping up the blood and applying salve to the wounds. Should you suffer from chronic fatigue syndrome, attention deficit disorder or an inferiority complex then this little pastime is definitely not for you.

A show with a difference is the Sydney International Wine Competition, at which I judged regularly for well over a decade. This consisted of two phases and had elements of both the show systems mentioned above. The first phase culled out the liquid junk while the remainder went on to the second stage. In this phase small groups of like wines were judged against a suitable dish, the idea being to eat a mouthful of food in between trying each of the wines. This fusion of chemistry in the mouth can certainly have a modifying effect on the appreciation of wines. A plain Jane may be given a facelift by the dish or a pert little number can seem like a street tart alongside refined food. It was about finding wines that shone with food, rather than just being good drinks. Each competition was a week of enforced haute cuisine organised by the genial, rubicund and generously proportioned Warren Mason and his master chef French wife, Jacqueline, whose culinary skills gave me new understanding of food addiction. In spite of adhering religiously to the rule of the six S's, it was always necessary to go on a prolonged post-competition starvation diet or lash out on a new wardrobe. Being a congenital miser, I opted for the former prescription. Emptying the spittoon buckets after this competition was not a task for the faint-hearted.

**HAVE YOU EVER WONDERED** who polices the police? It is an important question that receives a lot of media attention these days. An equally valid conundrum is who judges the judges? Our judiciary have to go through a long period of training in order to be accredited and appointed, but once they are bewigged they often appear to be a law unto themselves. Putting oneself up for assessment of proficiency, particularly if done in public, would not be appealing to 'Your Honour'. While being a wine judge is not remotely in the same league as being a legal egghead, the shells surrounding the egos can be just as brittle. How good is this self-important judge at telling one wine from another?

It was thus with some trepidation that Don Beaven, Graham Watson, Bill Smith and I formed a team and entered the National Wine Options Competition under the banner of 'The Physicians Wine Society'. Don, Graham and I had become competition wine judges but Bill had probably drunk more fine wine than the three of us put together.

It was a rain-lashed, wintry day and the room was cold as a morgue, or rather, a museum, for that is what it really was. We were in the Auckland Museum at the national finals. We had qualified by winning the Canterbury competition some weeks earlier and we were now sitting in a room with what seemed like 30 or 40 other teams, reduced down from the hundreds that had originally entered. We were all competing for the generous booty of prestigious wines that was displayed at the front of the room. We all had the same blind wine in our glasses, and we had to indicate the answers to the questions being asked by marking our individual examination sheets, of which there was one for every query. There were five questions to be answered on each of the mystery wines, which could come from any vineyard region of the world — four questions to be answered individually and one as a team. Grape varieties, methods of production, country, viticultural region, year of vintage, name of the winemaker and other related trivia were all possible brain-teasers.

The questions were being asked by the devilish Kingsley Wood, who was enjoying himself immensely. He grinned widely as he announced the correct answer to each question, after the papers relating to it had been collected. Slowly peeling away the layers of mystery surrounding each bottle built up a striptease-like tension as the competition progressed. Each of Kingsley's pronouncements was greeted by excited cheers and wails of agony. The room was a colourful sight, with many in fancy dress to match their clever and sometimes raunchy team names. More than a few had brought supporters, who sat around the walls sipping and adding their hubbub to the general party atmosphere. We felt pathetically tame beside the other teams' dashing monikers and gaudy splendour. We knew, however, that behind the general party atmosphere there was a lot of serious concentration and expertise amongst the rival teams.

We had come to the last wine of the afternoon. The scores and placings of the individual teams had been announced after each of the earlier wines was revealed. We were neck and neck with another team. Had the temperature in the room dropped even further or was I just in a cold sweat? As someone who had sat in judgement over many clammy examination candidates you would think I would have found it easy to tell, but I did not. I had to keep reminding myself that the result of our examination, or rather inquisition, was not really important.

'After all, we are supposed to be doing it for a bit of a laugh,' I told myself. 'Take a look at the festive atmosphere around us and relax.' As I looked up from my glass my eyes happened to light on the table of impressive prizes and I heard myself mumbling, 'Don't lose your concentration yet. There are only a few more moments to go.'

The answers to the first questions had established that the wine was a very good claret from an excellent Bordeaux vintage, and we now had to identify which of three famous châteaux it came from. We had only seconds left in which to come up with a team answer and we were divided.

'Let's go with experience,' suggested Don. 'We'll follow your instinct, Bill. You write down what you think it is.'

And that is how we won the New Zealand National Wine Options Competition and the judges were judged; more or less by fluke and on the coat-tails of a non-judge. I would not want to pretend that this was the only year in which the competition was held, but it was the only time we topped

New Zealand. Some years later, however, Chris and I had the satisfaction of seeing our vineyard and winery team, consisting of Lynnette Hudson, our viticulturalist Martin Tillard, and our sons Matthew and Edward, walk away with the same distinction. Unlike the boring old 'Physicians' team, they did not take themselves seriously and went along in party mood, colourfully dressed as their favourite pop group of the time, The Village People. They say that wine is clear proof that God wants you to enjoy yourself, and I am inclined to agree.

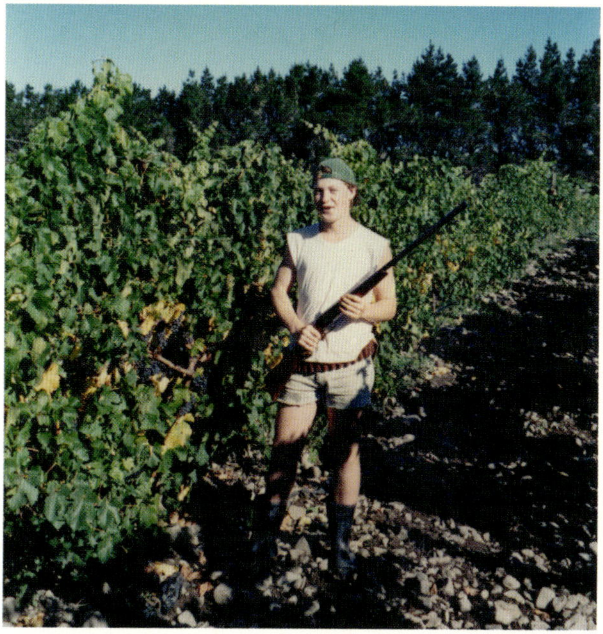

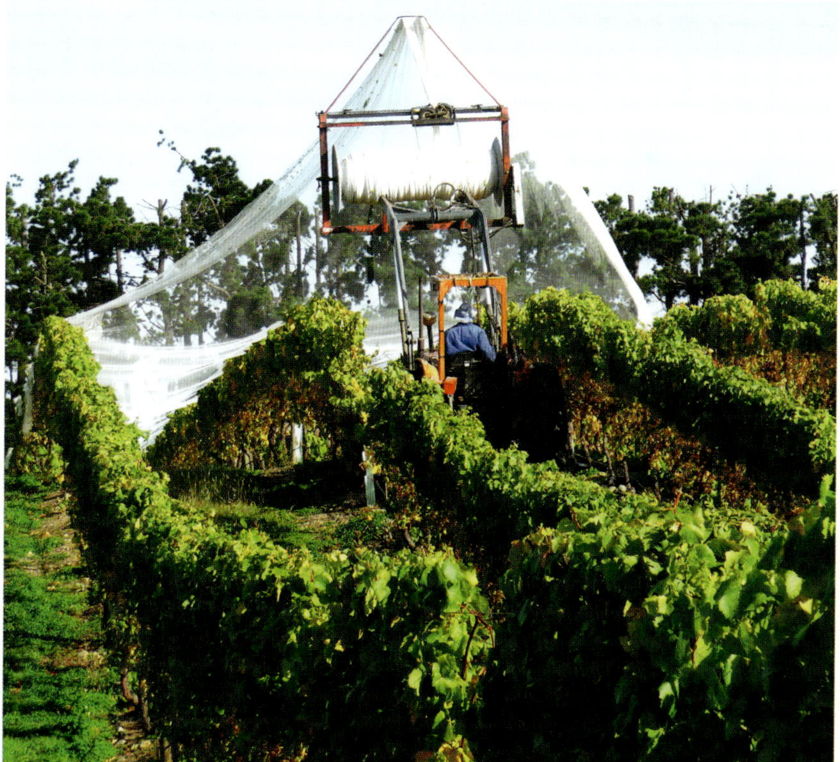

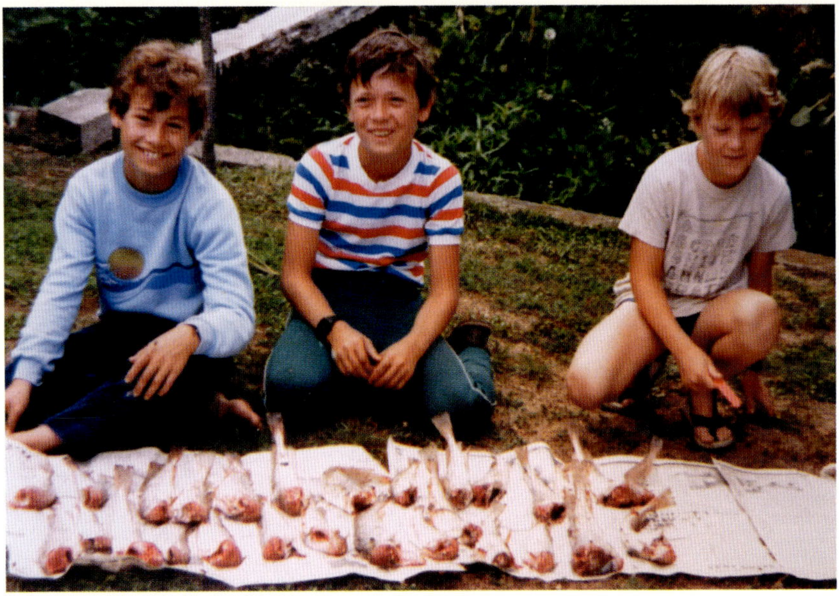

**PRECEDING PAGE ABOVE**
Paul bird-scaring in the vineyard, 1991.

**PRECEDING PAGE BELOW**
Taking the bird nets off the vines prior to harvest, autumn, 2012.

**ABOVE**
Michael, Edward and Paul with the daily catch of cod caught off the end of the Akaroa wharf, 1986.

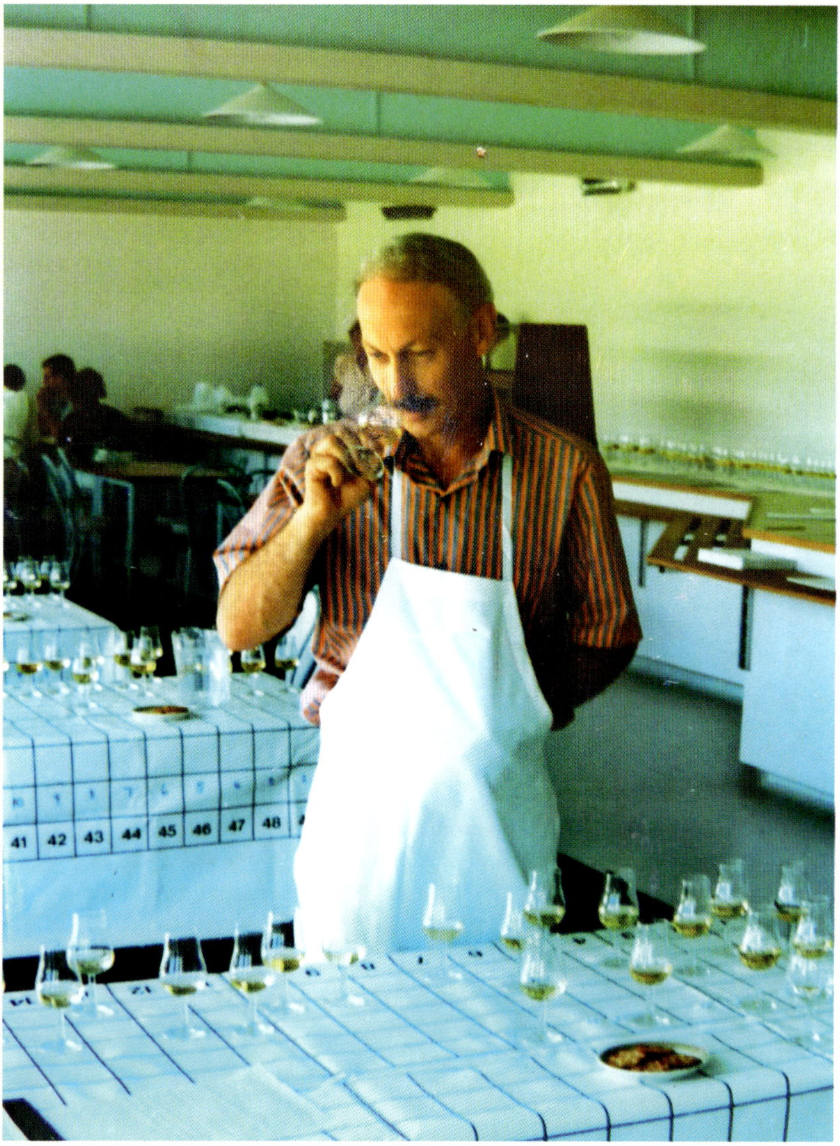


**ABOVE**
Ivan judging in a wine competition, 2000.

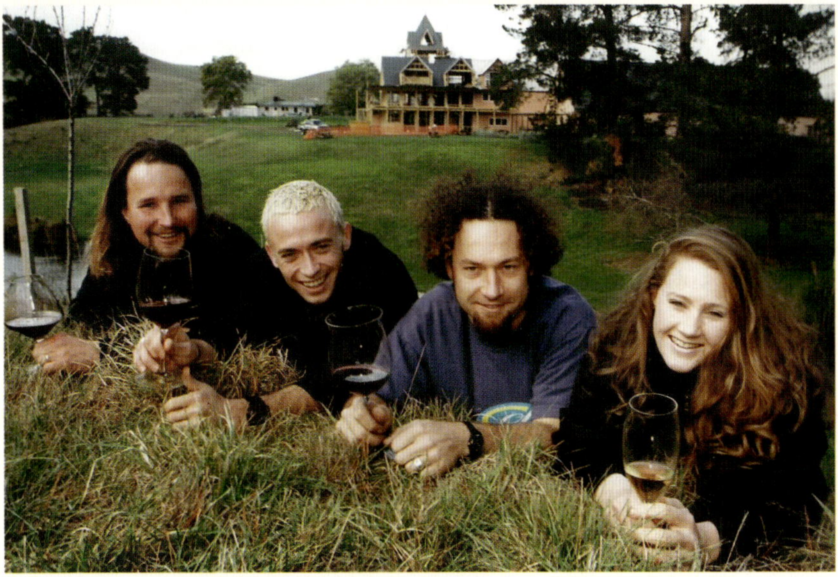

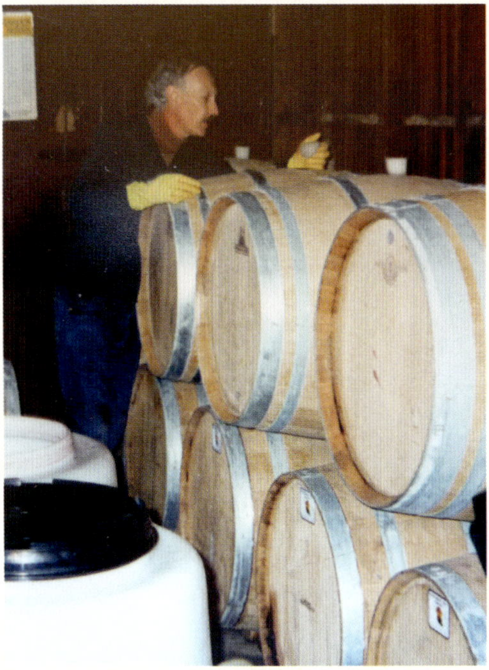

**ABOVE**
Winners of 1998 New Zealand National Wine Options Competition. From left: Martin Tillard, viticulturist, Edward, Matthew and Lynnette. Stage three of the Pegasus Winery under construction in the background.

**LEFT**
'Garagist' Ivan making the first vintage of Pegasus Bay wine in his garage at Christchurch, 1991.

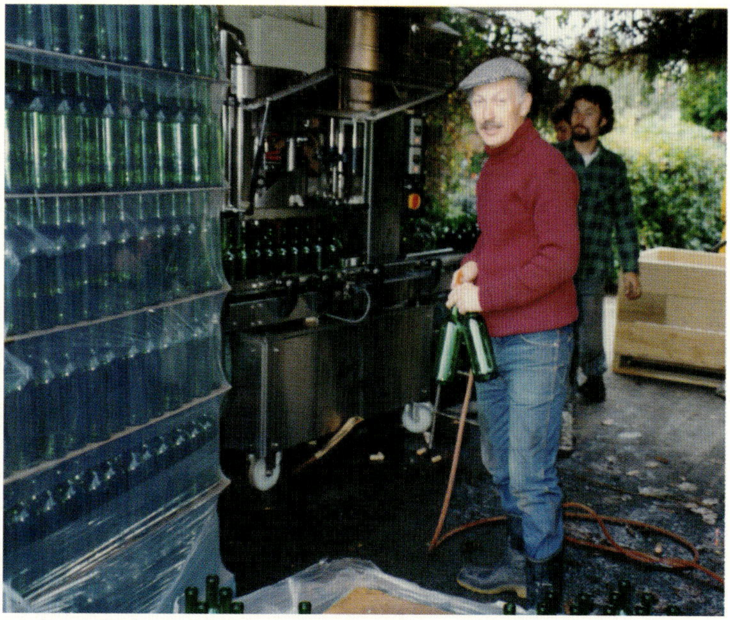

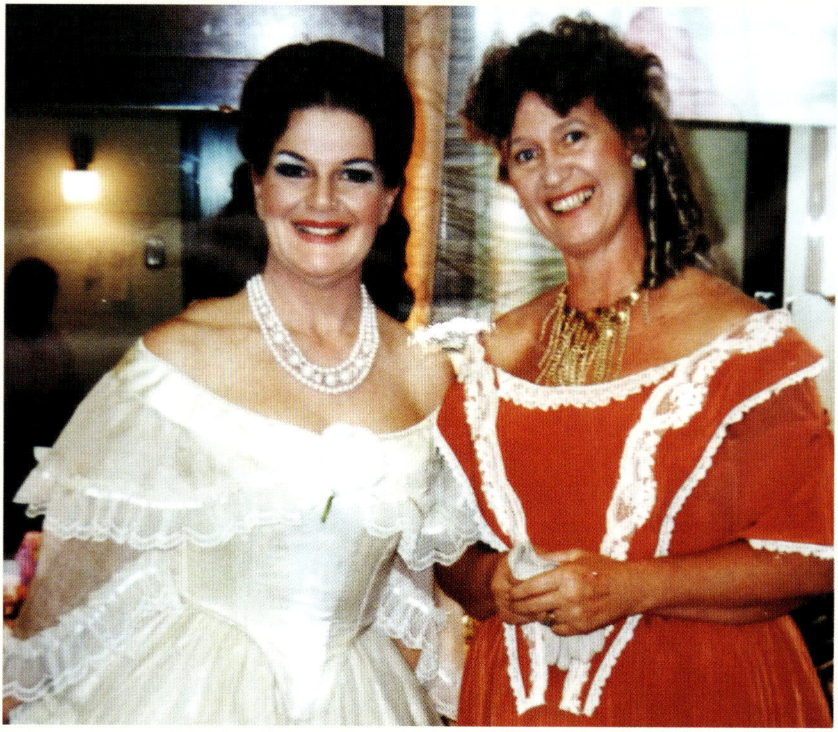

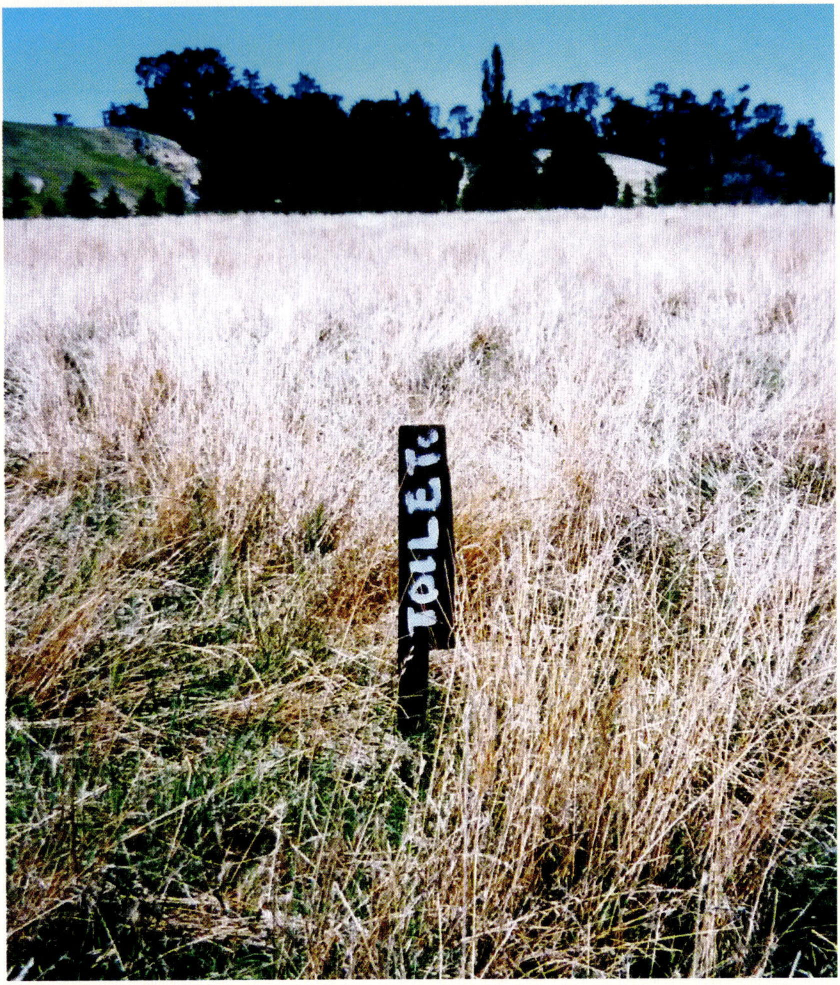


**PRECEDING PAGE ABOVE**
Ivan and Matthew bottling the first vintage of Pegasus Bay wine in the driveway of the house in Christchurch, 1992.

**PRECEDING PAGE BELOW**
Malvina Major and Chris (chorus girl) singing in the opera *Lucia di Lammermoor*, Christchurch, 1993.

**ABOVE**
The vital landmark that determined the exact site of the winery complex, 1992.

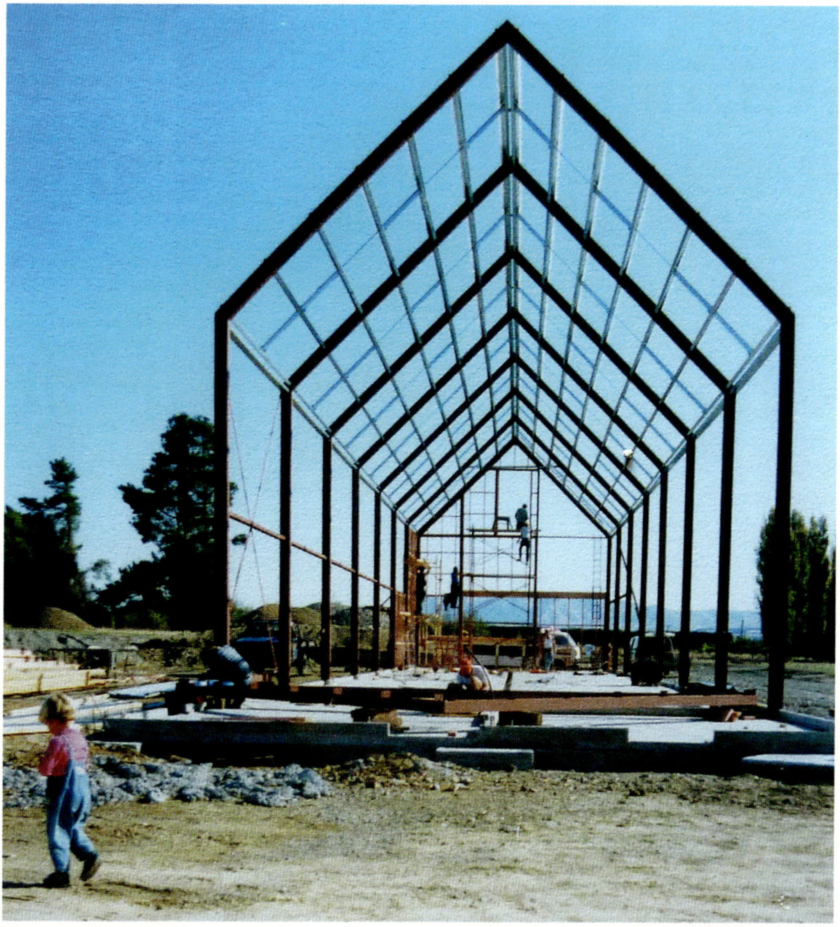

**ABOVE**
The first stage of the winery under construction, 1992.

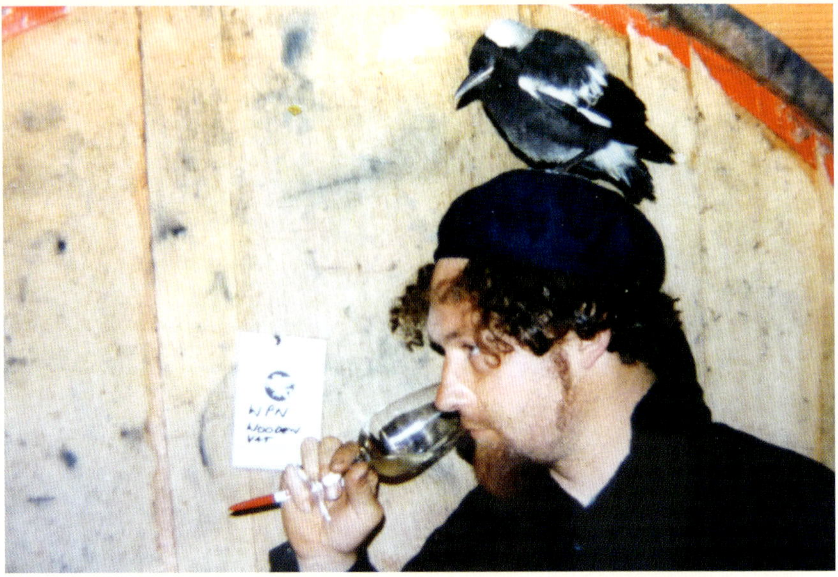


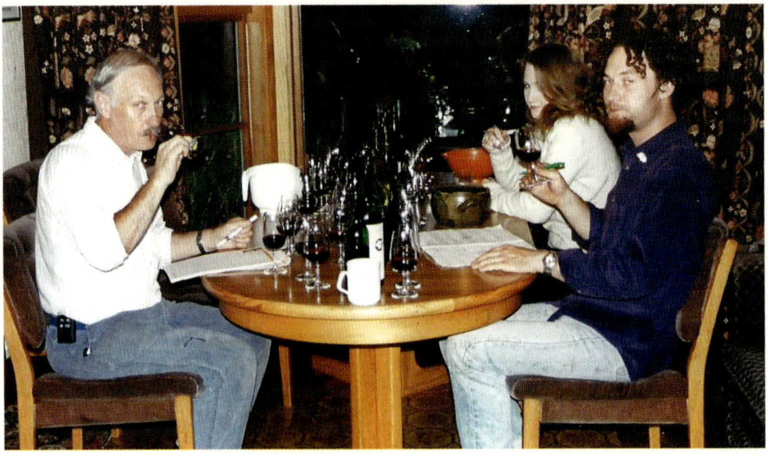

**ABOVE**

Matthew with the pet magpie he reared from abandoned chick, 1998.

**ABOVE**

Ivan, Matthew and Lynnette blending Pegasus Bay Pinot Noir, 1995.

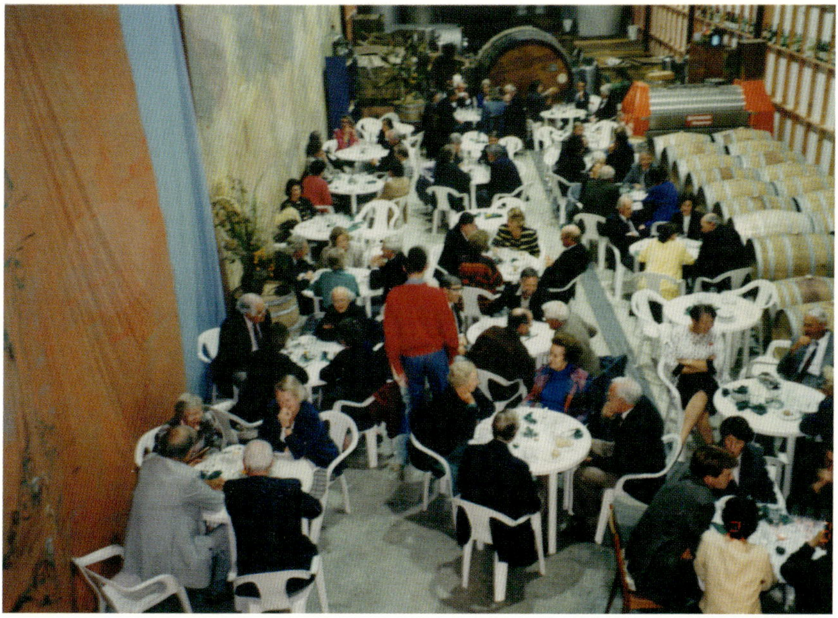

**ABOVE**
Dining in the first restaurant (in the fermentation hall) at Pegasus Bay, 1993.

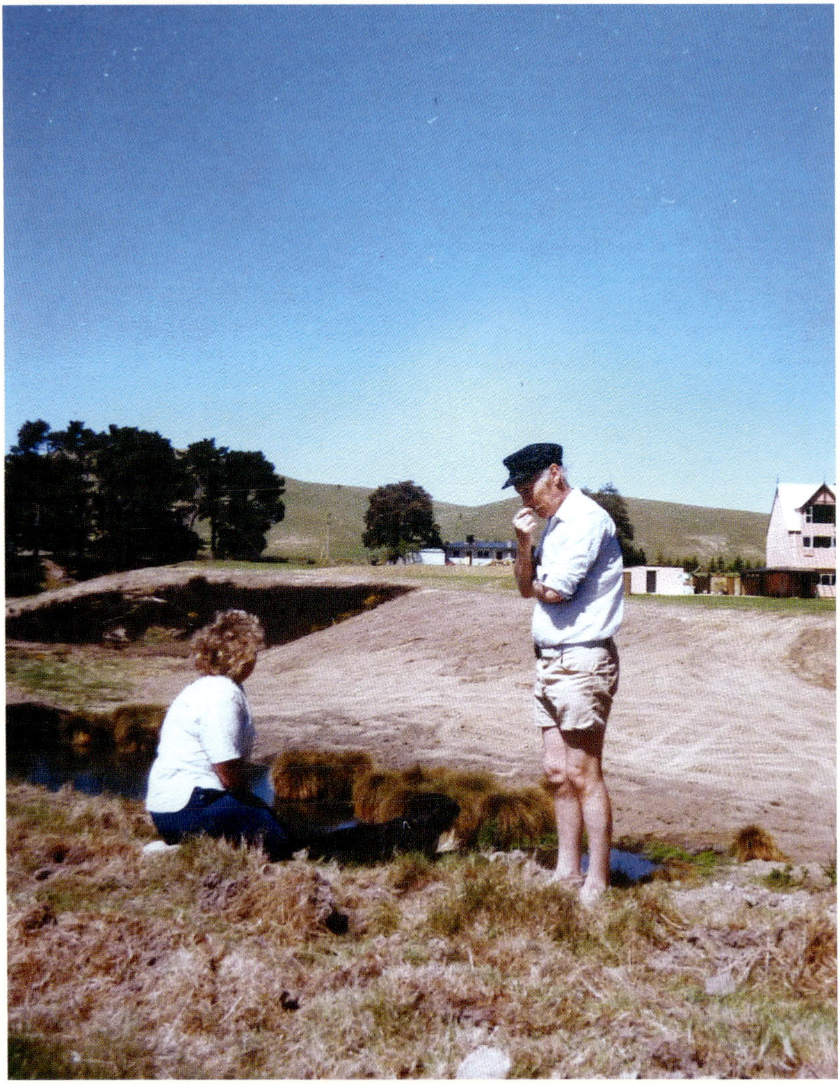

**ABOVE**
Chris and Ivan pondering what to do with the cleared gully and its environs, with stage one of the winery development in the background, 1993.

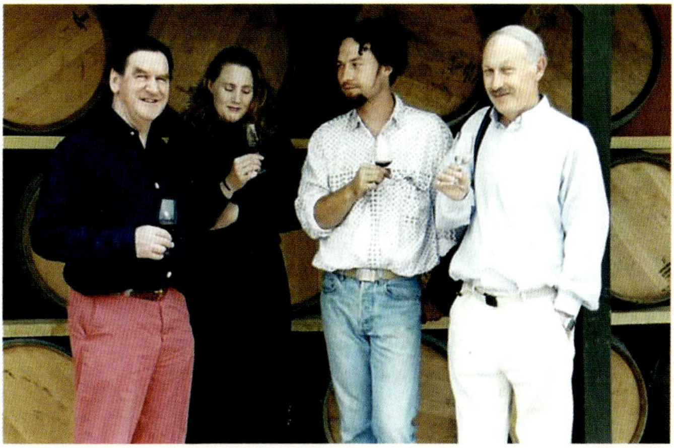

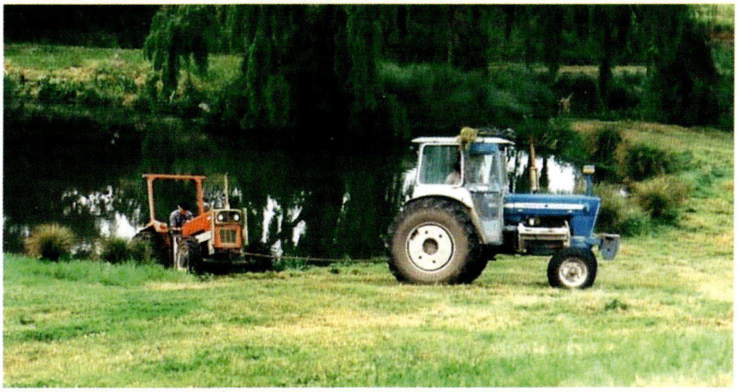

**ABOVE**
Hugh Johnson, Lynnette, Matthew and Ivan at Pegasus Bay, 1995.

**BELOW**
A bedraggled and shamefaced Ivan is pulled from the lake for the second time by good Samaritan neighbour, Graham Croft, 1996.

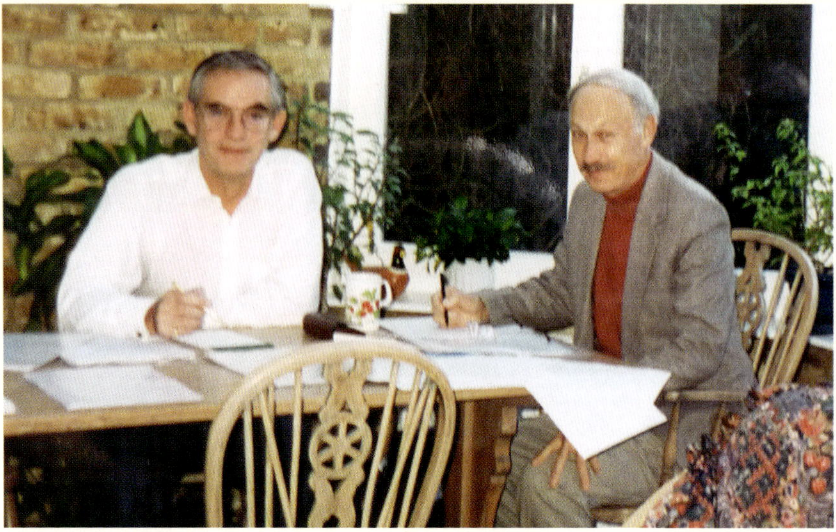

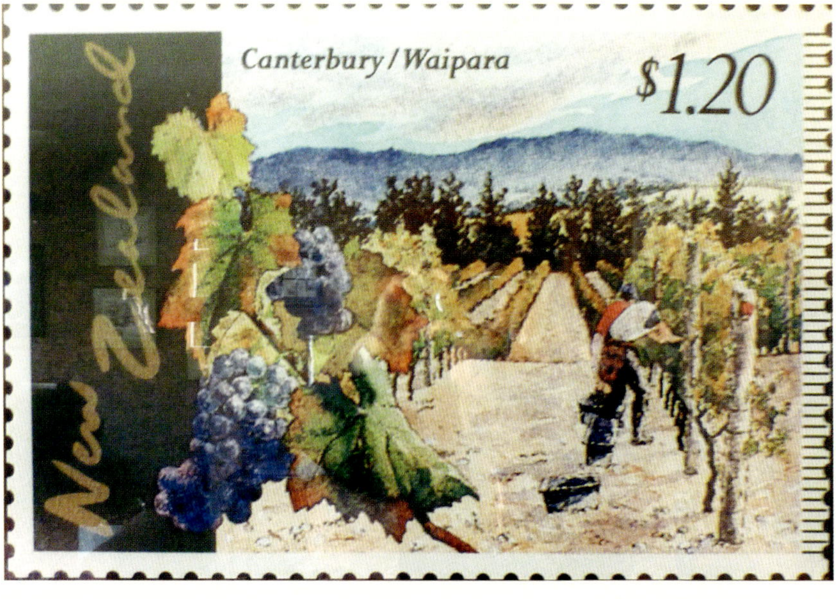


**ABOVE**
David Marsden and Ivan working on the movement disorder book at David's home in Ash, Kent, England, 1995.

**BELOW**
A New Zealand postage stamp featuring Pegasus Bay vineyard with Paul and friend picking grapes, 1997.

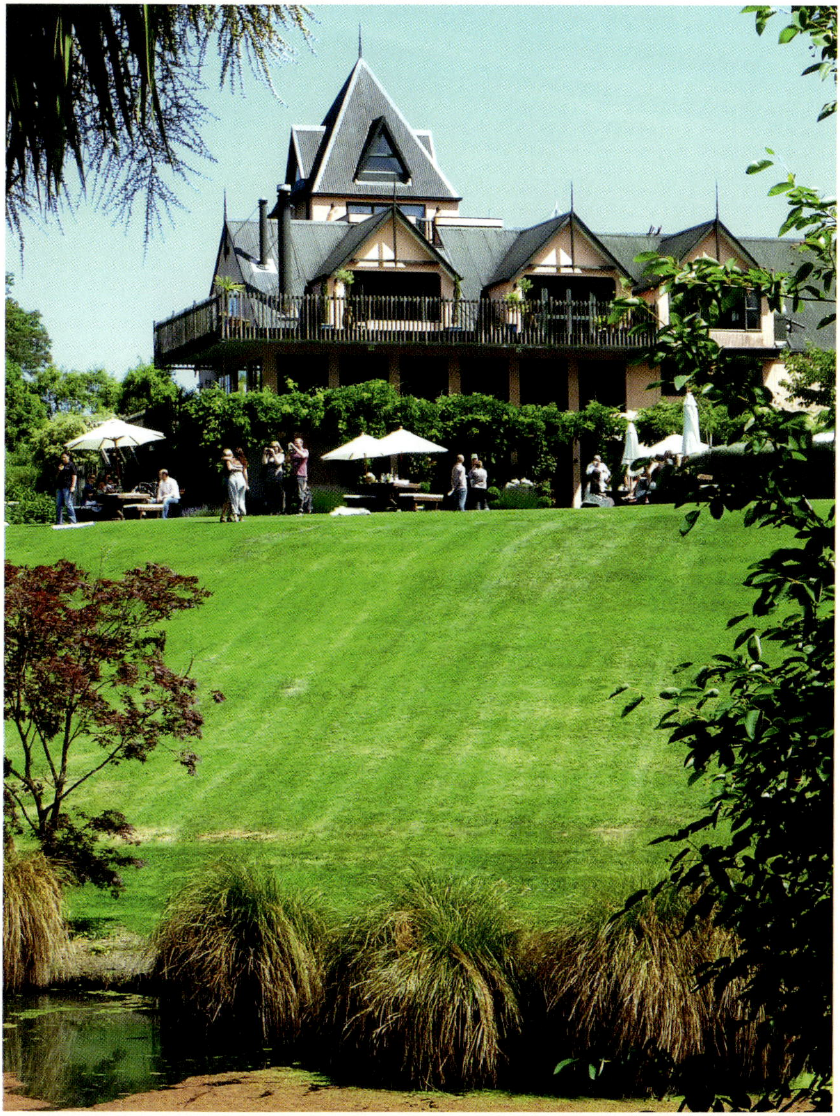

**ABOVE**
Pegasus Bay winery and restaurant viewed from the lake, 2014.

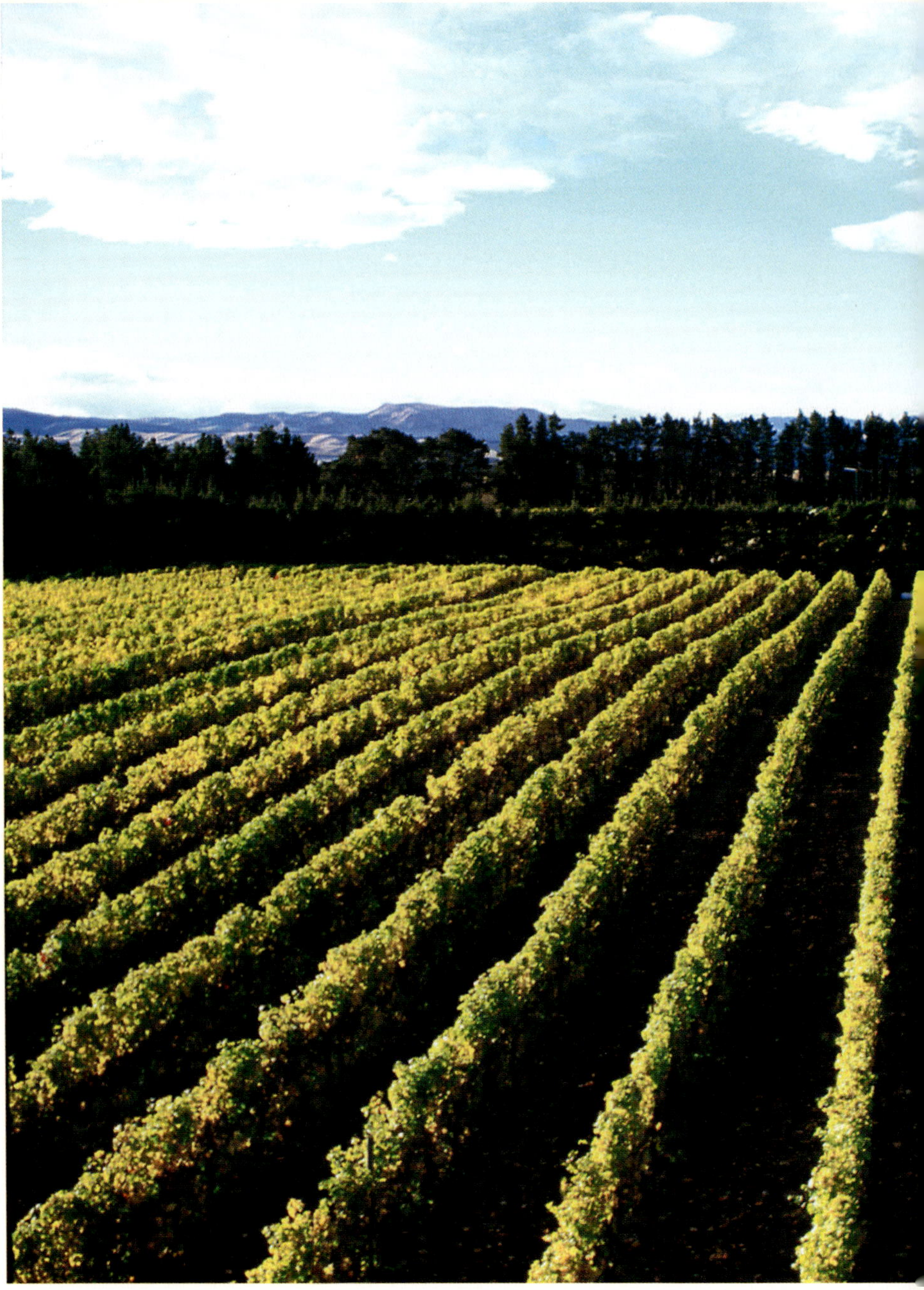

**ABOVE**
Pegasus Bay Vineyard, 2014.

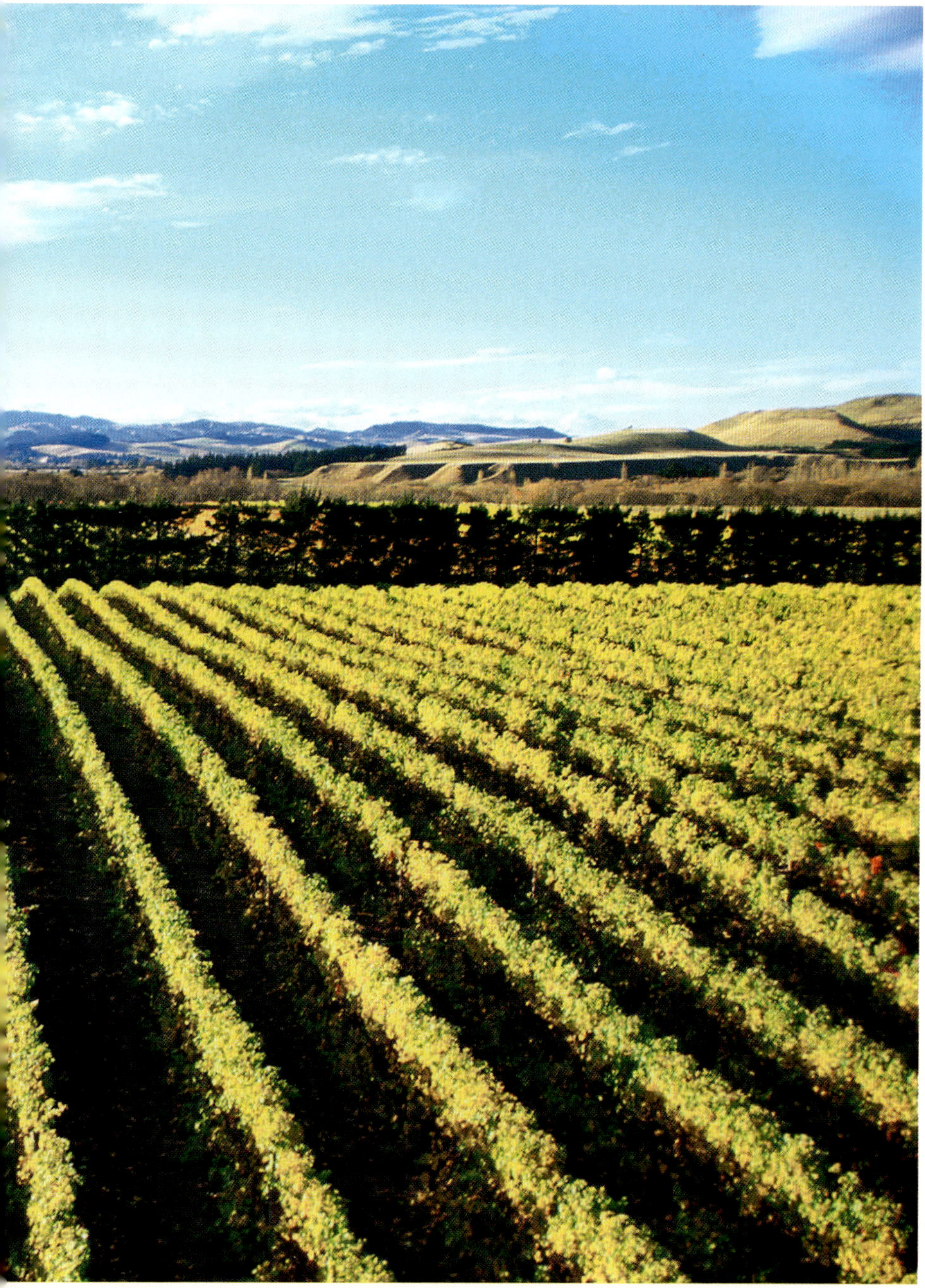

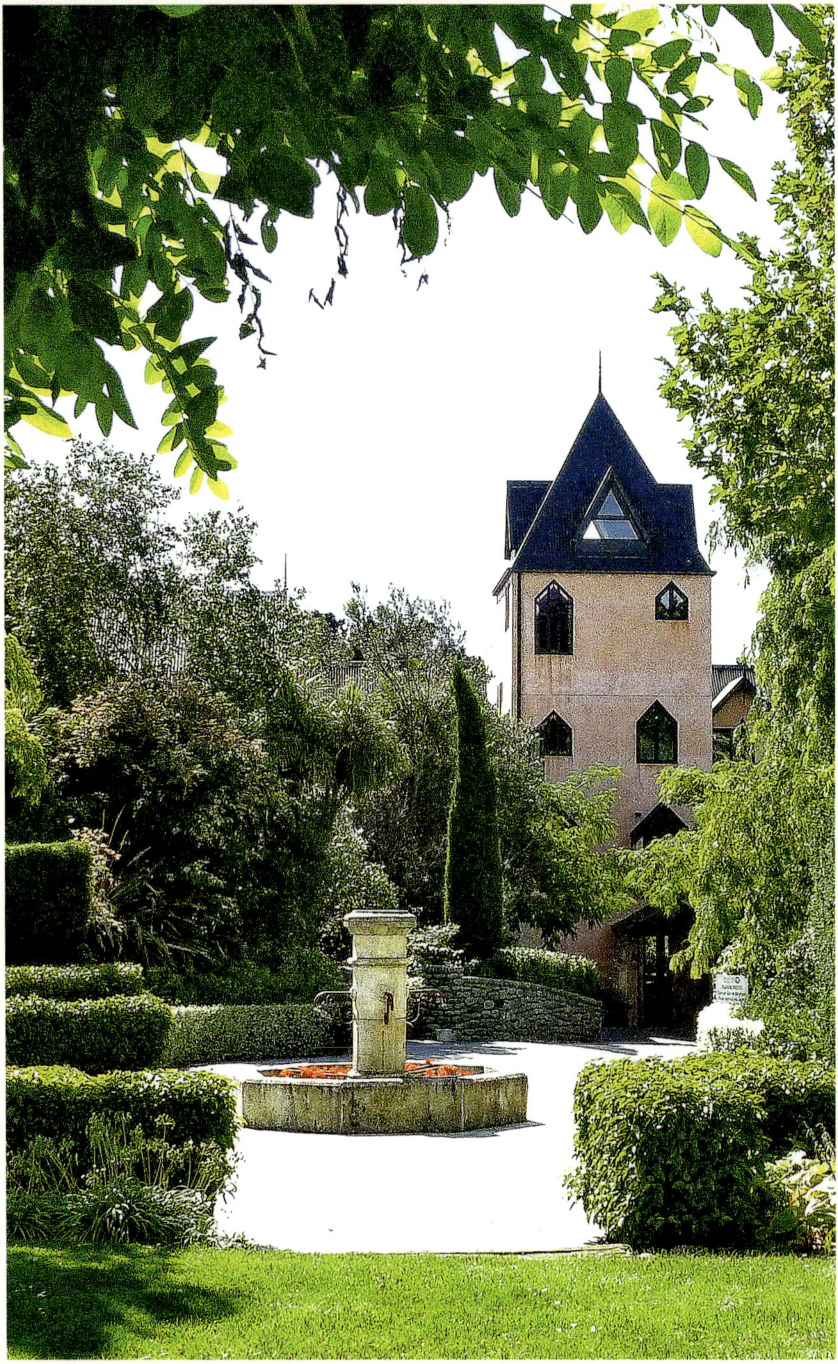

**ABOVE**
The entrance to Pegasus Bay winery and restaurant, 2014.

# CHAPTER 10

# *The* Worries *of a* Winemaker

## 1990–1992

**I HAVE NEVER BEEN QUICK OFF THE MARK**, and some would say that I am decidedly slow. A professional grape grower would weep with frustration and any conscientious bank manager would be at risk of a cardiac crisis if they were to review the financial accounts of our early vineyard days in Waipara Valley. Whereas occasional vineyards produce a small crop in their second year after planting, and any self-respecting vigneron expects some production in the third year, we got nothing until the fifth. This was largely due to the romantic twaddle we believed about making the vines struggle in order to produce top-quality wine, combined with the various ups and downs I have outlined earlier. These resulted from both misfortune and a substantial dose of mismanagement. In spite of us, rather than because of us, the vineyard eventually showed irrefutable signs of delivering a modest but respectable harvest. Although we had been given plenty of time to prepare ourselves, when we realised that this was actually going to happen it came as quite a jolt.

'Where will you make the wine?' Chris asked me one evening after dinner.

'We will have to build a winery, I guess, but there is no use in just throwing up some old shed. We will eventually need space for fermentation, barrel-ageing, bottling, warehousing and cellar-door sales. That's quite a big area, and because of the size of the tanks it will have to be quite high. It has to be carefully planned. We would need to make sure it is architecturally appealing.'

'What about an old church?' Chris suggested excitedly. 'We have always loved church architecture. It would be high enough, full of ornamental woodwork, and you've got a fetish for stained-glass windows. With falling congregations there are empty churches up and down the countryside. I have often seen them for sale, and if we bought a wooden one we could have it moved onto our vineyard site.'

'What a masterstroke. We would only need one to start off with but as we grew we could buy three others, put them in the form of a cross and connect them up where they meet.'

Unlike Mossad, the New Zealand Security Intelligence Service does not have a fearsome reputation. If it had, however, I am sure that Chris and I would have been taken in for questioning or worse as our behaviour became distinctly erratic and suspicious. Over the ensuing weeks and months we scoured Canterbury looking for suitable pickings. Without having had a 'road to Damascus' experience, and with little evidence of previous religiosity, we started visiting churches, sneaking in at the back of services, chatting up vicars and the like. We looked in the 'Properties for Sale' sections of the newspapers, rang real estate agents and did photographic drive-bys of houses of worship. In this day and age we would undoubtedly be taken for terrorists or religious fanatics and charged with loitering with intent or worse.

We were using a similar exploratory technique to the one that had found us our vineyard land, and eventually we accumulated an excellent picture of the local ecclesiastical architecture. At last we found what we were looking for, a lovely medium-sized parish church in good repair, with splendid woodwork and beautiful stained-glass windows. Age had withered the congregation and not spared the church elders, with whom we had a meeting; no, sadly, the church was not being used and yes, it was for sale and, oh yes, the price was right! Chris gave me a wink. We were beside ourselves with joy.

'And may I ask what you are going to do with the church?' asked a pleasant elder with a puce prune face and a bubbly wheeze that suggested the day of salvation was nigh for this respiratory cripple.

'We want to use it for a winery,' Chris answered cheerily.

It may have been our imaginations, but both Chris and I swear that we suddenly felt a breath of cold air pass through the church. Perhaps, however, it was the sudden alteration in facial expressions that changed the spirit of the atmosphere. Within the blink of an eye the venerable vendors had gone from happy and welcoming to sad and even hostile.

'I don't think any of us could countenance our House of God being turned into a factory, especially one which would be used for such a purpose. No, we would sooner let it fall into disrepair and ruin than allow that. Isn't that so, gentlemen?' asked the spokesman, giving a loud phlegmy cough as if to emphasise his point. The sombre-faced entourage nodded in assent.

'I'm sorry to have wasted your time, Mr and Mrs Donaldson,' the man apologised as he showed us to the door. 'Have a happy day.'

Depressingly, few of the other churches that we had lined up were available, and those that were proved less suitable. Nonetheless, we did have a couple of further meetings with pastors and priests of the parish, only to find that forward progress was difficult. They were either reluctant to desecrate their unused churches, or to do so without reference to higher authority, in spite of the first miracle. It was all becoming too complicated and we were running out of time. Our first harvest or *vendange* was looming.

'I'll bet the neighbours are gossiping flat-out. I'm starting to feel my ears burning,' Chris said with a mischievous smile. 'No doubt they will think one of the boys is in trouble.'

'Only one this time? Why would we be so lucky?' I asked as the police car pulled away from the front of our house.

The boyish-looking officer with the crewcut had been serious, although not threatening, during the interview. He had asked about our past. Had we been involved in previous shady dealings? Did we have any earlier convictions for drug offences, robbery, violence and so forth? In fact, had we had any previous brushes with the law? His older colleague looked down at his polished shoes solemnly. Chris had flippantly disclosed a parking fine, which did not evoke general hilarity. After the third degree the boys in black wanted to see the scene of the crime, or rather the proposed one. We showed them into the dark, fusty room. A shaft of light, in which myriads of dust specks danced merrily, penetrated the gloom. It illuminated a fat spider guarding its web and a black beetle scuttling across the floor, intent on fleeing from pressing business and narrowly escaping the full force of the law.

'This is the scene of the dust-up,' I said, spreading my arms to indicate the space, 'and believe me, it will be a good one.'

'It's quite clear that we can't build anything before the harvest,' Chris had earlier announced one evening. 'Why don't you use our garage?'

'It would make sense, and I could use the small winery I built on the back for Pleurisy Point as a laboratory,' I responded enthusiastically. 'But if you want to sell wine it has to be made in a legally registered winery. I'm not sure that I could get the necessary approval. I wonder what it involves?'

It turned out to be quite a messy business. First the police had to ensure that we were of suitable character to be entrusted with such a vital mission. We had not expected the long arm of the law to be bothered about where the action was to take place. We hoped that they were not going to report to the big wheels in the Health Department regarding the current standard of hygiene. After the constabulary departed we set about making the garage spick and span. We were not going to get caught out by that one again. Then we had a visit from an official of the city council, a sage-looking, bespectacled gentleman who was going to do things by the book, and in the council's book there were many conditions that had to be fulfilled. He ticked them off one by one, frowning intermittently, as though he was going to raise an objection, then looking frustrated as his point of concern evaporated. Eventually he conceded that all was acceptable.

Then an officer from the fire department arrived. He measured the access and satisfied himself that in the event of an inferno the hoses would reach the den of iniquity from the fire engine parked on the street. He was relieved to discover that wine is not inflammable and barrels of wine are not liable to spontaneously combust. We pointed out that, in the unlikely event of a fire, the wine leaking from the barrels might help extinguish the blaze. He wanted to be certain that we were not intending to distil spirits which, as we would understand, was quite illegal. Eventually he smiled, and he gave us a conspiratorial nod when we asked him if he thought we might pass the fire department's strict requirements.

There seemed to be a never-ending stream of officialdom that flowed in and out through our little garage, and the last of these was the scout from the Health Department, a sallow gentleman who looked so sombre that I suspected he was a teetotaller. I had met him on occasions in the pursuit of the other half of my life, my day job. He had always been pleasant enough, but, like so many of my colleagues who had gone into medical administration or public health, he inspired sympathy rather than confidence. I knew him to be a stickler for the rules. He ran the fingers of his soft, white, beautifully manicured hand over multiple surfaces, on each occasion subjecting them to subsequent close inspection. He was unable to find fault but his funereal mien remained and it was clear something was on his mind.

'Is everything all right?' I asked.

'It is satisfactory,' he replied, 'but I am worried about contamination.'

'Contamination from what?'

'From microorganisms.'

'What type of microorganisms?'

'I can't be specific. Microorganisms in general, I guess. I feel that where food is produced one cannot be too careful. One expects that all surfaces will be capable of being thoroughly hosed down. It would be difficult to hose the roof in here because you do not have a ceiling, and although the floor is concrete there is no drain in it. Dust might fall down from the roof and get into the vats.'

'But the vats are all covered, and once fermentation is over the wine has to be kept in sealed stainless-steel tanks or barrels. Maturing wine is essentially an anaerobic process because it readily oxidises and spoils in contact with oxygen. All the equipment has to be sterilised, including that used for bottling. At any rate, there are no pathogenic organisms that survive, let alone grow, in wine. Louis Pasteur, the discoverer of microorganisms, said, "Wine is the most healthy and hygienic of beverages." He advised drinking it instead of water, which is easily contaminated.'

'I'll tell you what,' the undertaker said, with an uncharacteristic look of relief which suggested that deep down he did not really want to bury my little project, 'I will do a little research into pathogenic organisms and wine. If I don't turn up anything it will be okay.'

We had to advertise in the local newspapers on more than one occasion to say that we had applied to have a registered winery on our property and to invite those with objections to contact the appropriate authorities. If we received objections then there would have to be a hearing in front of a commissioner, who would decide on the basis of the evidence provided whether or not we would get the necessary licence. We made the advertisement as small and inconspicuous as possible and had it published on Mondays, which was the day of the week the newspapers had the smallest circulation. We canvassed our neighbours and explained the situation, lobbying for their support. We had almost run out of time and the vintage was virtually upon us. It would have come and gone, leaving the grapes to rot on the vine, before a hearing could be convened. Chris and I were beside ourselves with anxiety.

'If you don't get a licence it won't stop you making wine here,' one cheerful, chubby, red-faced official had said.

'But it will stop us ever being able to sell it,' I had replied, 'and that is the whole point of the exercise. We wouldn't be able to drink it all ourselves!'

'Don't worry. I'm happy to help you out, and some of my mates would lend you a hand. We prefer beer, but we wouldn't say no to a good wine.'

Chris phoned with the news while I was in the process of conducting a clinic.

'We got it!' she said jubilantly.

That night we celebrated with a glass or two of special Champagne. We could start the harvest!

**ALTHOUGH WE HAD MADE A LITTLE WINE** in 1990, it was not enough to see the light of day from a commercial point of view. Our first real *vendange* in 1991 was a simple little affair but an exciting event for us, nonetheless. We had bought plastic crates and pairs of snips for our team of relatives, friends and helpful hangers-on, not to mention ourselves and our employees. We had to work over several weekends, harvesting each variety, not when it had reached its optimum, but when we felt it was good enough and the birds had still left us some berries on the vines. These were the days before we had nets and the pressure from our feathered friends largely decided when we picked. The volunteers' only reward was a decent lunch. On one occasion a Maori employee dug a pit in the earth, filled the bottom with stones from the vineyard, lit a fire and, when it had died down to become embers, doused it with water. She then proceeded to put in large slabs of meat and vegetables, which were in turn covered with wet sacks and earth. Later we all dined on a deliciously cooked hangi. There were shouts of joy when I produced bottles of a gold-medal Müller-Thurgau. Doubtless these would have been less enthusiastically received today, given this grape variety's disastrous fall in the fashion rankings. Nonetheless, I still cannot think of a better hangi wine!

Progress was slow and there was the inevitable snipped fingertip to test Chris's nursing skills and possibly add a little colour to the eventual red wine. We could not complain, however. We had a happy, largely unpaid crew and in the end we had a decent enough crop of grapes. These were ferried back to our new winery, the only legally registered winery in Christchurch. There, I hoped to turn it into saleable wine and perhaps gain a little income to help offset the financial haemorrhaging.

Making wine out of grapes largely involves watching over and controlling the action of yeasts, as they ferment the grapes' sugars and turn them into alcohol. Because the pigment resides in the skin and is extracted by the alcohol, it is necessary to ferment the berries to make a red wine. A white, however, is made only from the juice obtained after pressing. Fermentation releases carbon dioxide and heat. When making a red, the carbon dioxide bloats the grapes, causing them to rise to the surface where they form a 'cap'. This may dry out and needs to be regularly moistened by pushing ('punching') it back down into the forming wine with a plunger. It can be hard work, particularly on the abdominal and arm muscles. Eventually, the supply of sugar in the grapes is exhausted and the fermentation finishes. The so-called 'free-run red wine' is drained from the vat and the 'pressings' or 'press wine' is extracted from the grape remnants by using a press.

But making the wine is really only the start of the oenologist's task. The French consider it to be a bit like becoming a parent and, as any mum knows, having a baby is the easy part. The really hard work is in raising the child. The French use the term *élévage* for this phase of the winemaker's task. It means rearing, bringing up or training, and they apply it to children and animals as well as wine. As a father and a teacher of medical students I was well aware of the implications of *élévage* and I did not intend to shirk my responsibilities. When the euphoria of tasting the first free-run wine from our vineyard had passed, Chris and I were reluctantly forced to agree that we did not have a little angel but a cheeky young brat.

Having raised four sons we thought we knew a little about the business of *élévage*. Children need lots of rest, so we put ours into wooden barrels and left them to sleep. In the following spring and early summer it seemed as if the teenage years had kicked in. They became rebellious, and unless we were careful they were given to explosions without warning. In our winery we occasionally had bungs blowing out of barrels as our kids tried to break loose with a hiss and a roar. Like a teenager's ebullience, this rebellion was quite natural. It was due to the bacteria that convert one type of natural acid, malic, into another called lactic. This secondary or malolactic fermentation results in reduction in the acid level and it is essential for a red wine's stability. Thus, after this bout of exuberance, the wine and the teenager are expected to be softer, mellower and more stable. In spite of this, both need a further period of *élévage*, training and encouragement to help them achieve their full potential. It is only then that the little darlings are ready to make their social debut.

We were trying to make wine that would not only be ready to drink on release but would also cellar well for many years. As it was the product of a new vineyard we were uncertain how it would age. Wine is like a living thing and it gradually evolves in the bottle. We wanted our debutante to also be a sleeping beauty. We hoped that, if in years to come some charming Prince Purchaser stumbled upon a forgotten glass casket, he would not be shocked to find that his lips had really awakened an old hag! But *Sleeping Beauty* is just a fairy tale. Perhaps we were expecting too much — or were we?

In the mid-1990s a group of young Turk winemakers from the famous Saint-Émilion region of Bordeaux broke with tradition and began to produce a new-style red wine as a reaction against the classic clarets of the area. These were quite tannic, lean and hard, requiring years of cellaring before being ready to drink. These young oenologists made wines that were plumper, fruitier, more succulent and more immediately appealing. They did not need to be cellared for long periods, but could be enjoyed at or soon after their release. The pundits questioned whether the wines would disintegrate with age, but time has shown that they can stay the pace. They were very popular, although expensive, especially as they came from producers without well-established track records. Proprietors of prestigious châteaux, with centuries of tradition behind them, looked down their noses at their neighbours and turned up their snouts at such wines. They were called *Vins du Garage*, because they were generally made in small, humble premises rather than on grand estates. The winemakers became known as *garagistes.* Without knowing it, we had just become real *garagistes*, before anyone had ever heard of those cheeky little upstarts from Bordeaux!

**'CLINK, CLANK, CLUNK**, clink, clank, clunk, clink, clank, clunk, clink, clank, clunk …' went the bottling machine full-throatedly, emitting a discordant range of notes from tenor to bass. In spite of the racket it was no match for the ethereal soprano voice that floated above it, like a bird soaring over a herd of raging wild animals. One represented the brutish cacophony of industry while the other was a perfect example of fine art. Both, however, were music to our ears. We were bottling our *vin du garage*, the very first red wine from our own vineyard, and we were doing this in the driveway outside the garage in which I had made it.

Three years earlier, Matthew, or Matt, as he now liked to be called, had gone off to Roseworthy College in Adelaide to do a winemaking degree, making his and our lives more tranquil and comfortable. I had not seen him for three years, as he had worked in vineyards and wineries in Australia during his holidays, although Chris could not resist making an occasional trip to see our little lamb. While he was there the college winery was moved to Adelaide University and much of the Roseworthy equipment was put up for tender. As we were going to build a winery in Waipara Valley we tendered for some of the items. I subsequently heard from a mole on the college staff that our Matt had hounded the dean of the college for a decision, rather 'like a Staffordshire pit-bull in a fight to the death'.

The tactic worked, and we got everything we wanted, including some very large oak barrels, up to 5000 litres in size. These barrels had already seen a century of use, and Matt had to disassemble them, labelling all the parts in the correct order, for their transportation back to New Zealand. This was no small task. We subsequently had them thoroughly cleaned and reassembled by a cooper. Amongst the other spoils was an all-enclosed fully automated bottling machine, which we were now using in our drive. Both father and son had matured over the three years of their forced separation. They now worked together harmoniously as the latter instructed the former. The purple-faced young lady was fed into the gaping maw of the mechanical monster and a sleeping beauty came out the other end. But this was more than just a two-horse team, it was a family affair, and we all stopped to listen to the magical voice of Malvina, as it seemed to soothe the growling beast in the drive.

Chris and I had fallen in love with opera when we lived in London in the 1970s, and shortly after we returned to Christchurch she had joined the board of directors of the newly formed Canterbury Opera. Chris had been passionate about singing since childhood and now described herself as a 'chorus girl', as she also sang in the opera chorus. Malvina Major had been a bright star in the opera firmament, having pipped Kiri Te Kanawa in New Zealand's prestigious Mobil Song Quest. The two young ladies remained firm friends, however, with Kiri topping the next Mobil competition and becoming Malvina's bridesmaid. Both went to the UK for further operatic study and training. Kiri had remained there, while Malvina had sacrificed her glittering future for her growing family. She had returned to New Zealand to help fulfil her husband's dream of being a dairy farmer.

Although Malvina had become a farm girl, bringing up her young family in the backblocks of rural New Zealand, she did not for one moment forget her love of opera and the priceless vocal gift that she had so painstakingly cut and honed into a glittering gemstone. Even while she was about her domestic chores and farm duties she kept polishing the diamond, driven by a personal passion rather than by any expectation that it would ever again be shown in public. Her husband Winston's unexpected, sudden death at a young age from silent coronary artery disease forced Malvina to re-evaluate her situation. She could not do all his work on her own so she decided to relaunch herself and return to the stage. Shortly after this, Canterbury Opera was lucky enough to engage her for the role of Madam Butterfly in Puccini's celebrated opera of the same name.

Rather than stay for several weeks in the sterile environment of a hotel room, Malvina had opted to be billeted, and that is how she came to be part of our family and a firm friend. That was the first of several times that she was brave enough to stay in our madhouse while singing with Canterbury Opera. From day one she had slotted in as though she had always been there. Not only were we lucky enough to be able to hear her practising, but she also mucked in as one of the family, assisting with all manner of household and other chores. One night when Chris and I went out for the evening we left Malvina in charge of a foaming vat of fermenting pinot noir, with strict instructions that she was to punch the beast down if it started to make a break for it by climbing out onto the garage floor.

She was later to become Dame Malvina, and later still to morph into D-D, or Double-Dame, as we like to call her, as she was effectively knighted a second time when she was awarded the New Zealand Order of Merit, an honour that is restricted to just 20 living people. But in those days she was just Malvina, and her bedroom window looked directly out onto and was only metres away from the drive where we were putting our beauty to sleep. How she managed to keep singing at all is something that only she knows, and how her voice came to be heard over the cacophony remains a mystery to all. Perhaps there is not a scientific explanation. After all, in the opera Madam Butterfly does sing her child to sleep, and I like to imagine that Malvina's voice soothed the machine and was a lullaby for our 'sleeping beauty'.

Whatever the explanation, the fact remains that our first red wines, which came from the 1991 vintage, were bottled to the strains of her voice and they did develop well in the cellar. The pinot noir is still quite drinkable, but unlike our fairy-tale heroine it will not stay the pace for 100 years.

**I AM NOT SURE WHETHER** it was divine intervention that scuttled our plans to build the winery of the Cross of Four Churches, but after our failure to find what we wanted in the way of ecclesiastical real estate that had passed its use-by date, Chris and I eventually decided that we would just have to build something from scratch. For over a decade our garage had doubled as a winery, but it was abundantly clear that as soon as our Waipara Valley vineyard started to produce with a vengeance we would need something much bigger.

How should we proceed? A winery is a workshop or factory and, however romantically you may view it, it is essentially a shed or a combination of sheds. Many wineries look just like that. Although our piggy-bank told us that this was our only option, our hearts rebelled against it.

'We may be forced to build a shed,' said Chris, 'but let's find an architect who is prepared to sell his soul and tart it up; someone who could turn a plain Jane nun into a bathing beauty.'

We did not know any architects so we sought friends' advice as to one who might have individuality and flair. It was suggested we approach Trevor Ibbotson, who was passionate about wine and, as chance would have it, sometimes went to tastings that I regularly attended.

'He has put a swimming pool in his living room, has planted lawn on his roof, and his bedroom is completely covered in purple sheepskins: the floor, the walls and the ceiling!' we were told.

This gave me some misgivings but at the same time infected me with a sort of nervous curiosity. I spoke to him at the very next wine tasting and was both surprised and delighted by his response. He was clearly not one to muck about.

'I'll come around to your house tomorrow night, if you are free,' he volunteered, 'and we can get started immediately.'

Some would say that Trevor was eccentric, but I prefer to think of him as a character, a character from a bygone age. He cut a striking figure: tallish, lean and handsome in a rugged sort of way, with long white hair and a flowing Father Christmas beard. Although a Kiwi he had spent a number of years working as an architect in England and it turned out that he had also designed wineries in Australia. He was as keen as mustard about our project and listened intently to what we proposed, making suggestions and rapidly sketching to help us expand and consolidate our vision. Naturally, we worked with the aid of a good bottle of wine or two, and we all became increasingly animated as the night wore on. Trevor was very sympathetic to our cause, but he did not hesitate to tell us when he thought we were wide off the feasible or architectural mark. He had a happy knack of making the seemingly impossible work and he encouraged us to think big, although we pointed out to him that we might never be able to pay for it.

He would design the general outline of our vision but we would have to build it in stages, as finances permitted. Trevor would only prepare the detailed working plans of each stage when we were financially equipped to proceed with it. It would clearly be many years before we would know whether it would be possible to complete our dream. However, we would start where the winemaking process itself begins, with an area in which the grapes would be received and then fermented. In the grandiose scheme of things this would eventually become our fermentation hall, but to start off with it would also be for barrel storage, bottling, warehousing, a laboratory, cellar-door sales, a bedroom, a kitchen and a restaurant. Yes, we misguidedly decided that from the day we first sold wine we would also open an on-site restaurant to provide extra revenue for development. We knew nothing about restaurant economics and we were in for a rude shock.

It was late at night when we finally bade Trevor good night.

'Who can that be ringing the doorbell at 7.30 in the morning?' I called out to Chris, who was busy feeding four hungry mouths downstairs.

'You'll need to go and see for yourself. I'm too busy,' she replied.

'Hello, Ivan. Here are the plans. I hope they are to your liking. When would you like to go over them? Perhaps tonight?'

A dishevelled-looking Trevor, with a grin from ear to ear, thrust a thick bundle of documents into my hands.

'I don't believe this, Trevor. It is barely eight hours since you left.'

'Couldn't sleep. I like to get on to something straight away while it's fresh in my mind.'

'Thanks, Trevor. Perhaps Chris and I should go over them first and then give you a call to make a time.'

'Okay, but don't leave it too long as I might go off the boil!'

And that turned out to be how Trevor worked. Over the years to come we had many meetings with him and he would usually turn up on our doorstep with the plans the following morning.

'How did you like the plans?' Trevor asked by way of opening our next meeting as he folded back the front cover of his folio. On this he had drawn a fairy-tale version of the completed winery surrounded by beautiful, equally non-existent gardens. It looked as though he was trying to suck us in, but I soon came to realise that he inhabited a different space from other people. The task that we had set him was not just another job but a mission; one that allowed him to slip into a different world, a world in which he could let his imagination run riot. He was Don Quixote and there were windmills to be tilted at.

'The plans look exciting and very imaginative,' I said. 'Much better than we ever dreamed.'

'This looks rather imaginative as well,' Chris suggested with a chuckle, pointing to a nude figure who was coming through a doorway while playing bagpipes.

'In fact, there seems to have been a brainstorm of imagination judging by all these interlopers,' she added, indicating a number of other shapely young people in their birthday suits. They casually paraded or draped themselves all over the plans.

'Oh, they're just friends of mine who are there to help you out. They are giving you a feeling of the true scale of things. Their size is in exact proportion to the plans. They will show you at a glance whether the space you have envisaged is too cramped or too big, whether the ceiling is too low or the like. See this one here,' he said, jabbing his finger at a David that Michelangelo would have been happy to claim. 'You can see that he is going to become claustrophobic. We have tried to fit too much into that small space and he just doesn't like it.'

Trevor was correct. We could see immediately that several things that we had thought might work now looked inappropriate. We became used to these helpful and nubile figures romping or lounging over these and all of our future plans. We never knew what the humourless people in the various planning departments of the council made of these quirky figures. Perhaps they were too distracted by them to find the myriad minute breaches of obscure regulations in which such officials delight. Maybe they were put into a good mood after being unwittingly seduced by provocative shapes and they were enticed into a fantasy world that was far from their humdrum jobs. Whatever the explanation, Trevor's plans always seem to get approved without difficulty, but then, perhaps he was just a very good architect.

Things always take longer than you expect, at least that is my experience. I always overestimate my ability to achieve, and that particularly applies to projects of any magnitude. So it was with building the first stage of the winery, although I seemed to have been planning it in my mind for two or three years. But when I say this, I delude myself. Although I had plenty of input into the project, it was, as usual, Chris who was driving it forwards and not me. I sat on the sidelines criticising and making snide remarks, while she did all the hard day-to-day work, liaising with the builder, drainlayer, plumber, electrician, roofer, fire-safety officer, building inspector, council official and the rest. We were racing against time as the next harvest was looming and work on the site had hardly started, although Trevor had visited the site with us on several occasions in order to decide the exact placement of the building. The first visit was the most crucial.

'The most important thing to get correct is the location of the lavatories,' Trevor proclaimed seriously as he hammered a stake into the ground. It was small and painted white but proudly announced 'Toilets' in shaky black handwriting. 'Everything else hinges on this.'

He looked like an early European explorer who had just tumbled out of the deepest and darkest jungle in Africa. He was sporting a pair of tattered khaki shorts and battered jungle boots, while an old pith helmet completed the picture.

'Why?' I asked naïvely.

'Because the toilets will have to be on the southeast side of the restaurant that you intend eventually to build and they will have to fit very precisely into that stage of the project. You need to have them built now to serve your first building, but for several years they will be outside of and separate from it.'

There was a small gully, running from east to west, just north of where we intended to build, and its western half was covered in very tall trees. We wanted our future restaurant to have a view to the north, over the eastern half of the valley. Exact placement was crucial because we needed it to be close to the copse in order to get maximum shelter from the prevailing northwesterly wind but not so close that the restaurant would be shaded in the winter. By observing throughout the seasons Chris and I had decided that we had found the optimum spot. We had not, however, spared a thought for Trevor's unerring logic, which was now as inescapable as a steam train hurtling towards us in a tunnel. The only part of the future restaurant that would be constructed at this stage was the toilet block and all of our future development hung on what Trevor picturesquely described as 'the position of a dunny seat'.

'Although there are those who might find your reasoning distasteful, we are not going to let it put you in bad odour with us, Trev. Let's just accept that your cheeky little peg is important and use it as a theoretical basis on which to stake out the whole prospective site,' I said.

'Otherwise we won't have the building constructed in time for our 1992 harvest,' Chris added prophetically.

**IT WAS A BEAUTIFUL AUTUMN DAY,** warm and sunny with a light northwesterly breeze. The weather was perfect for the final day of harvesting grapes and the little crew of friends and family had worked well. If you surreptitiously watch any group toiling you will soon become aware that many seem incapable of talking and working at the same time. While I do not like to be sexist, I suspect that this afflicts men more than women. Perhaps it is just another example of males being challenged in the multitasking department.

There was much happy chatter and gossip that May day in 1992 and there were plenty of men in the team, but in spite of this the picking had continued at a surprisingly rapid pace. Perhaps it was because they knew they had to get the block finished by the end of the afternoon, and there was the additional temptation of a glass or two of wine at the end. Our bins, which were piled high on a battered old trailer, had been shuttled back and forth to the winery throughout the day, placing enormous strain on our decrepit tractor. Although Matthew and I had been picking earlier, we were now busy back at the winery processing grapes for fermentation; pressing the whites to get the juice and de-stemming the reds. We had been at it since early in the afternoon, when enough of the fruit had arrived to make it worth starting. It was now approaching dusk, but we still had quite a lot of work left to do. Matthew glanced up nervously.

'I don't like the look of those clouds,' he said. 'Were we expecting a southerly change in the weather?'

'The forecast said there might be one during the night, but I had not expected anything this early,' I replied anxiously, looking up at the menacing bank of cumulus clouds that hovered above us in the fading light.

Although we were standing on the concrete floor inside the winery we could clearly see everything that was happening above us because there was no roof. In fact, the 'winery' consisted solely of the floor and two partially completed walls that were joined at a corner. In spite of our best efforts, and those of our builder, we had not been able to get even a roof over our heads before vintage. We were totally vulnerable to the elements.

Suddenly there was a blinding flash and almost immediately an eardrum-rending explosion. Within seconds we were assaulted by a blast of freezing wind and heavy hail. Fortunately the stones were not massive, but they were being driven by the sudden release of the pent-up southerly gale that had been held back by the old 'Devil's breath'. The merciless stinging was all the worse because we were in shorts and short-sleeved shirts. Within seconds we felt frozen and our teeth were chattering. All we could do was cover the fruit and equipment and run for shelter. There would be nothing else that we could achieve that night.

It was a bleak scene that confronted us the following morning. It was grey but otherwise fine, and Matthew and I were muffled up against the cold. Fortunately our tarpaulins had stayed in place and the fruit was not damaged. We worked quickly amongst the builders' mess and we soon had the juice and the berries safely in vats. Then we were confronted by another problem. How were we going to start the fermentation at a temperature close to 0°C? If you have ever made bread then you will know that the dough has to be in a warm place in order for the yeasts to start working. As they metabolise the flour, they release carbon dioxide, which forms lots of little holes within the dough, making it swell up or rise. As wine is also fermented by yeast, the process would not start at such a low temperature. While the juice and fruit were probably safe in the near-freezing temperature, there was a risk of spoilage if the temperature rose and the start of fermentation was delayed. Once it was merrily bubbling away it would probably be quite safe as the carbon dioxide prevents oxidation.

We did not as yet have electricity to allow us to warm the vats. Many anxious days were spent watching our tanks and trying every trick we knew in order to encourage fermentation. I am sure that Bacchus was looking over our shoulder that harvest. Not only was our crop saved from the ravages of hail by a whisker, but about a week later, with my ear clamped to the side of the vat, I could hear the faint but blissful hiss of rising bubbles, even before they began to appear on the surface. Because our vats were small and effectively out in the open, we were worried that the fragile fermentation might be stopped by a frost. We ended up covering them with blankets and eiderdowns, tying them in place with rope and string. We hoped to keep them warm by retaining the heat that the yeasts' metabolism was producing. This was exactly the opposite to the cooling that is frequently required during fermentation in order to prevent a high temperature from killing the yeasts. This vintage of innovation had a learning curve that was close to the vertical!

**THE ERUPTION OF MT PINATUBO** in the Philippines in mid-1991 had dramatic consequences for the passengers and crew of a jumbo jet that was cruising over the Pacific at about 35,000 feet at the time. Passengers suddenly became aware of a flickering phosphorescent-like glow around the wings and the windows, and that the faint background noise of the aircraft's engines had suddenly tailed off. It was clear something was very much amiss.

The captain's voice broke the frozen silence as he informed the passengers that there had been a sudden engine failure. He would do his best to control the aircraft but it was starting to lose altitude. He asked them to help by remaining calm and not panicking. As the aircraft plummeted downwards for about 10,000 feet the petrified passengers did their best to suppress their terror and prayed for a miracle. Finally the crew managed to stabilise the aircraft at a lower altitude, and it was then able to limp to an airport and make an emergency landing.

This incident drew the aviation industry's attention to the dangers of tiny particles of grit and dust that are thrown to great atmospheric heights by volcanic eruptions. It led to the introduction of no-fly zones around and downwind of such events, restrictions that can remain in force for days or even weeks. This does not, however, reflect the true persistence of the dust and its widespread effect. The eruption of Mt Pinatubo spewed out a cloud of volcanic matter almost 20 kilometres high. It not only endangered the lives of the passengers on this flight, but it also spread a diffuse layer of dust high in the atmosphere. As a result of the air movement produced by the earth's rotation, this layer came to encircle the southern hemisphere for at least two years and led to 1992 and 1993 being cooler than normal south of the equator.

These years did not appear particularly cold in New Zealand, and we seemed to have the normal number of warm days throughout the spring, summer and autumn. What does it matter to us if the temperature on a particular day is 25°C instead of 26°C? We would probably be unable to tell the difference and just think that it was a pleasantly warm afternoon. We do not have a good appreciation or memory for comfortable ambient temperatures, although we do recall the extremes. By contrast, those brainless life-forms called plants retain an excellent memory or record of such differences because it affects their growth and development. Hence, scientists can tell what the climate has been like in bygone years by studying the growth rings in the trunks of trees.

Thus, although the growing seasons leading up to our 1992 and 1993 vintages appeared normal to those working in the vineyard, the slightly lower average temperature was day by day making its presence felt in the plants. The vines were, in effect, gradually adding up each day's dose of sunlight and finding they were being short-changed. They sulked and lagged behind their normal development. In fact, looking back over almost a quarter of a century of records shows that we have never had seasons in which ripening was more delayed.

Mt Pinatubo caused only a tiny, transient blip in part of the world's climate. It may not sound like a big deal when scientists predict that the average global temperature might increase by 2°C by the end of the century, but this experience highlighted for me just how massive such a change would be.

We were only able to ripen our fruit by leaving it on the vines until late in the season. This gave the fruit good flavours and concentrations of sugars but the acid levels remained higher than normal.

Wine with a high level of acid tends to be unstable in the bottle. Although perfectly clear and free of sediment when first bottled, over time the grapes' main acid, tartaric acid, joins with the wine's natural potassium and forms colourless crystals that appear at the bottom of the bottle. These so-called 'wine diamonds' are quite harmless, but some consumers think that they are pieces of glass and that the wine is unsafe to drink. The uninitiated may tip the entire contents of such bottles down the sink, destroying not only the wine but the winery's reputation. Because we were keen to avoid such a situation I decided to chill our 1992 sauvignon/sémillon wine in tank. This would encourage the excess acid to fall out as crystals there, rather than at a later stage in the bottle. The problem was that in order for this to be effective the wine had to be held at well under 0°C for quite some days or weeks. The trick is to have it cold enough to precipitate the excess acid as crystals but not so cold as to freeze the wine.

The only chilling unit I had at my disposal was a rather small and feeble one, but I thought it would be adequate. I had obtained it from an ex-patient, a jovial, red-faced publican who had allowed me to take it out of an underground beer cellar, so long as I did it in the dead of night. He could feel the hot breath of the receivers on the back of his neck.

This was to be the first of our white wines that I would bottle myself, as the tiny amount of our 1991 sauvignon/sémillon had been bottled for us by the Giesen brothers, who had a winery just south of Christchurch. Matt, who had returned to New Zealand at the end of 1991 after finishing his winemaking degree and who had been in charge of bottling our first reds, had now returned to Adelaide to do a postgraduate diploma in viticulture. I was intimidated by the thought of using our automated bottling machine without guidance, so I arranged to hire the services of a local commercial winemaker who had previously worked with such equipment. He would come at the end of the month, by which time I should have managed to 'cold stabilise' the wine.

I built a small airtight polystyrene hut around the wine tank and put the chiller head inside. A protruding thermometer encouragingly showed that the temperature of the wine was heading south. Then it stuck, or rather hovered, a little under zero. What should I do?

'Why don't you wrap some old eiderdowns around your little hut?' suggested the ever-practical Chris. 'They would give extra insulation and help get the temperature down further.'

I followed her advice and it improved the situation but not enough to be really effective. I then became desperate and piled all manner of insulating materials around and on top of the hut, holding them in place with a spaghetti-junction of string, wire and rope. The temperature restarted its erratic descent, and then we had the foulest bout of warm spring weather that you could imagine. The breeze blew from the northwest and we had a week of balmy days. Rotten little daffodils and irritating snowdrops began to open. The damned little unit was just not powerful enough to hold the mercury in place and the temperature began to rise. The end of the month was approaching rapidly and I was not going to be ready for my winemaker assistant. I became irritable and depressed.

'Ivan, it has snowed during the night!' Chris shouted from downstairs where she was preparing breakfast.

I rushed to the bedroom window and threw back the curtains. Sure enough, as far as the eye could see everything was covered in a thick white carpet: the rooftops, the garden, the trees, the paths and the road. I flew downstairs and fairly raced out to the winery. Salvation! Unexpected salvation! Snow at this time of the year was distinctly unusual. It was now below zero in the winery and the temperature inside the hut had plummeted. What is more, there was so much snow on the ground it was unlikely that it would thaw for several days, bringing us to the end of the month. If we could just hold the mercury where it was until then we might manage to pull this off. I ran inside to telephone my expert help.

'Ivan, I'm sorry but I'm going to have to call it off. I have so much snow here that I'm going to have to shovel it away to get out of the house. As you know, my wife and I also run a small shop and we expect business to be very brisk in the next few days as people stock up. To make matters worse, school has been cancelled and the kids are at home. No, I just can't do it.'

No amount of pleading would change his mind. By a stroke of luck we had managed to achieve what had seemed impossible, but we needed to be bottling before the weather and the wine warmed up. I felt deflated and angry. Should I try to bottle it by hand, a massive task, or should I try to use the bottling monster and risk slaying the growling dragon for all time?

'Why don't you phone Matthew?' Chris suggested. 'He is the one who really knows how to use that machine, and I'm sure he could take a few days off his course. We could fly him over from Australia today or tomorrow and he could be back there by the end of the week.'

And that was what we did. Matthew was delighted at the opportunity to play hooky and to have a break from his studies. He arrived the next day, while the snow was still crunchy underfoot and the air cut like a knife. Chris and I worked happily alongside the true professional, and within a few days he had crossed the ditch and was back in Oz. Perhaps it was this experience that gave him a taste for life as a flying winemaker because for many years to come that is what he was, disappearing to the other side of the world to work vintages in northern hemisphere wineries after he had finished ours.

And how did the wine turn out? Not too badly, in my opinion, although I know I am biased. When tasted alongside the 1991 sauvignon/sémillon, after being cellared for over 20 years, both wines were still alive. The 1991, coming from a hot year, was plumper and more rounded, while the 1992 was leaner and crisper but had more vibrant fruit. Neither showed that vegetal, canned asparagus or canned peas character that can be a feature of older wines made from sauvignon blanc alone, and neither had wine diamonds!

**POET T.S. ELIOT** wrote that naming cats was a very difficult matter. They had to have three different names. We were lucky as we only had to think up a single name for our vineyard and winery, nonetheless, we found that it was also *a difficult matter*, a very difficult matter. Being procrastinators by nature, Chris and I put it off as long as possible, which in reality meant during the development phase of the vineyard. We really did not need to have a name until we started to label wine for selling. This meant that for almost six years we just referred to our little endeavour as 'The Vineyard', without giving the issue a lot of thought. The possibility of ever getting a meaningful crop and having anything to sell seemed so remote that it was simply not worth wasting our time on the subject.

Then, seemingly all of a sudden, The Matter was almost upon us. We had a sense of rising panic and started to run off in all directions like headless chickens. We began to make long lists of potential names, which included pseudo-French, classical, romantic, Maori, shocking (i.e. attention-grabbing), family and many other categories. Terms such as Château, Domaine, Estate and the like were considered but rejected as seeming rather grandiose and inconsistent with the stark reality of our little patch of vines, growing on a piece of dirt that had so recently been the home of many contented sheep. We batted ideas back and forth between ourselves and the boys, but we could not come to any consensus.

Eventually we decided that we would each write down our six favourite names and see if there were any in common. Distressingly, there were not, but two general themes did emerge. These were that our name should contain no reference, however oblique, to claims of quality, and that it should refer to the place where the grapes were grown, the place that we hoped would stamp its identity and give its individuality to our wines. But what place was that? We looked at the map and found that there were many possibilities so we wrote several down on the back of an old envelope. We then tried to use each one for a week every time we referred to anything to do with the property. Each started like a racehorse bolting out of the gate and looked as though it was going to be a clear winner, only to lose its wind part-way around the course and end up being sent to the knacker's yard.

Was it the rarefied atmosphere, was it the wine, or was it the shedding of the constricting skin of stress? Maybe it was none of these things, but I was cruising at about 35,000 feet over the Pacific, on my way to London where I was to work with David Marsden on our book, when I did something that is very unusual for me. I discussed a personal problem with a complete stranger. I was deep in conversation with my next-door neighbour, a Maori gentleman called Kevin, when I sought his advice on naming our pet. I showed him a list of possible vineyard names and asked him what he thought of them. Perhaps he had other names that he might like to suggest.

Without a moment's hesitation he stabbed the page with his index finger, saying, 'That's it. That's perfect. It meets all of your requirements and, besides, it's a damn good name.'

It was like a 'Eureka!' moment; like suddenly picking out the face of a long-lost friend in a crowd of strangers. Why had we not settled on that earlier? I did not know whether it would be good from a marketing perspective, but who cared? It suited our moggy to a T.

When I met Chris at Heathrow a week later I could not help blurting out, 'The name has been decided ... but, naturally, only if you agree. It's Pegasus Bay.'

'I agree. I had come to the same conclusion myself.'

We then gave each other a belated hug and a kiss.

The white sandy arc could have been drawn by the sweep of a chalk held in a giant's hand. It starts at Christchurch and curves northward and eastward for about 50 kilometres, all the while framing the sparkling blue Pacific. The tumultuous waves that expend themselves by dashing upon this beach can have been generated thousands of kilometres to the east, occasionally as far away as South America. It was in 1809 that a ship was sent from Australia to chart and map these remote and wild shores. Before then, Maori waka had often crossed these waters, occasionally filled with bronzed warriors on their way to war. They may have known this stretch of their home sea as Kaiuau, O-ruapaeroa or Te Tai-o-Maha-a-nui, but with the coming of the Pakeha their names were to be forgotten and ignored. By contrast, the visiting survey ship sailed into the broad, swooping bay, with its magnificent backdrop of high snow-clad alps, did its work and carried on its way, leaving behind its name as a permanent record of its fleeting and inconsequential visit.

But Pegasus Bay is not always rough. Often, it is as flat as a mirror, as polished and clear as the mirror into which Perseus gazed as he cleaved the snaky head off the terrible Gorgon. It was from the rocks that were sullied by her blood that the wondrous Pegasus arose. The goddess Athena tamed the flying horse so that it would carry her through the sky, increasing her power and prestige. From the birthplace of Pegasus there flowed a spring of crystal-clear water and any who drank from this would be blessed by the Muse with the gift of music and words. So here we had a name that not only spoke of place but also reflected our love of music in general and opera in particular. With apologies to the local Ngai Tahu people and those who had gone before, we felt that it suitably expressed where we were from and who we were. We were glad to have finally named our vineyard, and its moniker gave us our label. We had killed two birds with one stone, something that our long-suffering anonymous pussycat was delighted about.

We were then faced with another mini-dilemma. The first stage of our winery had been built, wine was in the bottle, and we now had it labelled. Did we just open our cellar door and start selling wine or did we hold some sort of event to mark the occasion? There was not any agonising over this one. It was a no-brainer. It had been such a long haul to get to this stage that we felt we were in need of a good party.

And so a crowd of friends, colleagues, restaurateurs and wine-trade people gathered to celebrate the occasion, talking animatedly while devouring the wine and food with enthusiasm. Although there were a large number of people, the room seemed spacious, almost cavernous, not only because of its height but also because, apart from our guests, it was almost empty. We had built it to eventually take tall fermentation tanks, but at that stage we had only a small amount of equipment and only a few crates of wine. The only natural light filtered through the deep red and blue panes of a high window placed at one end of the building. Chris and I smiled knowingly when several people independently commented that it seemed like a cathedral. We had been frustrated by our failure to find a suitable church, but Trevor had sympathised with our plans and had improvised.

It never ceases to surprise me just how the simple clinking together of a couple of wine glasses will silence the noisiest of mobs, and within a couple of moments the room was silent. I said a few words of welcome and introduction, then Malvina, who was standing on a little landing two floors above, began to sing. Her magical soprano voice not only floated over the stunned crowd but seemed to hang suspended in mid-air above their heads, while at the same time insinuating its way into every little nook and cranny. Malvina persuaded Chris to sing also and together they performed the refrain as a duo. The uninterrupted space and insulated walls provided perfect acoustics, something we had not anticipated. After Malvina's performance, the Minister for Trade Negotiations, Philip Burdon, said encouraging but overgenerous words about the importance of new businesses such as ours before officially opening the winery and casting us loose onto the uncharted foreign waters of commerce. A few months earlier, the vineyard and winery that had first produced wine in the district had been put up for mortgagee sale. We were sure these treacherous waters were full of hidden rocks that were circled by sharks, including the well-known and greedy loan variety. We felt nervously happy.

Although it was November, overnight a southerly storm arrived, causing the mercury to plummet and bringing drenching rain. We had conscientiously cleaned up after the previous day's opening party, but it seemed unlikely that we would be rewarded with any customers on our first day of trading. Chris and I opened the cellar-door sales area and stared glumly at the horizontal water bullets that imploded on the winery. Then, to our amazement, we saw a lone, forlorn-looking shape trudging through the long grass, coming from the general direction of a neighbouring farm. A minute or so later the door opened and there stood a small hunched figure, bundled up in a shabby gabardine overcoat. The water cascaded off his coat and his old felt trilby, forming a large puddle on the floor. His shoes, socks and the lower part of his trousers were completely soaked through.

'Hello, Ivan,' a little voice said from somewhere beneath the brim of the trilby. 'I just thought I would come and see your new winery.'

'Greetings, Bill. How nice to see you. Let me help you off with your coat; I'll hang it up for you near the heater. But why did you come from the next-door neighbours' farm? Why didn't you use the main entrance?'

'I didn't see it. I thought I was coming to the main entrance but I must have walked right around the back of the winery and into the paddock,' Bill replied, peering myopically through his thick pebble-like glasses and looking rather sheepish.

'Sit yourself down here by the heater, Bill, and Chris will give you a glass of wine. I'll just dash up to the car park to see if the entrance sign has blown away.'

Surprisingly, the large sign with its bold writing was still in place and Bill's car was parked directly in front of it! But perhaps I should not have been surprised. Bill was a medical colleague who had never really found his niche or soulmate. Although he was now hurtling towards retirement age he still lived devotedly with his mother. He was a Kiwi but he spoke with the most frightfully proper of English accents and was forever reminiscing about famous — well at least in medical circles — figures whom he had met while training in the 'old country'. His very demeanour evoked sympathy, and it was very evocative that day.

I would have invited Bill to the opening but I had no idea he was interested in wine. Perhaps he was not, but merely curious to see what we were up to. Nonetheless, he was the most welcome of customers on that particular day — and we did have a few more. However, his was the face that launched a thousand ships, or rather bottles, for that was about the number we sold during the rest of 1992. We had launched our little craft and were on our way at last.

## CHAPTER 11

# Building *a* Business

### 1993–2012

**'I'VE MANAGED TO GET A REALLY PROMISING** young winemaker to help me do our next vintage, Dad,' Matthew announced enthusiastically one afternoon in the early autumn of 1993.

'Surely you won't need anybody to help you,' I replied, less enthusiastically. 'The vineyard is still in its infancy and we won't have very much crop. You and I seemed to cope quite well last year, and although I'll be busy at the hospital I can still make some time to come out to the winery and help you. We have started to sell some wine but we are still far from breaking even. We really can't afford to pay for extra winery staff.'

'But it would free you up, Dad, and it would give me extra time to make certain that I do things absolutely perfectly. You have always said that you want to make the best wines possible, but I'm not very good at organising things. This is a very organised type of person who could make certain that the work programme over vintage runs smoothly, that we return the empty picking bins to the vineyard promptly, that we press off the red ferments at the right time and all that sort of thing. It's vital to have things done just at the right moment if you want to make the best wine.'

'Perhaps next year, Matthew, when we will have more grapes and, hopefully, more cash,' Chris chipped in, backing me up.

'But it won't cost a lot. This person only recently completed the Lincoln viticulture and oenology diploma and was top of the course, but doesn't have a lot of experience so we wouldn't have to pay very much. Besides, it will only be for a few weeks.'

'Okay, Matthew. You win this time, but just make certain that it is not for too long,' I said regretfully.

‘Thanks! You won’t regret it. She did last vintage with Danny Schuster and he said she was a great worker.’

‘She?’

‘Yes, her name’s Lynnette.’

And that is how the beautiful, charming and very talented Lynnette Hudson came into our lives. Everything that Matthew had said was correct — well, almost everything. Lynnette did not leave at the end of vintage, and after a number of years Chris and I were privileged to have her become our daughter-in-law. Without a doubt, Matthew had planned it from the very start and it really would not have mattered what we had said, he would have found a way to get around us.

Lynnette was not the only new long-term arrival for the vintage of 1993; there was also Ruissec. From the start, this young lady displayed a rather changeable disposition, but she was reasonably well-behaved. Whether the wine eventually got to her, I am not certain, but after a while we noticed a change in her temperament. She became more excitable, impulsive and attention-seeking. We never saw her sneaking wine but we suspected it. Alcohol, however, is volatile so perhaps she just breathed it in from the atmosphere and absorbed it into her system. If you have ever visited a winery and strolled among the vats, tanks and barrels, you will no doubt be aware of the strong, sweet, heady aroma that is typical of such establishments, and ours was no exception. I have never seen any scientific studies measuring the blood-alcohol concentration of individuals who have simply inhaled such deliciously aromatic air, but I suspect that it may not be zero. After all, the level of wine in watertight wooden barrels gradually decreases, which necessitates topping them up every few months, hopefully with the same wine. The amount of wine that is lost in this way is known in the trade as ‘the angels’ share’, and it is quite considerable.

Perhaps, on the other hand, Ruissec’s behavioural change had nothing to do with wine and was either genetically determined or she had experienced some traumatic life experience before she came to us. I guess we will never know because unfortunately she died. At first, when her behaviour became flamboyant, we tolerated it. Then she started to display uncalled-for aggression, but only when she became excited. Being a neurologist, who fancied himself as a movement disorder specialist, I felt she had developed stereotypic behaviour or a mannerism, although I have no doubt that a psychiatrist would have called it a fetish. Whatever the exact diagnosis, the result was socially unacceptable and I felt she would have to go. I gave an ultimatum that was greeted with howls of disbelief and objection from the family.

'You can't have her just going around biting ladies' bottoms willy-nilly!' I pronounced in support of my proposal.

'She is not doing it willy-nilly; it's only when she is excited to see someone,' retorted Chris. 'She is trying to attract their attention.'

'And it's not really a bite, it's just a little nip,' added Matthew.

'A little nip you call it? It seems more than a nip to me. She actually punctured the skin of Norma's bottom — although that may just be hearsay as I didn't inspect the wound myself. Perhaps that time her action was justified, as the owner of the buttocks in question is not known as a great dog-lover,' I said by way of signalling vacillation.

'You can take my word for the nature of the injury, but it was minor,' Chris stated firmly. 'It was certainly not something that Norma would like her son-in-law peering at. None of the women who have been bitten have suggested that Ruissec should be put down, so she cannot be too threatening.'

'Well, if it happens once again she's a goner. You will have to keep her tied up, find another home for her, or she will be on Death Row.'

Maybe Ruissec had been listening outside the door or maybe there was a secret pact of silence about all future such indiscretions. Whatever the explanation, she never again caused me any grief, except when she died full of years much later. By that stage she had long become accustomed to having a mini-partner in crime, Growler, who was even more mischievous. He was said to be a long-legged wire-haired Jack Russell terrier, if such a breed really exists. Growler looked identical to Milou, aka Snowy, in the Tintin comics and it proved impossible to stop him barking every time Graham Croft came to the winery, even though our neighbour was a 'good guy'. Naturally, his behaviour would trigger off the same reaction in Ruissec; such are the incomprehensible vagaries of dogs. It seems, however, to be an unwritten law that all self-respecting vineyards and wineries have to keep pet dogs. If you do not believe me, just Google it; people have even written books on this human fetish!

It seems a given that a winemaker would have a good palate, just as you might imagine that it was an immutable law that rugby players and soldiers are brave. As a vigneron and medic, let me assure you that this is not the case. In fact, I believe that the percentage of professional rugby players and soldiers who are terrified of hypodermic needles is far in excess of that in the general population. Similarly, in my view, many winemakers do not have good palates. Even with training, they may have trouble distinguishing a decent wine from a rotten one, let alone from a very good one. There seems to be something innate in the ability to define and appreciate all of the nuances in wine, good and bad, and I believe the same applies to food.

By happy chance, Matthew and Lynnette both had excellent palates, or perhaps I deluded myself about that solely because theirs usually seemed to be in concert with mine. We thus took to blending all wines as a trio. Our system was to make our wines in small batches, keeping the grapes from each picking and from every parcel of our vineyard separate, even if they were the same variety. Thus, the wines from all the fermenting vats and tanks were matured individually, so that when it came to deciding on the final blend for a wine that was to be bottled we had very many choices on how it would be assembled. For example, when blending our pinot noir we might have 20 or more different batches of wine, each of a different volume, which could be considered for the final assemblage or blend.

First we would taste samples of all the different batches and make notes about them. It was always surprising how different these batches could be, even when they were made from the same clones of grapes and when fermented and matured in identical ways. Then we three tasters would use measuring cylinders to make up small amounts of the blends that we each felt might be the best, and these three would be carefully evaluated and criticised. This, like all of our tastings, was done blind, with the code indicating the exact blend concealed underneath our tasting glasses. From there on the winning blend would be gradually refined, adding a little bit of this or removing a little bit of that, the aim always being to make the best wine possible, even if it meant excluding a significant part of the volume available.

One batch may add aroma but lack the body that another could provide. Excessively drying tannins could be mellowed and made velvety by a portion that would be too soft and flabby by itself. These barrels might give fruitiness, while those might add structure. In this way we would generally creep forward, but not infrequently stray sideways or even fall back a pace or two. It may sound like a lot of fun, but let me assure you, like judging in a wine competition, it was actually a lot of hard work. It might take a dozen or more sessions, each of an hour or two, before we could come up with a potential final blend. Then we would always make up two or three bottles of this and take them away to re-evaluate over a meal. We were very conscious that palate fatigue was an ever-present risk that could influence our decisions, so we took every precaution to avoid it.

Not all winemakers make wine like this. There is a school of thought that fermenting all the various parcels of what will be the final wine in one big tank allows the various elements to marry together better. If, however, it does not work out as intended, then you have disastrously burnt your bridges behind you.

The path that we chose had a significant disadvantage, however. It almost always turned out to be a jigsaw puzzle with too many pieces and we were frequently left with excess wine to dispose of.

**SHOULD YOU FANCY YOURSELF** as a restaurateur let me give you a warning: there is many a dream that becomes a nightmare. It is not that we have had this problem ourselves but we know others who have and, like the wine business, there is a lot of hard work attached to running a restaurant. It was never our goal to be restaurateurs *per se*, but we felt it would generate much-needed income to help support our money-hungry vineyard and winery. How wrong we were! Nonetheless, from the day that we opened our winery tasting room and started to sell wine, we also opened a winery restaurant.

A secondary aim was to showcase our wine with food, and in this the venture was successful. Although Chris and I were chronic 'foodies' and Chris had taken a semi-professional course at a cooking school in London, we had zero experience in the restaurant business. We had a few chefs apply to our advertisement in a local newspaper, but how did we select one? We decided that if the proof of the pudding was in the eating then the proof of a chef was also in the dining. Edward had demonstrated an interest in cooking from the time he was a small boy, when he would raid our tree and make lemon meringue pie for his friends after school, so the job of making the choice fell to him and Chris. I was glad to plead pressure of work as an excuse to leave it to the experts. The job went to a young English chef, Colin Cutler, not because they particularly liked his raunchy open steak sandwich on a bed of raspberry coulis, but they admired his imagination and flair. We also employed a young local woman, Kate Ensor, to look after front-of-house. She waitressed and ran the tasting room and cellar-door sales.

It was our intention that our budding establishment would be open every day to maximise sales, and therein lay a serious problem that we had not adequately thought through. Both our chef and our front-of-house needed days off, and when these occurred who had to fill in? Chris, of course; the task fell on her broad shoulders. It was not something she relished, but she did it. Sometimes, their days off coincided, and then she hated the job because both the job and the food could so easily turn to custard.

'It was just chaos today,' she whimpered one evening over a soothing glass of pre-dinner bubbly. 'Customers would turn up at the cellar door and I would welcome them. Invariably, they would want me to conduct a tutored tasting of the range of wines. Then they would order lunch and I would have to rush upstairs and put on my chef's hat in order to cook it.'

Our cellar-door sales and tasting room was on the ground floor, where in our grand plan the kitchen was finally to be sited, and our kitchen was directly above, where it was intended that our laboratory would eventually go. Above that was a bedroom that Chris and I used when we stayed on-site.

'Then I would need to become the waitress and rush downstairs to serve it to them,' Chris continued mournfully. 'By this time the next lot of customers were waiting to have a tutored tasting. When I had completed that I had to clear the tables, give out the invoices, collect the money, cook more meals and be the waitress again, and so it went continually throughout the day. Between times, I tried to put the dishes, cutlery and glasses in the dishwasher and then, when they were clean, take them out. At the end of the day I had to clean out the whole place and prepare for tomorrow. I'm absolutely exhausted.'

'It sounds simply dreadful,' I sympathised.

'Dreadful! It was worse than dreadful. It was Fawlty Towers and I was Basil Fawlty!' she said, sounding completely at the end of her tether.

She was, of course, referring to the famous BBC production of the same name, which starred John Cleese. We did not then know that Cleese was actually a wine buff who would later do TV programmes on wine. Nor had we any inkling that he would one day come to our winery and that we would give him one of the tutored tastings that Chris was complaining about.

'What are we going to do?' I asked.

'Well, I could run the cellar door when Kate has her days off, but I can't do Colin's job at the same time. If we are going to be open every day then we need another chef, but there is not really enough work for two. Besides, we had quite a lot of trouble sorting out one chef and I don't fancy doing that again.'

It was then that we had a brilliant idea. Edward had left school and was at a loose end. Why not see if he wanted to train as a chef? He could perhaps become an apprentice to Colin Cutler and at the same time do a part-time chef's course at the local polytechnic. It would cook two birds in the one dish. And that is exactly what happened. Edward was as keen as strong Dijon mustard, and he and Colin hit it off like apple and tart being flambéed *ensemble*. Edward later found his chef's qualification gave him a travel ticket and he was able to gain further experience of international cuisine in top overseas restaurants, all of which was to stand him — and us — in good stead.

But it was never our intention that Edward would remain a chef, however noble that profession might be; no, we had always thought of him as *chef de marketing*. There are those who think of marketing as a science and treat the subject as such. They head university departments, conduct surveys, write books, publish articles and the like. Then there are those to whom marketing is a business. They are consultants, who advise clients on appropriate logos or labels, on how to position themselves in the market, how to attract customers and so forth. And then there are those who themselves have a natural flair for marketing. They are not just good at selling things, they are attuned to the times and tides of the marketplace, they have a feel for what is appropriate in different situations, and they are sensitive to the needs and wants of individual customers.

It was in this last-mentioned way that Edward was gifted. From an early age he was a people person, a good mixer and an easy conversationalist, and he had a talent for organising others. More often than not he was the ringleader of the children's neighbourhood games and, as he cruised through adolescence into his teenage years, he turned these skills in a blatantly commercial direction. As a lad he would set up a stall at the gate of our house in Christchurch and sell anything that was available: tadpoles, frogs, lemons from our tree and suchlike. Sometimes his brothers would find that their favourite comics or books were missing, and under duress Edward would confess that he had sold them.

Not long after we had planted our first vines at Pegasus Bay, Edward organised his brothers and friends to plant a vegetable garden in a little sun-drenched hollow at the foot of the vineyard where a small spring bubbled forth. He then set about selling the produce to neighbours. Finally, when his miserly parents refused to buy him a car, he paid a team of school friends to collect and bag-up pine cones from our vineyard shelter-belts which he then hawked around the suburbs and sold at a not inconsiderable profit. In this way, Edward circumvented his parents' desires and purchased an old jalopy.

'That boy could sell French letters to nuns,' Chris had said when we were discussing Edward's job.

'I agree,' I replied, 'although I don't know that analogy is necessarily appropriate. I have never seen a study which has shown that the task would be very difficult. They might be inclined just to make a compassionate purchase in order to help out a poor young man.'

We, and Edward, agreed that training as a chef would be a stepping stone and that, as we did not really have enough work for two chefs, he would also cut his professional marketing teeth by promoting our wines around Christchurch for a couple of days each week.

We never really understood why people bothered to come to our restaurant in those early days, but we were very grateful for their support, not a small amount of which came from my medical colleagues. We had a pretty cheap and crummy set of white plastic tables and chairs, which reflected the light dreadfully if it was sunny enough to sit outside. When it was cold the customers had to retreat into the winery and sit at the same tables scattered between the barrels and wine tanks. Because of the wine, we wanted the building to be as insulated as possible, which meant a minimum of window space. Hence, the only natural light filtered through the vivid blue and red window placed high in one end of the room. We were thus forced to use the strong overhead winery lamps to provide light, producing an ambience that was more industrial than romantic. The space was so large that we needed to use an enormous gas heater to provide warmth. This looked like a jumbo-jet motor and made a not dissimilar noise, a cross between a deafening roar and a whine. We had to point it well away from our tables and customers in case it melted or burnt them, respectively. Initially we would apologise for the rather quirky restaurant surroundings, but people seemed to really enjoy themselves so that we eventually adopted an unrepentant attitude.

Things were somewhat improved a few years later when we built the next stage. The restaurant was then moved into a space that was intended eventually to be used for bottling, and at least there were more windows to provide a modicum of natural light. Our gradually increasing staff felt that all their birthdays had come at once when several years later we decided to bite the bullet and provide them with a purpose-built restaurant. Because we had had a bad rush of blood to our heads and had asked Trevor Ibbotson to design it with a tower, we refrained from cracking any Basil Fawlty jokes. Having now run a restaurant for over 20 years, however, we have had many Fawlty experiences.

While every chef is an individual, my observation is that they generally fall into two categories: the 'calm' and the 'excitable'. While a head chef of the former type usually makes for a happier kitchen team, this does not always result in better food, although it tends to do this. A subcategory of the excitable is the 'Dr Jekyll and Mr Hyde' syndrome. Most of the time, such specimens appear so calm, cool and collected that you could easily misclassify them as calm. This refined outer appearance, however, conceals inner tensions. When the lurking werewolf does occasionally appear it usually does so instantaneously, and often when the restaurant owners are not around to see the transformation.

Another subcategory of the excitable is the 'surly'. Surly chefs are most decidedly a menace. You do not need to be a psychoanalyst to know that they are as hot and explosive as a dish of prunes heavily laced with chilli, and it is always a relief when they finally pass out of the system. We have sometimes found that working for us can act as a catharsis and bring a revelation to an inwardly unhappy chef. We have had more than one who has seen the light and gone over to the dark side, retraining in viticulture or winemaking.

'What's the matter, Edward?' Chris asked as Edward put down his mobile phone, quietly cursing under his breath.

It was the first time in over a decade that all of the family who were involved in the business had gone away together. We had just arrived at our hotel after flying to Wellington to attend a pinot noir conference, at which there would be a lot of influential international media and wine-trade delegates. It was especially vital that Edward be there. A few years earlier he had given up being a chef, but part of his brief was to manage the restaurant and kitchen.

'That was Jason on the phone. He says Kevin has just disappeared. He doesn't know where he has gone, but he thinks that he may not be coming back. Kevin was talking on the phone and then he just suddenly walked out, taking all his knives with him. Apparently that was an hour ago and he hasn't returned.'

Jason was the sous chef, a timid, monosyllabic man, and while he was meticulous and conscientious, he was painfully slow in the kitchen. He worked under the supervision of Kevin, the head chef, who had proven to be satisfactory, if not exceptional, at his calling. We had not previously experienced any significant problems with him.

'Do you think Jason will be able to cope by himself?' Chris asked.

'Not a chance,' replied Edward; 'we're catering for a wedding reception tonight and another one tomorrow afternoon. Unless I do something immediately it seems we will have total disaster on our hands! Even if I can get another chef to help out he won't know the kitchen or the menu. I'll have to go back on the next plane to supervise, if not to cook.'

Fortunately, the local dial-a-chef was able to oblige and under Edward's eagle eye we were pulled back from the brink, although his presence at the pinot jamboree was sorely missed. It was a fortnight later that Kevin reappeared in the restaurant, without forewarning or explanation, looking as bright as a button and ready to start work again. He had even brought his knives with him. It transpired that an argument with his girlfriend had triggered a need for him to 'clear' his head. We sympathised, but it was clear to us that it had been so thoroughly cleaned out that it was now completely empty and devoid of reality.

When we got around to building our restaurant proper, we realised that it was vital to have a separate tasting room. Before that, people wanting wine tastings had locked horns with those who were looking for meals and they had formed a tight scrum around a single counter.

Tasting-room clients tend to fall into one of two categories. The first are casual drinkers; good-natured souls who enjoy a glass of wine but are not fussed about the details. The second group are wine geeks, like me, who want to know what type of yeast was used, the temperature of fermentation, whether the wine has malolactic and so forth.

One day the nubile young maiden who looked after the tasting room informed me that something strange was happening. A series of young men had come to the tasting room on different days, but they all seemed strangely similar. They did not seem to fit into the second category, in that their wine knowledge appeared scant to non-existent. However, they wanted to know in detail how our wine was made. They were all well-dressed, clean-shaven and neatly coiffured, and our young lady wondered if they had delicate eyes because they all wore dark glasses, even though the tasting-room illumination could euphemistically be described as romantic. She found it somewhat unnerving as they all spoke with strong American accents and they invariably purchased a bottle of the same Pegasus Bay wine. The trend continued and eventually some of these young Yanks staggered out carrying cases of the aforesaid beverage. We were delighted to serve them, but what on earth was going on? Were we under surveillance by the CIA?

It soon became clear: Bill Clinton was to grace our little isles with a visit, and our wine had been chosen to be served at the upcoming state dinner. We imagined that the President's security men first fed Pegasus Bay wine to mice then, if they survived, to monkeys, possibly followed by prisoners. At last they may have taken a sip themselves before finally giving it clearance to pass the President's lips. A few years earlier our wine had been served to Queen Elizabeth when she visited New Zealand, and we were amused, although she may not have been, when we realised that cheeky little drop had not been subject to the same rigorous scrutiny. But then, Brits seem rather more relaxed than their transatlantic cousins when it comes to matters of high security. We were delighted when somewhat later we received an order to supply wine to Buckingham Palace.

Even though officials of the People's Republic of China do not have a reputation for slackness in matters of security, they also did not seem to subject our rough product to such close surveillance before it was served to their president when he visited our shores. But then you never know what really goes on behind the scenes. Now these people all have one thing in common, besides their greatness: namely, that they have survived their encounters with the Flying Horse!

No matter how good a restaurant thinks its wine and food might be, its reputation will ultimately depend on its customers' experience, and this is to no small extent in the hands of the front-of-house staff. Edward's background in the restaurant business proved to be invaluable, not only in attracting chefs and other kitchen personnel but also in selecting the *maître d'*, waiters/waitresses and tasting-room staff. We were blessed in having caring, considerate and professional people. Yes, he knew how to pick them, but when he hired Belinda Keys as *maître d'* he may also have had something else in mind. If so, he did not let on to us about that. Belinda came with extensive restaurant experience and a BA thrown in for good luck. She had all the qualities mentioned above, along with a gentle personality and a very special sparkle. The inevitable followed, and in due course Chris and I were delighted to have a new daughter-in-law. With the arrival of children Belinda took over the job of restaurant manager, allowing Edward to concentrate fully on marketing.

It was Chris who answered the telephone one night when its ringing interrupted our late dinner.

'Ivan,' she called, 'quickly pick up the phone in the other room. It's Belinda, and she has something special that she wants to tell us.'

'Something fantastic has just happened,' said a very excited Belinda. 'Pegasus Bay restaurant has just been named by *Cuisine* magazine as the best casual-dining restaurant in New Zealand.'

'Congratulations!' we shouted nearly simultaneously. Then I asked Belinda, 'What does that actually mean?'

'Well, there is a silver-service restaurant in Wellington that they have judged to be the top restaurant in the country, while we have been judged the top "Casual Dining" restaurant. They only have two categories, and as we only serve lunches in a vineyard setting we've come under the "Casual" category. Imagine that! They have only named two top restaurants in the entire country and Pegasus Bay restaurant is one of them!'

*Cuisine* magazine, which was New Zealand's top wine and food publication, had just announced the winners of its first country-wide restaurant evaluation. Belinda and Edward had had a sneaking suspicion that something was afoot when they were telephoned by the magazine a few days earlier and asked if they were intending to go to the awards dinner in Auckland. They had apologised and said that they could not manage it. However, the caller had been keen that they make every effort to attend or at least send a representative. They thought they might have gained some minor award, and were completely stunned when the results were announced.

That was in 2005. In the following years several other categories were added to the *Cuisine* restaurant awards, including 'New Zealand Winery Restaurant of the Year', in which Pegasus Bay was named the winner each year from 2008 to 2012. Thus, for six years the restaurant was named the best in its category.

In 2014 it was awarded a coveted 'Chef's Hat' in the *Cuisine Good Food Guide* and named as the Best Regional Establishment in the Christchurch Hospitality Awards. This has shown a remarkable consistency, especially given that over this period we had four different head chefs due to circumstances beyond our control, including earthquakes. It underscores that a restaurant's reputation rests on a team effort and throughout this period Belinda and Edward have consistently striven for the highest standard. Chris and I have felt overwhelmed and overjoyed by their successes.

**A WINERY IS A WORKSHOP** and, just because you attach a restaurant to it, the result is not necessarily pleasing, at least from an aesthetic point of view, and in this we had a problem. Hence, Chris and I had decided from day one that the environs, the setting of our madcap venture, were all-important. Essentially, where we intended to site our buildings, we had a fairly flat paddock. This was divided on its northern side by a small funnel-shaped valley that had its spout to the west and its wide mouth on the east, where its south bank formed a north-facing natural amphitheatre. The floor of this gully was choked with broom, gorse, blackberry and other such exotic nasties.

We felt like explorers in the upper reaches of the Amazon jungle when, one sunny summer morning, Chris and I set off to try and penetrate this wilderness. We were armed with slashers/machetes, a pruning saw, an adequate supply of sticking plaster, and morning tea. We were both wearing waterproof footwear as we suspected there would be hidden marshy patches, and if it had not been for the thorns we would doubtless have been sporting shorts; for the effect, if not out of necessity. The going was quite tough, but after an hour or so we had hacked a little path to about where we thought the centre must be. We were delighted to find several pools of limpid water, which were closely surrounded by brambles and scrub and were home to frogs that croaked noisily before making a sploshing getaway. There were a number of mature trees in our little valley, including some very old pines at the periphery and willows at the centre.

We sat on a fallen trunk and celebrated our success as intrepid explorers with cups of tea and biscuits. We felt that our wilderness had potential and that the gully could become an attractive focal point in front of our future establishment, but first it would have to be sanitised. We would need to clear it of all the unwanted journeymen, those roguish plants that had just arrived uninvited from afar, decided to stay, put their roots down and then fought desperately with their neighbours, trying to strangle them in a chaotic battle to the death. We knew that this little town of vagabonds had enticed all other sorts of riff-raff to take up residence, including rats, ferrets, possums and the like.

But what should we do with the valley after it had been cleared? We felt we needed to make a statement, something that would be immediately impressive, and we hit upon the idea of creating a great dam on its east side and flooding the whole gully. The resulting large lake would have its shore right in front of our restaurant. An additional advantage was that it would use up quite a lot of the three hectares of bare land that would otherwise surround our future buildings; a blank space that was becoming frighteningly larger every day in our equally blank minds. We applied to the authorities and were eventually granted permission to install the dam and create the lake, although not without objections and further legal sparring with the ever-pugilistic Farmer Jones.

As soon as we had acquired the property we had started to plant trees, bushes and shrubs, by which I mean that Chris would decide what would go where and she would acquire it, while my input was solely in the brainless form of hole-digging. She wanted to get as much growth as she could as soon as was practicable while avoiding potential building places, which somewhat limited what she could do. Once the building site had been firmly established with our architect, Trevor Ibbotson, however, she bent my back double in a renewed frenzy of planting.

Chris had always been keen on gardens and garden design, but her increasing enthusiasm for the topic was now bordering on an addiction. Mealtimes seemed to revolve around the scientific names of plants and where they would be best situated. Meanwhile, as the planting continued I could see that the garden-free area was nearing extinction and I was secretly looking forward to being made redundant from my casual gardening job. Then something happened that delayed any thoughts of immediate retirement. Chris realised that she did not have space for the ambitious garden that she really wanted. How rapidly that seemingly vast empty space had shrunk!

'It's a disappointment,' she said, 'but I guess I'll just have to make it smaller; cut my coat to suit the cloth, so to speak.'

'Why don't we forget the idea of having a huge lake?' I disbelievingly heard myself say. 'By building it we will really destroy the valley, and it could be made quite picturesque. We could still have a series of smaller interconnected lakes or ponds in its floor, and you could let your imagination run riot on the rest.'

'Yes!' cried Chris. 'We would then be able to use the natural amphitheatre for concerts, opera and the like. If we flooded the gully it would really be destroyed.'

'Just like all those Egyptian temples in the upper Nile after the Aswan dam was built?' I enquired in jest.

'They weren't destroyed, silly. They were saved by being relocated, but we can't relocate the valley, which is actually a treasure for us. It will just die a watery death.'

We thought about it for all of a further millisecond. It seemed such an obvious thing to do, but it had escaped us. It would be more complicated and a lot more work than just building a large dam, but in the end it would be much better. My lower backache would be a small price to pay.

'Do you know what the worst thing about this will be?' Chris asked.

'No, I don't. I don't think there is any downside.'

'Yes, there is,' said Chris. 'We are going to have to apply for a new permit to build those small lakes and I know somebody who is bound to submit 101 objections!'

Chris did not just plant her garden willy-nilly, she planned it very carefully, although the plan was living and had to be able to adapt to changing circumstances as the development progressed. She wanted the general impression to be park-like but at the same time to have multiple intimate spaces; secluded gardens that would surprise and delight the eye and areas that had particular themes. These needed to be created around public parking, an entrance to the winery, a restaurant potager, a small orchard and appropriate screening of winery work areas. The garden plan would also need to accommodate the changing seasons.

Her garden was clearly not something that could just appear overnight. As it turned out, it would take her many years to develop it, but, as every gardener knows only too well, a garden is never finished. This is part of its fascination and joy. Chris drew much of her inspiration from visiting gardens in New Zealand and overseas, including that of Hugh and Judy Johnson, who had about five hectares of superb garden around their Elizabethan house in Essex. Hugh's book *Wine* had been responsible for starting Chris and me on our downward vinous track many years earlier, and it was wonderful for us that they had become friends.

Later Chris established an extensive biodiversity trail with the help of Lincoln University as part of the Greening of Waipara Project. This was successful in restoring indigenous vegetation to the Waipara Valley and attracting native birds. At the opening of the trail, we were presented with a pou, a richly decorated traditional Maori carving, to symbolise our family's attachment to the land.

Even established gardens require a huge amount of maintenance, including plenty of back-bending weeding, which I tended to avoid. I was an expert at criticising from afar and, like most grown-up boys, I was prepared to help out with the mowing, especially as we had a large rotary mower which was towed behind an old tractor. It seemed a bit of fun rather than hard work. I had driven tractors on a few occasions before we started our vineyard, so naturally I regarded myself as quite an expert. Late one Sunday afternoon I noticed that Chris had left a strip of unmown grass along the edge of our newly formed ponds, which was at the bottom of a grassy slope in front of the restaurant and winery. For some inexplicable reason it irritated me.

'It looks messy,' I complained. 'It should be easy enough to mow right to the edge of the lake. After all, the mower is mounted well behind the tractor and you would only have to back gently towards the water with the slasher blades whirling over the edge. It would make a perfect job and the tractor wheels would remain firmly on the bank.'

'I'm not going to do it. It's too dangerous,' Chris retorted. 'You will just have to put up with a bit of long grass around the edge of the lake.'

'There's no danger,' I said emphatically. 'I'll show you how it's done,' and so saying I swung myself up into the driving seat and turned the old orange tractor so that it was facing up the grassy slope with its back towards the pond. I then slowly started reversing towards the lake with the mower blades whirring at top speed. It was making a perfect job, and I called out proudly, 'See what an expert can do!'

I do not know whether it was the bonnet of the tractor rearing up in front of me, the falling sensation or the water rushing around me that was the most frightening. One second I was proudly demonstrating my clearly superior tractor skills, and the next I was unceremoniously hurtling backwards into the water. My initial thought was that I might be crushed beneath the heavy contraption. When the waves settled my white knuckles were still clinging to the steering wheel, my lower half was wet and I could see that I was well and truly in hot water, so to speak, although I was freezing cold. An oily slick was slowly spreading its attractive rainbow-coloured pattern across the surface of the pond. Worst of all, there was Chris high and dry on the bank, looking concerned but faintly triumphant.

'What a great way to measure the depth of the lake,' she called out, 'but it might have been easier with a stick.'

We had never really been certain of the depth of the pond and I was now very relieved to find that it was not deeper, at least near its edge. The tractor's motor was dead, however, and would not respond to my attempts to start it. There was no option other than to get off the tractor, ignominiously flounder to the bank and haul myself up onto the grass, where I lay panting in a muddy wet heap.

I clearly needed to get help to remedy the unfortunate situation that was all of my own making, and for this I turned to my next-door neighbour; no, not Farmer Brown, who was to our east, but Graham Croft, whose farm was immediately to our west. Graham and his wife Angela had been very helpful on multiple past occasions and I was confident that he would come to my assistance. Angela told me that he was ploughing a field a little way off, so I traipsed off in that general direction.

'What an earth have you been up to?' Graham asked with a broad smile, and on hearing my feeble explanation he burst into a fit of laughter.

'This is the first time I have heard of someone trying to mow a lake, but then I guess you have to be pretty smart to be a doctor so you probably know a trick or two that I don't.'

I felt not only acutely embarrassed but also guilty at interrupting his work. He unhitched the plough and told me to get up behind him. On reaching the lake he expertly backed his more powerful tractor down the slope, then he hitched two strong chains around the front of my beast. Slowly but surely he drove back up the lawn and pulled my sad-looking, dripping machine onto dry land. To my surprise, Graham was even able to jump-start it from his own tractor, and my machine was able to slowly creep away with me at the helm, my head hanging low.

It is said that criminals often revisit the scenes of their crimes and I suspect that this is particularly true of psychopaths. I do not profess to know why this should be, but I suspect they get a morbid thrill out of reliving their damnable experiences. To this day I do not know why I foolishly revisited the situation of my misdemeanour, but let me assure you it was not because I wanted to relive my damnable experience. I think that it was just because I was too stubborn and proud to accept that I was wrong; that I had made a bad mistake. It was surely misfortune rather than misjudgement, and I would be extremely prudent and vigilant the next time, when I would emerge victorious. I had merely backed too close to the lake, closer than I had needed.

The following weekend, when no one was around to watch, I put the tractor in low gear and started to climb the fateful slope with the mower's slasher blades whirring madly. I only had to put the tractor into reverse and then, ever so gently and slowly, back down towards the lake, with its ever-so-tempting fringe of ugly long grass. As everybody knows, to change from a forward gear into reverse requires the vehicle to come to a standstill, otherwise the gears will not engage and you are in danger of damaging the cogs or, at worst, stripping the gearbox. Should you have driven a tractor, especially an ancient one, you will know that the gears do not always engage easily and it can take a moment or two for the cogs to mesh properly. During this brief but critical time the clutch pedal has to be depressed, but it should not be a problem on a hill because you only have to apply the brake to stop the vehicle running backwards. All this assumes, however, that your brakes are in excellent working order.

It was only when I felt the tractor start to run back down the hill, in spite of the full force of my body weight upon the brake pedal, that I realised that my brake pads were still wet and hence ineffective. I had a strong sense of *déjà vu* as I stupidly hurtled backwards into the water. It was almost an exact replay, except that on this occasion the tractor had gained considerable momentum and I suspect that the old girl may even have had a long-dreamed-of *Chitty Chitty Bang Bang* moment of flight as it leapt from the Rive Droite towards the Rive Gauche. If so, any such orgasmic sensation of lightness of being must have been as brief as my feelings of terror and mortification were long. With a tsunami of impressive proportions she bellyflopped into the water, but this time she threw herself further into the pond than on the previous occasion. The waterspout had soaked me, but the faithful old lass had stayed upright and I was still alive and well, apart from a very painful ego.

Chris, who had heard the commotion, came running and stood aghast and dumbfounded. She helped me up the now slippery bank and I went off again in search of my ever-tolerant Good Samaritan neighbour, who split his sides laughing while I ate a large second helping of humble pie. What a grand tale he would have to tell the locals! I had finally learnt my lesson and it was the last time I attempted to demonstrate to Chris my superior tractor skills, but it was not the final time that I would mow the lake.

Just about all palaces, châteaux, manor houses and the like have water features, including ponds and lakes. Such a tradition stretches back millennia. They can be focal points in magnificent gardens and engender feelings of restfulness, peace and tranquillity. Sometimes exotic water plants entice the eye and provide special interest and beauty. When you gaze on a pond or lake you feel an inner sense of harmony and at peace with yourself and the world, unless you happen to be the gardener. Everybody knows that gardens are a lot of hard work, but few people realise that owning lakes and ponds can be just as demanding and arduous, especially if they are shallow and do not have a strong flow of water through them.

To our dismay, we found out the hard facts of aqueous life quite early on. First of all, duckweed began to appear on the surface. This can be attractive in little patches but if left unchecked it will soon cover the whole surface and your lake will look like a lawn. These little floating plants, not much bigger than a pinhead, cling onto the feet of water birds and are easily transported from one waterway to the next. One day you do not have duckweed and the next you do; it is as simple as that. We initially tried to rake the patches of weed to the side and just remove them, but the majority of the weed was well out of reach. I then got into my bathing suit and tried to cope with the stuff that was tantalisingly floating in the centre, but it proved to be too much for me alone. I asked one of our vineyard workers, a strapping young he-man, to give me a hand. We made slow but steady progress as we floundered about and directed thick mats of weed towards the bank, where Chris was removing it from the water. Suddenly a bloodcurdling scream of sheer terror rent the air, then I heard a frenzied splashing noise. I swung around to see my he-man desperately making for the shore, where he rapidly dragged himself up the bank and stood shaking with fear, his eyes bulging.

'What's the matter? Are you hurt?' I enquired with concern. I wondered if he might have cut himself or stabbed his foot on some sharp piece of wayward metal lying in the mud.

'Get out! Get out immediately!' he shouted. 'There are eels in the lake! Huge eels!'

'I know that, but they're quite harmless. They don't have big teeth. In fact, they are rather like coarse sandpaper — perhaps a little sharper, but they won't do you any harm. Come on back into the water and I will make sure they don't hurt you. They are really quite lovely fish and you can make pets out of them,' I added consolingly, trying to encourage him to keep on working.

'I'm not getting back in that lake again, not with all those damned eels in there; they're downright dangerous. Not for all the tea in China will you lure me back in that water!'

'Have you had a bad experience with an eel before?' I enquired.

'No, and I'm not about to. They're ugly-looking brutes.'

And so I had to continue on alone, fuming to myself at how strange it was that some people have a morbid fear of eels, just the same way that others are paranoid about spiders or mice. There is no accounting for some people's reactions. Was it because eels resemble snakes? Now, coming from a snake-free country I could understand serpentophobia. Then I recalled that I feel distinctly uncomfortable with heights, a salutary reminder that I should be more charitable and tolerant of other people's little quirks.

**'YOUR PRESENT IS IN THE GARAGE, DEAR,'** Chris announced on Christmas morning. 'I hope you like it.'

I did not need to remove the newspaper wrapping to know what lay concealed beneath, but when I did, I was delighted. There was the most lovely-looking snub-nosed wooden dinghy, sporting a new coat of glossy white paint and complete with a set of varnished oars.

'You shouldn't have, darling. However did you guess?'

'I just thought about the delightful rotocrumbler that you gave me for Christmas several years ago,' Chris said, 'and then I had a little retaliatory bout of inspiration. Now you can clear the weed on the ponds any time you want to. You will be like Toad of Toad Hall. You chaps are all the same; you just love mucking about in boats.'

After several days of splashing around in the lake in my bathing suit it had become eminently clear that this was not a practical method and that we would have to think of some other way to clear the weed. Chris had come up with the final solution. It was a masterstroke.

'There are some people floundering about in the lake, fully dressed,' a concerned diner informed Edward one Sunday afternoon. 'I wonder if they're all right. They may need help.'

'I'll come and see,' our son answered, and hurried to the top of the grassy slope that looked down to where Chris and I were struggling about in the muddy water.

'They're a couple of old eccentrics,' Edward said. 'They sometimes go for a swim in the lake. Don't worry, they'll be all right,' he added as he turned to go back into the busy restaurant.

By the time we reached the bank a crowd of fascinated customers stood gawking at us and a couple of them offered to help us up onto the grass. Chris and I were absolutely soaked and liberally smeared with mud. We feebly made light of the matter and hastily made off, feeling enormously embarrassed.

I had found that while it was easy enough from the dinghy to collect the weed, it was not much fun having it all sloshing around my feet inside the boat. Accordingly, I put the weed into plastic grape-picking bins, which I floated alongside the dinghy. It was slow and awkward work because when I had cleared one small area I then had to row to the next, dragging the picking bins behind. Chris, quite correctly, thought that it would be quicker with two people and nobly volunteered to sit in the back of the dinghy, holding on to the picking bins and helping with the detestable green harvest. Physics had never been her strong point at school, particularly the science of flotation and displacement. In addition, she was not used to small boats. In spite of several warnings about the potentially disastrous consequences of sudden movement and imbalance, she reached over to one side and tried to pluck a heavy crate of wet weed up into the little craft. The stern on the starboard side of the ship tilted dangerously low and, in slow motion, we began to ship water. The *Titanic* gradually slipped below the surface but the band did not play on, and the captain and his crew were the first to desert the ship.

Once the surface was largely free of duckweed another problem emerged, one that is common to most ponds with muddy bottoms that are less than a metre or two deep. The floating duckweed had blocked the light and prevented water weeds from growing up from below. These had their roots in the mud and now pushed vigorously upwards to reach the surface where they became entangled with the trivial amount of remaining duckweed. This meant the duckweed could not now be moved on and just started to proliferate again. I had seen how council workmen dealt with this problem in small streams and rivers. They had cut the bottom of the weed with a scythe-like blade, allowing the weed to float to the surface, from where it could be removed. This seemed too much like hard work, so I decided to try to mow this weed underwater using a rotary lawnmower. I removed the motor and its rotary cutting blade and attached them to an inflated inner tube. The motor was up in the air and the cutting blade was well below the surface of the water. After two or three anxious tugs on the starter cord the motor spluttered into life.

'Success! Success at last!' I shouted as Chris and a small band of similar disbelievers looked on.

'But why are the inner tube and the motor whirling around so fast?' asked an observant Chris. 'I thought it was the rotor blade that was supposed to be turning.'

I had forgotten that a helicopter needs to have two sets of rotors, the small one on the tail stopping the cab of the helicopter from spinning around.

'Easily fixed,' I shouted above the din. 'We'll tie it to the back of the boat and I'll just row around the lake.'

And that is how we came to mow our lake weed, although we eventually found it easier to tie two ropes, one to each side of the inner tube, and to pull the Heath Robinson contraption back and forwards across the water with Chris and I standing on opposite banks, each holding one of the lines. There was, however, one remaining problem that we were unable to solve and which limited the device's usefulness. The slasher blade and its connecting rod kept getting entangled in a thick mat of weed that would eventually prevent the cutting and could stall the motor. It was clear that I would never make a living as an inventor and that I had better stick to neurology and winemaking.

One member of our family who found the lakes irresistible was Ruissec, that naughty girl who liked to play up and tease us. Any time she was feeling hot she would plunge in and swim about. It made no difference to her whether the weed had been cleared or not. Usually she would emerge looking like an enormous, dirty Monster from the Black Lagoon and proceed to shake her soaking, weed-covered body over the nearest bystander. She was a bright girl, and apart from the water her other great love was rabbit. Like most modern girls she adored mixing her pleasures, so when she caught a bunny she would dive into the lake and drown it, before proceeding to savour its delights.

**'HELP! HELP! SOMEBODY HELP ME.** I'm desperate. Help!'

The petite waitress who thought she heard this faint cry from afar initially wondered if it was genuine. Had it really been a voice? Perhaps it was just one of the restaurant customers. Was it just somebody fooling around? She was in the middle of serving a group at an outdoor table and she vacillated, but eventually thought she should go and investigate. She excused herself for a moment and wandered around in the garden. Where had the noise come from?

'Help! Help! I can't last much longer.'

There it was again, and it definitely was a voice; a cry for help that was coming from somewhere in the gully. The waitress began to run down into the valley in front of the restaurant, and then she realised the desperate plea was coming from near its western end. It was there that she found Chris.

It had been threatening all afternoon. The sky had started as a leaden grey and there was the smell of rain in the air. Now billowing cumulus clouds, with white heads and black bellies, were arriving from the south. Chris had been mowing lawns all day, but had moved as far away as possible from the restaurant to avoid disturbing the diners. She was in a patch of lank grass that had not been cut for some time and she was keen to get it finished before the promised downpour started. Since my fiasco with the tractor in the lake, I had been banned from mowing, not that I had ever done very much. I agreed wholeheartedly that Chris's tractor skills were much better than mine; something that was quite hard for a bloke to accept. I had been relegated to looking after a couple of wine writers, and at that moment I was giving them a tasting in the winery.

Still mowing, Chris passed beneath the shelter of a willow tree, just as there was a large crack, a bit like thunder. Instantly the tractor stalled, stopping dead, and at the same time a huge branch came crashing down, thrusting Chris sideways and pinning her against the tractor's roll-bar. This frame of heavy steel, the so-called 'safety-bar', had caught on the low-hanging bough as she had passed underneath, and the force had ripped it from the tree. Chris's neck was pinned between the bough and the roll-bar and it was a miracle that she was intact. The further descent of the large curved branch had been halted by the front of the tractor, on which the branch was now resting. She could not extract her head from the narrow gap and her windpipe was becoming compromised by the swelling. If the tractor had not stalled she would have been headless, brainless or simply dead.

'Quickly. Please run and get Matthew and tell him to bring a chainsaw,' Chris managed to whisper.

Matthew arrived post-haste and began the rough but delicate task of cutting his mother free. He had to saw close enough to her head and neck to remove the major part of the bough but also had to leave sufficient gap to avoid further injury. Eventually she was liberated.

'Thank you, Matthew. Now I know what it is like to be the lady who is sawn in half in the magician's box. You were an expert, but I don't want to be in your next performance.'

I did not arrive on the scene until the whole show was over, which was probably just as well as I am sure Matthew had behaved in a much calmer way than I would have done. From that time on Chris was much more tactful about my tractor-driving skills and much more restrained in the exercise of her own prowess. In fact, she bought herself a ride-on mower, which was not only safer but made a superior job of the lawn.

Not long after we built the first stage of our winery, the conductor of the Christchurch city choir, Brian Law, offered to give us a family of peacocks from a flock he had on his own property. The more we thought about it the more we liked the idea. We had delusions of grandeur and could picture the majestic birds strutting graciously over our sweeping lawns. They would be the prop that would turn our winery into a stately home. Moreover, Farmer Jones had peacocks that he kept cooped up in a cage. How splendid it would be to have ours wandering free about our property. It would be a stunning comparison with the fate of our neighbour's miserable birds. It was magic and so simple. It was easy to maintain them, Brian assured us. You simply brought them onto the property in a large cage and kept them there for several days until they became accustomed to their surroundings.

'Scatter plenty of their food on the ground around the cage and then quietly open the door,' he advised. 'The birds will come out and will start to feed. They will stay in the vicinity of the cage so long as you continue to feed them there. I would suggest that you do that for a week and then gradually move their feeding spot to where you want them to live. They will look after themselves and will roost in the trees at night. Once they are established they will just stay around your gardens.'

They duly arrived, a cock, a hen and their chicks. How lovely they looked, the cock resplendently dressed in his richly iridescent plumage, the hen less showy but more homely, and their cute family. They would be jewels in the crown. We did everything according to the rule book, and after the prescribed time we spread liberal amounts of food in the immediate environs of the cage, which was in the most remote part of the gardens, the furthest removed from Farmer Jones's property. The birds slowly emerged from their temporary home and started to peck at the food and scratch in the earth. Over the course of the day we could see them adjusting to their surroundings.

All was well, they had made the transition. It was a success.

You may be aware that peacocks have a strange cry, rather like a cat mewing, but much louder and more strident.

'Meow! Meow! Meow! Meow!'

The previously irritating but now welcome sound awoke us early in the morning. We had heard it often enough before. It was Farmer Jones's peacocks ... or was it our very own? We rushed to the window, and there they were in all their shining splendour on our lawn. But what were they doing? They seemed to be hurrying in the direction from which those damnable screeches were coming. They were making with all speed towards Farmer Jones's! We rushed downstairs and tried to stop our family of peacocks, but to no avail. They were determined to answer the call of nature, the call of their kind.

We peered over the fence and there they were, excitedly lined up outside Farmer Jones's peacock cage. We checked their feed and there was a surfeit left untouched where we had fed them. Throughout the day we patiently waited, but the only sign we saw of our flock was our lonely cock, sitting on the high bough of a tree adjacent to Farmer Jones's property. We tried to entice the bird down with food but he would have none of it. His lady love and all of their brood had been seduced into life in a harem. The cock cried repeatedly throughout the day but without success. Chris telephoned and spoke to Farmer Jones's wife. No, she had not seen any peacocks, and if we got back our brood would we please make certain that they never strayed onto the Jones's property. They did not want their birds to be upset or perhaps catch some deadly avian disease from ours. We really should keep our birds in a cage so that they would not annoy our neighbours.

'Meow! Meow! Meow!'

The sad cry of the rejected cock continued intermittently throughout the night. It was closer than our neighbour's cage, and it came from the direction in which we had last seen our cuckolded friend. We looked for him at first light, but by then he too had disappeared. Our neighbours insisted that they had not seen beak nor plume of our feathered friends, but we could not help but imagine that there were more birds in their cage than we had ever seen before.

Subsequently, we did not regret the loss of our peacocks. Friends who have had them have told us that they are very messy birds, leaving their not inconsiderably sized calling cards in most inconvenient places, including on roofs, where they like to perch. For a long time we had been trying to attract pukeko, and finally these attractive but cheeky little native swamp hens adopted us. In keeping with Chris's biodiversity section of her gardens, featuring indigenous plants, pukeko seem much more appropriate. I like to imagine that these feisty natives would not have fancied sharing our little abode with stuck-up peacocks.

**OUTDOOR CONCERTS IN NEW ZEALAND** are always knife-edge affairs. Our weather is so changeable that even over the warmest summer period heavy wind or cold rain can interfere with proceedings or lead to their cancellation. Nonetheless, from early on it was our policy to hold charity concerts in our natural amphitheatre, as people lounged about on the grassy slope and picnicked while listening to great music. Chris and I favoured operatic concerts, complete with an orchestra, and amongst others we were lucky enough to have Malvina Major perform for us. On one such occasion Geoff Chard, an Australian opera singer, was in full flight, or should I say 'bull fight', part-way through the toreador's song from *Carmen* when the weather took over. There had been a gentle, warm northwesterly breeze in the morning, but by the time the concert started in the mid-afternoon the wind had strengthened. Suddenly, the 'Devil' blew his fiercest and the stage tumbled around poor Geoff, who had to use his best bullfighting skills to avoid serious injury. He narrowly escaped with his red cape flapping behind him, but, like the true professional that he was, the show carried on until the last note had been played and the last word had been sung. Just as the concert finished, the weather changed. The bulging southerly clouds that had sneaked up from behind suddenly rent and discharged their raging flood. The crowds fled to their cars.

Not unsurprisingly, our boys favoured concerts that featured their type of music, and under their watch there was a not-too-subtle change in the style of events. They tended to have a more 'modern' and even 'contemporary' focus, usually with the volume knob turned well clockwise. Were not these pop bands very expensive? we enquired.

'Mum, Dad, just remind us how much it costs to hire a symphony orchestra?'

We retired in silence.

**'DO YOU THINK THERE** would be a position for me in the business if I was to come back to New Zealand?' Paul asked tentatively.

I gave Chris a sly wink. We had hoped for some years that Paul might join us, as we both felt that we badly needed his services. Neither of us had any formal business or accountancy training and we had just grown into our individual roles, coping as best we could. I kept an eye on sales and stocks, and I was responsible for the forward-planning of production. I would tell Matthew when and how much of the different wines would need to be bottled and the weight of grapes that were required for each vintage. Chris oversaw the office and warehouse, coped with the vagaries of Customs and Excise, attended to the books and produced budgets. Together we coped with the finances and produced a regular business plan. We were, however, flying by the seats of our pants and we often felt out of our depth, which must have been very obvious to our long-suffering accountant, David Brown. We had left our children to decide for themselves what they wanted to do with their lives, and had tried not to put any pressure on them to feel responsible for or committed to the lifestyle, or rather the life sentence, that we had chosen for ourselves. We did not know then that Matthew and Edward had secretly spoken to Paul and had encouraged him to join us.

'There is probably not enough work in looking after the lakes and making sure the eels are in good condition to keep an aquatic zoologist in full-time employment,' I quipped. 'It might have to be combined with keeping an eye on the business side.'

Paul had a BSc (Hons) specialising in aquatics zoology, and he had been part-way through his PhD in the same topic when his supervisor quit his job, leaving our youngest-born in the lurch. They say that a university education is not an insurmountable handicap to obtaining a job in the real world, and our son was clear proof of this tenet. As jobs in aquatics zoology were thin on the ground Paul had embarked on a banking career, taking up a position in Wellington. He later felt he needed to see the big wide world and went to Ireland for his first dose of overseas experience. There he continued in banking before going to London, where he extended his already considerable computer skills by working for an IT company. Like most Kiwis on their OE, however, he eventually began to feel the tug of the home ties, and he now wanted to settle in New Zealand.

After further discussion Paul decided that he would enrol for a Master of Business Administration (MBA) degree at the University of Canterbury, which he would pursue part-time while feeling his way into his new role in our business. And this is how our general manager happened to end up having degrees in both zoology and business administration and how he and his delightful wife Rachel came to live in a neighbouring suburb.

When Paul joined Pegasus Bay he gradually took over the business and management duties that Chris and I had been doing, relegating his outmoded but delighted parents to governance. It proved impossible, however, to totally stop them poking their noses into forbidden territory, so an amicable form of armistice, known as flexible governance, crept into place.

'How about giving me a hand by washing out this old vat, Paul?' asked Matthew late one afternoon. 'Lynnette has gone into town and I'm alone. I need to leave shortly in order to meet her and I want to fill it up with wine before I go. It would be a great help and it will only take a few minutes.'

'But I've got my suit on, Matthew, and I'll almost certainly get it wet.'

'Be a pal. I'll give you a low-pressure hose and a brush so that if you're careful there should not be a problem.'

'You said something similar when you asked me this morning to collect that old pump that you had repaired in town. I ended up getting dirt all over my trousers.'

When Paul began working at Pegasus Bay he wore smart clothes, suitable to his elevated new role. It was not long before he discovered that he was called on to do all other sorts of tasks that were not in his hypothetical job description; he found that he was not infrequently called on to muck in. As a consequence, his attire became distinctly casual, if not scruffy. In spite of what the MBA had so vehemently taught, the boundaries between management and shop floor had also become blurred. Paul had to put up with the unhappy prospect of encroachment on his managerial position from both sides, but after all, where is the family that does not have a bit of give and take, or should I say, shove and push!

And what about our remaining son, our second-born, Michael, the one who had made a break for it, evaded our evil clutches and managed to escape? As a child, teenager and adult, Michael was always the placid one. He left our little nest at 17 and went to the University of Otago in Dunedin, from where he graduated four years later as both BA (majoring in anthropology) and LLB. He was ideally situated to be the lawyer in charge of a dig, but, instead of following this obvious opening, he went into a law office in Wellington and subsequently was admitted to the bar. Given his ready banter and quick way with words, Chris and I felt that he had a bright future ahead of him as a barrister.

I do not know if the soul-searing revelation came upon him as a Road to Damascus experience or if it arrived more gradually. Surprisingly, Michael found that he did not really like dealing with criminals and pretending that they were good honest folk, nor did his pulse race when he scribed the last will and testament of an elderly widow. Before long he joined a group of young lawyers who were involved in the legal and management side of the telecommunications industry. When, several years later, he moved to London, he continued in the same field and has done so until this day, although he now lives in Ireland. As a youth he worked in the vineyard, like his brothers, and this apprenticeship has clearly stood him in good stead as he still likes a bottle of decent wine. Fortunately, we see him often and we are able to recommend the tolerable product of a vineyard that we know. He is also very obliging and has said that he is always ready to lend a helping hand in the event of an embarrassing oversupply of produce.

# CHAPTER 12

# *The* Curious Incident *of the* Cat *in the* Night-time . . .

'AND THE LORD SAID, "LET THERE BE LIGHT!" and suddenly there was light. It shone all about them, at them and through them; or rather me, because I was the only one there. I don't know how to explain it. It sounds absolutely crazy, but I suddenly realised that I was blind. No, blinded! A very bright light was shining directly in my face so that I could not see a thing. Otherwise, everything was pitch-black … or so it seemed, and those pseudo-religious thoughts just kept going through my brain.'

'Where exactly were you, Simon, and what were you doing there?' I asked, prompting him to go on.

The 53-year-old sitting in front of me looked totally perplexed. He passed his hand through his tousled mop of greying hair and looked at the floor, as though hoping to find inspiration there. After a few moments' silence he looked directly at me. He looked as though he was on the verge of tears.

'That's just it. I had absolutely no idea. I looked down and saw that I was in a prisoner's striped uniform. Slowly it dawned on me that I was wearing my pyjamas and that the right trouser leg was ripped. I was standing in front of what seemed like a searchlight and it was raining. I was cold, shivering and soaked to the skin. Then I noticed blood was trickling over my right foot. It was from a long scratch on my shin and I was barefoot!'

Simon started to sob gently and his wife, Yvonne, reached over and patted his hand.

'Were you otherwise injured?' I enquired. 'Was there any evidence of a blow to your head: a bruise, a bump, a cut or a sore spot?'

'No, otherwise I was fine, except for not having the slightest idea where I was.'

'What did you do then?'

'I looked around me and slowly became aware that I was in a yard … It seemed to be the yard of some type of factory and I was standing directly in front of one of a number of bright security lights that were shining on the building. There were several piles of equipment stacked about and some of the lights were directed on these.'

'How had you got there, Simon?'

'I didn't and I still don't have the foggiest notion,' my patient replied desperately. 'It's terrible … but I just don't know. My last memory is of going to bed, and everything seeming perfectly normal.'

'That's right,' Yvonne agreed. 'Simon seemed absolutely normal when he came to bed, and I didn't wake up when he must have left. I didn't know anything was amiss until there was a loud hammering on the door.'

I wondered if Simon had been caught in the act of committing a burglary. Was he just feigning amnesia in an attempt to get off some criminal charge? How best to approach the possibility?

'How did you get home, Simon?' I asked.

'I found that the factory yard was surrounded by a high fence topped with barbed wire. The yard gates were closed and padlocked. I had to scale the fence to get out and that's when I cut my left arm … here,' he said, indicating a livid scar. 'I was lucky not to damage anything more vital on top of that bloody fence!'

For the first time in the consultation a brief flicker of a smile illuminated his unhappy face.

'I could see that I wasn't far from a busy road and I managed to flag down a passing taxi.'

'A passing taxi! You were lucky to get anybody to stop for you in that state. You must have been very persuasive to get a lift,' I said admiringly, adding, 'What a golden tongue!'

'To start off with the driver was suspicious and he took a bit of persuading. I didn't tell him that I didn't have any money until I got home.'

'That's the first thing Simon asked for when I opened the door,' Yvonne chipped in. 'He just rushed past me and into the warmth. He asked me to pay off the taxi driver, and I was only in my nightie.'

'So the police have not been involved at any stage?' I asked.

'No. Why should they have been?' Simon asked in surprise. 'I hadn't done anything wrong.'

'You might have been charged with breaking and entering,' I suggested.

'Breaking and entering! I thought I had been kidnapped.'

'Yes,' said Yvonne, 'Simon thought that he must have been abducted, but when we thought about it, it was simply unbelievable. Nobody could have come into the house and taken him from our bed. The house was locked and I would have woken up. Besides, there was no one with him when he came to his senses. He was alone in the factory yard.'

'How had you got in there, Simon?'

'I must have climbed over the fence. The gates were definitely locked and there was no other way to get in. I went back there a couple of days later and looked all around the place from the outside. There was no gap in the fence that I could have got through and that fence was damned high. They clearly intended to keep people out. I wouldn't like to climb over it in the daytime, let alone at night.'

'It's a complete mystery,' said Yvonne, frowning and adding yet a few more wrinkles to her generously lined but pretty face. She appeared older than Simon, but they looked equally worried.

'You may not be a cat burglar, Simon,' I quipped, 'but by the sound of that high fence you're definitely a cat.'

'It's not only his getting over the fence that's a mystery, but how he got there. The factory is three or four kilometres from our house. Our car was in the garage and neither his shoes nor his slippers were missing,' said Yvonne.

'Was there any reason for you to have gone to that factory?' I asked.

'None,' they responded virtually simultaneously, while Simon added, 'It was a joinery shop and I have no interest in that sort of thing. I'm completely useless when it comes to using tools and I have no need of woodwork.'

Then I posed the obvious question: 'Has anything similar ever happened to you before?'

'Nope,' replied Simon, while Yvonne shook her head in confirmation.

'Had you taken any drugs, medication or alcoholic drinks that evening?' I probed.

'Definitely not!' Now it was Simon's turn to shake his head.

'What about the door of your own house? You said it was locked when you went to bed. Was it still locked when you came home, Simon?'

'No, it was unlocked, with the key still in the lock on the inside. We always leave it there after we lock the door and go to bed, just in case we have to get out of the house urgently during the night,' said Yvonne. 'Simon banged on the door when he came home, not realising that it wasn't locked.'

It was a fascinating story that suggested a prolonged period of automatic activity for which there was no memory. Such a state is sometimes proffered by the desperate defence to explain unsavoury criminal behaviour for which the accused professes to have no memory and hence claims diminished, if any, responsibility. Psychologically based fugues usually occur in emotionally charged situations, and interpretation of their true nature is often confounded by drugs or alcohol. I had tossed such a possibility out of the window early in the consultation.

Possible neurological causes of Simon's little escapade are relatively restricted and three immediately sprang to mind. The best known was somnambulism, or sleepwalking, which usually starts during childhood and is often restricted to this period. It occurs during the deepest stages of sleep when the person apparently rouses and wanders about with eyes open in a trance-like state, mumbling, fumbling with objects and the like. Sleepwalkers have little, if any, recollection of these events when they eventually wake up. The activity that a somnambulist undertakes is usually simple and purposeless, although rarely more complex behaviour has been reported. It seemed unlikely that this was parasomnia, which is what somnambulism and similar sleep disorders are called.

Another possibility was transient global amnesia. This disorder occurs in adult life, often in the middle-aged or elderly, and it is typified by a telephone call that I received one Saturday morning from a friend about her husband.

'I wonder if I could ask you to come and see Will, Ivan?' Annabel asked, sounding very distressed. 'I think he must have had a stroke. He's wandering around the house and he seems completely confused.'

'I'll come straight away, Annabel.'

When I arrived at their house, Will, who was an older medical colleague and good friend, greeted me at the door, with Annabel peering anxiously out from behind him.

'What are you doing here, Ivan?' Will asked, looking perplexed. 'I'm just about to leave to go to my consulting rooms.'

'I won't hold you up but I just need to have a short talk to you, Will. Annabel telephoned me and said that you seemed a little confused. Do you mind if I come inside?'

'Come in! Come in! It must be important to come here first thing on a Friday morning,' he said, stepping to one side and waving his arm to bid me enter. He was his usual gentlemanly self and dressed in a suit, fashionably set off by a tie of declamatory but subdued hues. His wavy blond hair was immaculately coiffed.

We went into their tastefully furnished lounge and sat down.

'Why have you come, Ivan?' Will asked again.

'Annabel said that you seemed confused, so I have come to talk to you and examine you, Will.'

The physical neurological examination was perfectly normal and all of Will's motor and sensory functions were intact. Throughout the examination he kept asking why I had come, in spite of my having explained the reason several times. I then embarked on a series of tests to evaluate Will's mental functions. He was completely orientated, in time and place, except for thinking that it was Friday. He knew who we were and where we were. His general knowledge was excellent. He had no sign of motor or sensory aphasia, so that his speech was unimpaired, he had no difficulty in finding words and he followed complex instructions without difficulty. He was not dyslexic or dysgraphic and could read and write normally. He performed mental and written calculations with ease, frequently beating me to the correct answer. There was no evidence of apraxia, so he fully understood his own and others' body images and could correctly manipulate and construct objects in three-dimensional space. In short, Will performed perfectly on a wide range of bedside tests of neuropsychological function, except for those related to memory.

Between neuropsychologists there are many areas of debate about memory, but it is generally agreed that there is a fundamental difference between short-term and long-term memories. The mechanisms underlying their formation and retrieval seem quite different. Generally speaking, what is referred to as 'short term' is really what a layperson might think of as 'ultra-short term'. The mechanism underlying this allows us to remember a new telephone number that we have just read or heard and to dial it. A minute or so later this combination of digits has disappeared into thin air, never to be spontaneously recalled again. For something to be remembered for longer than this it has to be committed to the 'long-term memory'. This will occur automatically if something is very unusual or is especially significant to us, but otherwise we may have to bang it into our stubborn brains with repetition. Thus, we may remember the details of a personal tragedy or success until our dying day but, as every student can testify, we have to repeat intricate or boring stuff many times when swotting, only to forget it shortly after the examination.

Will's short-term memory was excellent. He could repeat long strings of numbers and words without a problem. It was his short-term memory that was enabling him to reply sensibly to my questions. He could not, however, put new material into his long-term memory store and subsequently retrieve this. Thus, when asked to remember a few simple objects he had no memory of these only a few minutes later. In fact, he did not even remember being asked to remember them! Will's memory for things in the more distant past, events that had occurred months or years earlier, was unimpaired, Annabel corroborating all the details that her husband provided in answer to my questions. 'Distant memories' are already in the long-term memory store, and this confirmed that Will's problem was not in accessing or retrieving his existing long-term memories but was a failure in forming new ones. Will was not confused but he had amnesia, and it was not just a loss of memory for one particular event or set of circumstances. It was a complete inability to form any new memories and was thus global. He had a form of global amnesia.

Neurologists and neuropsychologists had hypothesised from the histories of patients who had experienced so-called 'transient global amnesia attacks' that the problem was solely one of failure to form new long-term memories. No one, however, had actually had the opportunity of performing neuropsychological tests during such a bout because of their brevity and infrequent recurrences. I subsequently published my findings in the neurological literature as the first direct confirmation of the actual nature of these enigmatic episodes.

They usually commence without warning and last about an hour, although they can be shorter or longer, some going on for several hours. The patient may experience a period of so-called 'retrograde amnesia', so that they may not be able to recall a period of hours or even days before the onset of the attack, even although they behaved quite normally throughout this time. During the attack itself they appear confused and keep asking the same questions over and over again, in spite of being repeatedly told the answers that they cannot remember. They can, however, perform quite complex and difficult pre-learnt tasks, and I have had other patients who have continued to safely drive motor vehicles, suddenly finding themselves at strange destinations with no memory of how they got there. Even after the event has passed off there is no memory of what happened during it, suggesting that the problem is mainly one of putting new information into the long-term memory, rather than just a difficulty in retrieving it. The latter is more common in the forgetfulness of the elderly who, if given a clue or a prompt, frequently recall the correct memory. Most transient global amnesic attacks occur only once, and if they recur it is usually only on a few occasions.

I explained the situation to the justifiably worried Annabel and the bemused Will, predicting that his memory would return to normal over the next few hours but that he would be left with a permanent island of complete amnesia for the event itself and probably for a short period before its onset. This proved to be the case, and fortunately Will never had another attack.

Each and every one of us depends on our limbic system for our memories, and of central importance in this system are the temporal lobes of our cerebral hemispheres. One temporal lobe lies just beneath each temple, a little above our ears, and its memory pathways are connected to other important limbic structures that are tucked in behind our eyes. We thus effectively have a limbic system in each cerebral hemisphere, but they pretty much function in unison. Amnesia is due to a malfunction of the limbic system and, like disturbed brain function elsewhere, it can result from a variety of pathologies.

Most of these, such as a brain tumour, do not cause damage that is restricted to the limbic system and they are thus accompanied by other neurological and neuropsychological symptoms and signs.

Years earlier at Queen Square, I had looked after a young woman who, months before, had suffered from inflammation of both temporal lobes due to herpes simplex virus encephalitis. This little nasty, which normally contents itself with making our lives miserable and our appearance uninviting with its trademark cold sores, occasionally finds its way into the brain where it loves to wreak havoc with the temporal lobes. The result is commonly fatal, but if treatment is successful a full recovery is possible.

Fortunately, Jennifer's life had been saved, but unfortunately her life had been ruined by this so-called simple virus. She was a rare example of selective damage to the limbic system with pure amnesia. Jennifer performed perfectly on all tests of neuropsychological function apart from those related to memory. Her IQ, or intelligence quotient, which is measured by ability to solve problems, was in the superior range and her short-term memory was fine. Her memory of her life prior to the encephalitis was intact, but from that point onwards she could recall nothing. She played the violin beautifully, but unless new music was put in front of her she went over her favourite tune time after time because she could not remember that she had just performed it. She could carry on a perfectly normal conversation and we would chatter away happily. When I left the room for just a minute or two and then returned she would introduce herself again because she had no memory of ever having seen me. Jennifer was trapped in an Alice in Wonderland-like world where everything, even the most mundane and routine, was unfamiliar and novel. That grubby little cold-sore virus had left her with permanent global amnesia.

Simon's nocturnal jaunt could theoretically have been due to an attack of transient global amnesia, but his basic personality and behaviour would not be expected to change just because of inability to form new long-term memories. In spite of her amnesia, Jennifer was still the same sweet, retiring little lady that her relatives said she had been prior to the encephalitis. Simon had unlocked his door, wandered far afield and scaled a nasty fence that night, whatever other unrecorded hanky-panky he may have got up to. Giving him credit for not being a professional cat burglar, I assumed that his behaviour had been distinctly atypical, purposeless and confused, although clearly his motor activity had been coordinated and complex. What else could cause such a clinical picture? What else could cause such a relatively brief and focal derangement of brain function with complete reversion to normal? What, for that matter, causes the transient disturbance of memory that is seen in transient global amnesia?

The answer to the last question is uncertain, but the most popular theory is that it results from a temporary decrease in blood supply. The inner sides of both temporal lobes derive blood from a single vessel, the basilar artery, which splits into two in order to supply the right and left sides. Thus, impaired blood flow in one vessel can result in a bilateral ischaemia (impoverished blood supply) and have a devastating effect on memory. But while blockage to a blood vessel in the brain may be temporary, it can also be permanent and it then causes a stroke. When I saw Will I could not be certain that he had not had a stroke and that his amnesia would not be long-lasting. I knew, however, that the statistics were on my side, because, although a stroke in the basilar artery territory can produce amnesia, there are usually additional symptoms and signs due to damage to other surrounding parts of the brain.

In addition, if such sudden-onset global amnesia is due to reduced blood flow to parts of the limbic system, then there is something peculiar about this because it seldom produces or is a harbinger of a stroke. In this it is unlike most other forms of transient cerebral ischaemia or blockage in blood flow. In other words there seems to be a relatively benign distinct clinical entity of 'pure' transient global amnesia, although what causes it remains uncertain. Arterial spasm or increases in cerebral venous pressure, slowing arterial blood flow, have been hypothesised.

**BUT THERE IS A THIRD ENTITY THAT** can cause a brief disturbance in brain function and this is epilepsy. It is due to an abnormal electrical discharge caused by many nerve cells firing off simultaneously. There is no suggestion that this underlies 'pure' transient global amnesia, but one type of epilepsy can cause a similar clinical picture. I wondered if this might have been the cause of Simon's problem.

The best-known type of epileptic event is the so-called *grand mal* seizure. Jeremy Porter had suffered from such attacks since he was a teenager, although he had been free of them for more than 20 years. As is often the case, he was afraid to stop his medication for fear of a recurrence of the seizures and because of the legal requirement to discontinue driving for a prolonged period if his therapy was altered. Like most of us, Jeremy regarded driving as essential for life, rather than just being essential for life as we know it. It subsequently transpired, however, that Jeremy had become rather sloppy in his tablet habits, taking them when he remembered and not infrequently missing doses.

'Please tell me what you remember about what happened, Jeremy,' I requested.

'I don't really remember any of it,' said the worried-looking middle-aged gent, mopping his balding head with a handkerchief. 'One moment I was driving along the street and the next thing I knew I had hit this old guy. Luckily, I missed his wife. Janice can fill you in,' he added, nodding his head towards his equally anxious-looking wife.

'I had never seen a fit before,' Janice explained. 'Jeremy had grown out of them by the time I met him. I didn't think that he needed to keep taking all those tablets. They didn't seem to be doing him any good.'

As Jeremy had not had any seizures during all the years of their married bliss I wondered what sign of 'good' she had been looking for, but I restrained my curiosity and gave her an encouraging smile.

'I was looking out of the passenger window when I heard this strange noise. It sounded like something between a grunt and a cry, a type of strangled cry. The car suddenly accelerated and I turned to see Jeremy staring straight ahead ... but with his head slightly tilted back so that he was looking towards the sun visor. His arms were straight and looked stiff. I think his legs may also have been rigid and pushed on the accelerator. Then there was a jerk, immediately followed by an almighty crash. We had gone onto the footpath and smashed into a brick wall. It was a mercy that we weren't both killed.'

'Were either of you injured?'

'I thought Jeremy must have hurt himself badly and that he was dying because he was unresponsive. I was screaming and shaking him at the same time. Then he started to jerk all over and I realised that he must be having an epileptic fit. I thought it must have been brought on by the crash. Perhaps he hit his head.'

'Was there any sign of an injury to his head — a cut or a bruise, perhaps?'

'No, but he had wet himself, although I didn't notice that until later on when I helped him get out of the car.'

'How long did the jerking last?'

'It seemed an age but it was probably only about half a minute. Jeremy then seemed to go into a deep sleep. He was breathing very heavily.'

'Were there any other injuries?' I prompted. My suspicions had been well and truly aroused and they were rapidly racing towards what seemed like an unavoidable conclusion.

'No,' Janice replied.

'What about the old man?' interjected Jeremy with a somewhat sheepish look. 'He was hurt, wasn't he?'

'I wasn't counting him. That's not what the doctor meant ... was it, Doctor?' Janice said, her rosy face becoming scarlet. 'It's not that I meant the old man didn't count.'

'Tell me about him,' I encouraged.

'The car must have hit him after it mounted the curb. Whether he was thrown over the fence or just tumbled over it, I don't know. It was really just a low wall. He ended up in a pile of bricks but he was unconscious. The owner of the house had come rushing out to see what all the noise was about and he immediately telephoned for an ambulance. The old man was taken off to hospital. I think he had a head injury but I am not sure how bad it was. His wife had been walking with him but she wasn't hurt. A second ambulance took us to hospital.'

By coincidence I had seen the elderly couple several weeks earlier at the request of their family doctor. Mr Higgins had regained consciousness by the time the ambulance reached the hospital and, although he was shaken up by the event, he seemed to make an otherwise uncomplicated recovery. The tall, aristocratic-looking old boy had been discharged the following day. Since the event, however, the elegant but self-effacing Mrs Higgins had noticed that he was forgetful and uncharacteristically short-tempered. Their blissful retirement had suddenly been turned into something of a trial.

'And all because of that man, the driver,' Mrs Higgins had told me. 'I am scared that he might have changed the whole course of our lives. He seemed to be having some sort of fit in his car, immediately after the accident. I rushed over to tell him off for being so careless, but he was unconscious and twitching. Perhaps he banged his head in the crash. I turned to see if Martin was coming to remonstrate with him, then I realised that Martin had been hurt. The driver must have been out to it for five or 10 minutes, but he had come round by the time the ambulance arrived. He seemed very groggy and I wondered if he had been drinking, but it was only 10 in the morning!'

A brain scan had excluded the possibility that Mr Higgins had any surgically treatable injury inside the head, such as a blood clot. He had, however, suffered from concussion, which is not desirable at any age and is particularly liable to produce permanent problems in the elderly.

Jeremy had had a typical *grand mal* seizure. A test taken when he was in the emergency department of Christchurch Hospital, shortly after the accident, had shown that the concentration of anticonvulsant medication in his blood was well below the level that is normally needed to prevent epileptic attacks. When I tackled him about this he readily admitted that he took his medication only intermittently.

'Taking antiepileptic medication irregularly can cause great fluctuations in its blood concentration. This in itself may trigger epileptic turns, particularly if the blood concentration suddenly falls to a low level. You may be better on nothing than just taking the therapy irregularly,' I warned.

A few years earlier I had seen a 10-year-old boy who had been prescribed an antibiotic. Unfortunately, the pharmacy had dispensed the wrong medication, giving him antiepileptic tablets. Jason had taken these for two days and then his parents had stopped them because he had become drowsy and uncoordinated, typical side-effects in someone unused to the medication. The following day, as the high blood concentration of the medication would have been rapidly falling, he suffered his first *grand mal* seizure. It is a curious thing, but many antiepileptic medications can trigger seizures if used incorrectly.

Jeremy decided that, although he might opt for a medically supervised gradual withdrawal of his antiepileptic therapy in the future, for the present he was going to start taking it regularly once again. Even this single *grand mal* seizure had proved to be catastrophic. Above all, traffic regulations required him to be seizure-free for a prolonged period before he could recommence driving. How would he survive!

But *grand mal*, which is a French term, just means big sickness or attack. In spite of its name, *petit mal*, which means small sickness or attack, can be just as devastating. This is particularly so if it involves *absence*, which again is a fancy French term that signifies being 'absent', as in lack of awareness. Most absence attacks consist of complete loss of consciousness without a disturbance in posture. Affected people usually just stare straight ahead and look blank, appearing to be daydreaming. Often they sit or stand still, although they may walk about or make fiddling movements.

Any of us can be made to have an epileptic attack if the brain is stimulated sufficiently in a particular way. Some people are more susceptible to this than others, and they may be viewed as having a lower threshold to epileptic seizures. In patients with epilepsy, seizures occur in the absence of any apparent stimulation. In simplistic terms, epileptic absence attacks that begin in childhood usually involve the whole brain and can be thought of as being caused by an inborn reduction in the brain's threshold to seizures. Absence attacks that commence in adult life usually result from a focal area of irritation that has developed in a brain with a normal seizure threshold. Unlike most childhood-onset absence seizures, in which the abnormal electrical discharge during the attack involves the whole of both cerebral hemispheres, adult-onset absence seizures are caused by an electrical discharge that is restricted to a temporal lobe and its limbic connections.

The temporal lobes and limbic system have functions other than just memory, and thus focal temporal lobe epileptic attacks may produce a number of symptoms apart from absence. These functions include smell, taste, emotions, and sensations from visceral organs so that the affected individual may experience a variety of hallucinations that relate to these during a temporal lobe epileptic seizure. There may also be a sudden strong sense of *déjà vu*, that everything is strangely familiar and has occurred before. Such episodes are called complex partial seizures because of the complicated nature of the symptoms and the fact that the epileptic activity only involves part of the brain. Perhaps the most dramatic of these are visual or auditory hallucinations in which the individual may see a scene, a situation, other people or the like. He or she may hear voices, music or other sounds. These experiences have a dreamlike quality and probably represent jumbled memories, perhaps long forgotten or intermingled. Most commonly they are stereotyped, so that the same hallucination recurs in each seizure. Usually they are vague and poorly remembered, so that the sufferer can give few precise details. A patient might know that in his seizures he seems to be at a wedding but not who is getting married, that there are flowers on the table but not what colour they are, or that another guest talks to him but not what is said. Occasionally it is possible to obtain a clearer picture of the hallucination, and I have one such rare example that was given to me many years ago. It hangs on the wall of my living room in mute testament to this man's illness.

Clifford was an amateur painter, quite a dab hand at watercolours, and he liked to indulge his passion when his busy job as a journalist allowed. He had started having brief visual hallucinations several months earlier. He found these strange events disturbing and they gradually became more frequent. For no apparent reason he would suddenly see a face, which he described as looking like 'Captain Cook with a halo', as though the sun was shining from behind his head. The visage was surrounded by clouds and the torso was replaced or overlain by a golden honeycomb. It was dreamlike in quality and Clifford found it difficult to explain. Being an artist, he decided to paint his hallucination as best he could; after all, 'a picture is worth a thousand words'. His wife said that during these episodes he would stop what he was doing, stand or sit immobile and stare straight ahead with his eyes open. Sometimes he would also make chewing movements. As is typical, he was unresponsive and afterwards had no memory of anything that had been said or had happened around him during the seizure. The episode would last for up to 10 minutes. Sadly, investigations showed that Clifford had developed an inoperable malignant tumour in his temporal lobe, and although his seizures responded to antiepileptic medication he was dead within a year.

Most commonly, complex partial seizures are felt to be unpleasant, frightening, or have no emotion associated with them. Occasional patients have seizures that are pleasant, and in rare individuals they are intensely pleasurable. Mary's attacks were an extreme example of this. Now in her early thirties, she had suffered from temporal lobe epilepsy since her teens and it had rent the social fabric of her life. She described her seizures as being like 'a hundred orgasms all rolled into one', and there was no way she wanted them to stop. She had been an attractive, if not glamorous, blonde, who had three children from several long-term relationships. She was now like an ancient ship, wrecked on the reef of fate and old before her time. A pallid complexion, thick rouge, smeared lipstick, tousled hair, grubby old clothes and scattered bruises suggested that she might be an alcoholic or drug addict from skid row. Tom, her current partner, seemed an uncomplicated type. He had been living with Mary for two years while trying to run his plumbing business, but it was all becoming too much for him. He seemed devoted to her and was doing the best he could for her children, none of whom were his.

'The trouble is that Mary just won't take her medication regularly, Doctor,' Tom said despairingly. 'She will promise me that she will take her tablets and everything will be okay for two or three weeks. Then she'll start neglecting the kids. I'll come home from work and find the house in a mess. The kids will be running around, kicking up a hullabaloo, and Mary won't have prepared a meal or given them anything to eat. She won't even have done the shopping. She will be lying gaga in the bedroom having those damn seizures of hers. She prefers them to any orgasm that I can give her. She's bloody well addicted to them! When I go through her medication, I'll find that she has stopped the tablets yet again. I love her and I want to stay with her and the kids but I can't take much more. Unless things improve I'll walk out, just like the other blokes.'

'I'll definitely take them this time,' Mary chipped in pathetically, looking desperate. 'Just give me one more chance, Tom; one more chance for me and the kids.'

'Okay, Mary. But this is definitely your last chance! One more slip-up on this and I'm gone!'

I renewed Mary's prescription and once again arranged for her to have psychological and social help, but I did this with a heavy heart; hers surely was the mother of all addictions.

Sometimes epileptic seizures can last much longer than those I have referred to and they can occasionally go on for hours, days or weeks. This is referred to as *status epilepticus*. When it is due to temporal lobe epilepsy it can result in quite complex automatic motor activity, although this is generally without apparent aim or purpose. A person does not seek out and kill his worst enemy as the result of a complex partial seizure, in spite of what the counsel for the defence might claim. Along with some form of parasomnia and transient global amnesia, a very prolonged complex partial seizure had to be considered as the cause of Simon's nonsensical nocturnal ramblings and, given the details of the event, it was perhaps the most likely explanation. In addition, a number of neurologists have written about the peculiar religiosity that is sometimes seen in people with frequent temporal lobe epileptic activity, and Simon had made a rather jumbled attempt at a religious quotation. It was probably a red herring but it made me wonder. Simon, however, had not had frequent epilepsy; or had he?

'Have you ever experienced any other strange episodes or sensations that you cannot explain?' I asked him. 'Perhaps feelings rising up through your body or sudden peculiar smells or tastes? Have you ever seen or heard things that are not really there or had strong feelings that situations or experiences have happened before? It's what we call *déjà vu*. Perhaps you have suddenly found yourself somewhere and not known how you got there? Have you ever had a blackout, a faint, a convulsion or a loss of consciousness of any type?'

'No, I haven't,' Simon replied without hesitation.

'What about your little hot flushes?' Yvonne chipped in.

'They're nothing. They're just part of me. I've always had those,' Simon said with a hint of exasperation in his voice.

'I've told him that I don't think it's normal for a man to have hot flushes,' his wife said, casting Simon a sideways glance.

'Tell me about them, Simon,' I requested.

'Well, I've had them for as long as I can remember. They seem to come in bursts. Perhaps I'll have six in a day and then I mightn't have any more for a week or a month. They're quite irregular and nothing seems to bring them on, although they might occur more if I'm under stress. I just suddenly get a warm feeling in my tummy and it sweeps up towards my face.'

'How long does it take?'

'The whole thing can't last longer than a second or so, and then I feel completely back to normal.'

'Do you ever lose consciousness or become unaware of what's happening when they occur?'

'Never.'

'He sometimes seems a bit vague when he has one,' Yvonne volunteered. 'If I'm talking he might ask me to repeat what I have just said.'

'And if he's talking?' I prompted.

'He just seems to hesitate and looks a bit flustered, but he can usually pick up on what he's saying within a few seconds. He looks a bit vague, as though he's thinking about something else, as though he's daydreaming.'

'Naturally I am thinking about something else. I'm thinking that I'm having another flush, of course. What do you think I would be thinking about?'

Simon was becoming irritated, and he added, 'I'm not some sort of hormonal freak. It's just part of me. It's normal!'

'Simon, I don't want to upset you, but this is really important. I think that these might be brief epileptic attacks and that you might have had a much longer one that made you confused on the night you climbed the factory fence,' I explained.

'What if …' Simon started to speak, then his speech suddenly stopped and he was looking straight ahead.

'Africa!' I shouted and flung my hand towards his face, stopping just in front of his eyes.

Simon did not flinch or bat an eyelid, but almost immediately turned and looked at me as though I was crazy. What was I doing with my hand in front of his face? Was I going to assault him? I lowered my hand slowly so as not to upset him further.

'What did I say just then, Simon?'

'You didn't say anything,' he replied, 'but I just had one of my hot flushes.'

'What did I say, Yvonne?' I asked.

'Africa,' she replied, looking excited.

'What's that got to do with anything?' Simon looked quite puzzled.

'It shows that you were actually unconscious, and I'm sorry to tell you that you have epilepsy,' I explained, 'but the good news is that we can put you on treatment that will probably control the hot flushes and prevent any recurrence of the strange wandering or anything similar.'

Investigations showed that Simon had a small area of hardening in his right temporal lobe, and this anomaly had clearly been there since childhood. It was probably the brain's equivalent of a birthmark or a scar. An electroencephalogram showed that he had occasional spikes and surges of electrical activity over that part of the brain. His hot flushes disappeared with anticonvulsion treatment and there were no further nocturnal episodes. Although his absences had extended back as far as Simon could remember, they were due to a focal lesion irritating the brain and not to the reduced threshold to seizures that underlies most childhood-onset absence attacks.

The curious incident of the cat in the night-time was not atypical of the problem patients who walk through the door of the neurological consulting room. But before I tell you about a few other curious customers of mine, let me apologise to Mark Haddon, the author of the celebrated *The Curious Incident of the Dog in the Night-Time*, for plagiarising his title. The book is about another fascinating neurological problem, the *idiot savant* or wise idiot. This uncommon disorder is related to the more frequent Asperger's syndrome or autism. The 'idiot' may appear simple, and indeed many have a low IQ, but there are a few whose IQs are normal or in the superior range. Such *idiots* usually have marked difficulty with social interactions, problems in interpreting others' emotions and the like. They often have obsessional tendencies and may build up vast knowledge on particular subjects. Some can perform the most amazing and complex mental calculations.

Unlike the pump that controls our circulation, the filter that fills our bladder, the bellows that supply us with oxygen or the pipework through which we absorb our food, our brain is what sets us apart from all other creatures on this planet. It is the world's greatest supercomputer and responsible for our thoughts, dreams, emotions, behaviour, activities and achievements. The brain's normal activity and its derangement interact to produce myriads of fascinating problems, each one of which is individual to the patient with his or her unique set of symptoms and circumstances. Therein lies the endless fascination of neurology. But let me tell you about just a few more of my many puzzling patients.

**'IT'S WHEN I RUN, DOCTOR**, that's when it's worst. It's really starting to drive me crazy.'

Keith did not strike me as a crazy type, but then you could never tell. He seemed to be obsessed with sport, so maybe his outdoor he-man appearance was just wallpapering over cracks in a fragile personality. He came off a dairy farm and had a somewhat suntanned, bullish look.

'And within a few minutes of it starting I begin to get a headache. Unless I stop, it becomes a pounding headache. I can't allow it to continue like this, you know. I've got an important game in a couple of weeks and I have to train. As I am I couldn't even do the first 10 minutes; I'd be sidelined!'

'Tell me more about the headache,' I prompted. 'Where does it start and what exactly does it feel like?'

'All over my head and it's bloody awful! It feels as though my head will explode. It's worse than a dozen hangovers. I thought it might be the piss so I gave it up. It's made no difference.'

'How long does it take to settle down if you stop running and just rest, Keith?' I asked.

Keith had seemed uncomfortable from the time he had entered the consulting room. I had put it down to the unfamiliarity of the situation, but now he looked on the verge of tears, possibly due to reliving the experience of one of his bouts of head pain. He sniffed loudly through a nose that proudly bore evidence of previous battles, lost or won on the rugby field. He sniffed again and looked about in embarrassment so I pushed a box of tissues across my desk towards him. He gratefully pounced on it.

'About five or 10 minutes, I guess. It doesn't last long, but then it never really goes away. I always seem to have a dull head these days. I never had headaches until a month ago.'

In my mind I had been running through possible causes of Keith's exercise-induced headaches. At 28 years of age he could easily have developed his first migraine symptoms, and in some people attacks can be precipitated by exercise while, somewhat perversely, in others physical activity will relieve them. It is all very much an individual thing. Then there is a condition called cough headache, in which a cough or straining, such as at the toilet, can cause a severe generalised headache. It can be a symptom of blockage to the flow of the cerebrospinal fluid from the head to the spinal canal, which normally occurs at these times. This can also be triggered by sudden exercise. But then there are a hundred and one causes of headache. I needed more details before I got carried away trying to make a diagnosis prematurely.

'Do you get any other symptoms with the headaches?'

'Only splashing.'

'Splashing?'

'Yes, but I get that at other times as well. I told my doctor about it, but he said I must be imagining it, or perhaps it was coming from creaking in the joints in my neck.'

'What do you mean by "splashing"?' I asked, thinking that Keith must have gone soft in the head. 'Perhaps his brain has turned to mush and is just slopping about inside his skull,' I thought to myself uncharitably.

'It's just ordinary splashing, like you might hear if you shook a can of paint that was only half full.'

'Do you mean that you hear it?'

'Yes, and it comes at other times, such as when I shake my head. Sometimes when I turn over in bed I can hear a bubbling, but it doesn't last long. I guess I must be imagining it and I have stopped paying it any attention. It's not the noise that bothers me or prevents me from playing rugby, it's the headaches, and I need to get rid of them before the next game!'

'How long have you had these splashing noises?' I persisted gently, trying not to irritate him by harping on about something that he thought was irrelevant.

'About three weeks. Not as long as the headaches. I'll show you,' Keith said, shaking his head vigorously from side to side. 'There, you see, that's what it's like. You must have heard that.'

'No, I'm sorry but I didn't hear anything.'

'I might have heard the bubbling,' volunteered Eva, who until that time had sat silently; 'I'm not sure.'

I was uncertain whether the buxom Eva, who was oozing cheap perfume, was Keith's wife or partner, but it was irrelevant. The concerned young lady seemed absolutely genuine and was corroborating what Keith had said.

'Yes,' she continued, 'sometimes when it is quiet in the night and Keith turns over in his sleep.'

'Keith, could I listen to your head with my stethoscope while you do that shaking?' I asked, assuming permission and moving behind him to put my stethoscope in the centre of the top of his head, at the vertex.

That was how I heard the splashing, which could mean only one thing: Keith had air in his head as well as cerebrospinal fluid.

'Did you suffer a bad head injury not long before these headaches started?' I enquired.

'I did get a fair knock during my last major game. It was a sort of a head butt, done on the sly while the ref wasn't watching. It made me see stars, but I've had worse so I didn't think much about it,' Keith said, blowing his nose vigorously on another tissue. 'Damn cold, don't seem to be able to shake it off.'

'When did it start?' I asked with rising excitement.

'About the time the headaches kicked in. I thought they must be due to sinusitis and the doctor gave me a course of antibiotics. It didn't do any good.'

'You mustn't blow your nose, Keith. Just wipe it. It's dangerous to blow your nose because you must have a fracture high up inside it. This crack in the bone is between the inside of your nose and the space below your brain. It's the cerebrospinal fluid that surrounds your brain that is leaking out and air must be replacing it inside your head. If you blow your nose it might force germs into the cerebrospinal fluid and cause you to get meningitis. It is surprising that you haven't had that already.'

I saw Keith in the days before brain scanning had been invented, but a simple x-ray showed that the top half of each of the large fluid-filled spaces inside the cerebral hemispheres, the lateral ventricles, were filled with air, with cerebrospinal fluid below this. There was also air over part of the surface of the hemispheres. He had adroitly performed his own air encephalogram!

A neurosurgeon opened the front of Keith's skull and carefully eased the right frontal lobe of the brain upwards, exposing and then blocking the leak. This solved the problem of the air-head rugby player — well, almost solved it. Keith missed his important match. Neurosurgeons can work wonders, but miracles take extra time.

It may seem surprising that Keith's skull had been fractured without his losing consciousness, but this is not a rare occurrence. Fortunately, Keith had no evidence of brain injury, but it is possible to sustain considerable brain damage from a blow to the head without blacking out, and significant persisting disability can follow an apparently simple concussion. All head injuries are bad news; well, almost all. They say it takes the exception to prove the rule, and on rare occasions a patient may appear to be improved. Such was the case with Thomas Peters.

Tom was not a big man, in fact, he was puny, but he was feared by his wife and children, even though they were physically larger than him. When he was not laying bricks he spent his time laying into them, often boozed to the eyeballs. After he knocked off work each day he headed straight to the pub where, although he was a bricklayer, he generally got plastered. When he arrived home half-sozzled, dinner had to be on the table and woe betide anyone who spoke while he ate his meal, watching his favourite soap opera with the volume knob turned strongly clockwise. Industrial deafness was said to be the problem, but it was an industrial accident that turned out to be his making, or his undoing, depending on your point of view.

A load of bricks was being swung by a crane onto a building site when the pallet hit the side of Tom's head, sending him sprawling in an ungainly heap. If he was unconscious, then it was only for a brief period; perhaps not more than 30 seconds. By the time the crane driver reached him, Tom was rolling on the ground groaning and clutching his head. Shortly afterwards, he was able to stagger to his feet with assistance. The dutiful husband and respected father was kept in hospital overnight and then returned to the bosom of his concerned family. After a few days he went back to his job, but within a week he had been laid off because he seemed incapable of doing the task. In spite of several further attempts at rehabilitation he proved to be unemployable and spent his days at home. He could still lay bricks, but he was slow, slapdash and unreliable. Now Tom sat for much of the day watching television, not the soaps but sport.

'His memory's no good and he forgets what's been happening during the programme, so he can't follow it. Before long he becomes bored and changes the channel. But sport, that's perfect. It's full of action, there's no plot and you don't have to remember anything because they keep telling you the score. Sport on TV is great for brain-damaged people,' enthused Maud, Tom's rather frumpy and overweight wife. 'And Tom's a changed man. He's so placid and quiet; no more arguments. He does what I tell him and he's become a thinker. He often just sits in one place for an hour or two at a time, staring into space. Don't know what he's thinking about 'cause he never says, but he must be thinking deeply to keep occupied that long.'

Tom had clear evidence of major frontal lobe damage causing a personality change, in addition to his faulty memory, but this seemed to suit everybody, including Tom; everybody, that is, apart from the taxpayer, who had to foot the bill for Tom's early retirement.

But if there are persisting sequelae following apparently mild head injury the clinical picture is usually quite different. The patient is discharged from hospital with a clean bill of health and returns to work within days or a week or two. It is often months and sometimes years before they are referred for further evaluation. Their story is just about always the same. Joe's memory for new events is defective so that he now forgets things at work, leading him to make mistakes. He is more irritable and has difficulty controlling his temper, especially when his mistakes are pointed out to him. Because of arguments he has lost his job. Joe's personal life has become a mess. He shouts at his wife and kids and may be physically violent. He intermittently feels light-headed or dizzy and suffers from headaches. His headaches may be triggered by noise, so the family have to keep quiet. No one, apart from those with whom he is closely associated, realises that Joe has a problem because he looks fine and on casual acquaintance he behaves perfectly normally.

Joe's life may be completely ruined, without recognition or compensation. His wife and kids have taken off, he cannot hold down a job, he has fought with his best friends and he has been in court for assault. If he had lost an arm in a work-related accident he would have been handsomely compensated and could get on with his life; by comparison, the amounts handed out for Joe's type of brain injury are trifling. Like diamonds, Joe's brain damage is forever, but unlike them it is worth peanuts.

Even if Joe had sustained relatively mild concussion and did not have the persisting problems mentioned above, he probably would have shown some transient evidence of brain dysfunction on careful neuropsychological testing. In other words, he would not have been able to think so clearly for some days, weeks or months after the event. If he was lucky the test results would return to normal and his symptoms would disappear. Now, should Joe be unlucky enough to have similar mild concussion at a later date, it would take longer for his neuropsychological test results to return to normal than on the initial occasion. In other words, there was some persistent brain damage from the first incident, even though it was so subtle that it appeared to have cleared completely on the highly sensitive neuropsychological tests. Repeated concussions can be additive and lead to gradually accumulating neuropsychological defect, which is why neurologists take even repeated minor head injuries in contact sports seriously.

**IF THE SUPERCOMPUTER INSIDE** your head does not like having even an occasional unintentional knock, what is its response to receiving a regular pummelling? This can be seen by examining the brains of boxers. There have been a number of scientific studies showing that boxing is very bad news for the brain, which is not rocket science; after all, the aim is to knock your opponent senseless, and the brain's consistency is rather like a thick jelly. These studies show splits, cavities and scars in the brain as well as general shrinkage of the cerebral hemispheres and dilation of the lateral ventricles. This leads to a variety of neurological symptoms that can become progressive, even if the individual stops boxing. Gradually increasing dementia is one of these. Jerks, tremors and even a syndrome like Parkinson's disease, which Muhammad Ali developed, are other manifestations of abusing the brain. All this confirms what you already know: you will not improve your computer's performance by kicking it around.

A single serious head injury usually has a tragic outcome, but there are rare exceptions, and such was the case of David Asher. Almost half of David's 30 years had been spent in psychiatric institutions. He was diagnosed as having schizophrenia in his mid-teens, and in spite of the best therapy available and a very caring, supportive family, his multiple attempts to live at home or in the community had been failures. David's parents had given up hope of his ever having a stable life, but, with the consent of the mental hospital in which he had been a long-term resident, they had taken him home for a weekend. It was late on Sunday afternoon when they discovered that he was missing. The Ashers contacted the hospital but, no, David had not found his way back there. The police were sympathetic and would do all they could to assist, but there had been no reports of a young man of David's description behaving strangely.

David's conscientious parents were beside themselves with anxiety and guilt. Why had they not been more vigilant? It was Wednesday afternoon when they received a call from the neurosurgical ward at Dunedin Hospital, where David had been admitted. The Ashers never did find out how their son came to be in a car with several other young men when it failed to take a bend and rolled into Lake Wakatipu, hundreds of kilometres away from where he had disappeared. Fortunately, the water was shallow, but unfortunately, the drop had been considerable. David was unconscious when he was admitted to hospital and tests showed a large extradural haematoma. The blood from the adjacent fracture was lying between the inner bony surface of David's skull and the leathery dura mater. Beneath this lies the much thinner arachnoid membrane, from which it is separated by the subdural space.

It was bleeding into this subdural space that had caused the stroke-like symptoms in the elderly patient of my Iranian house officer, Jay, and it was bleeding into the subarachnoid space between the arachnoid membrane and the outer surface of the brain that had been suspected in Claire Adams-Pinker, whose case I described in Chapter 1. Although all three types of haemorrhage involve bleeding between the skull and the surface of the brain they tend to produce different clinical pictures, and David's was typical of an 'extradural'. It formed such a large swelling that it was severely compressing and deforming the underlying brain. Urgent surgery removed the blood and David's life was saved, but was it worth it? His life had been miserable before the accident, and what would he be like with brain damage added to his deranged psychiatric state? Mr and Mrs Asher waited anxiously at his bedside. David was their only child, and although he had been a trial they loved him dearly.

David regained consciousness on his second post-operative day, but was groggy and did not seem to recognise his parents. Over the ensuing four or five days he surfaced and began to take an interest in his surroundings. He was overjoyed to see his parents, in spite of their distraught appearance. He talked to them and to the hospital staff, trying to find out what had happened because he had no memory of his little jaunt through the countryside. It took some time for David's parents to realise what was the matter; he was not hallucinating! In fact, they could carry on a normal conversation with him, and with the exception of the island of recent memory loss he seemed mentally normal.

David's unconventional cure for schizophrenia appeared permanent, or should I say long-lasting, because I did not follow him forever. But he attended outpatients for several years and did not require any medication. The young man was able to live independently in his own flat, and he had taken up his old hobby of painting, now on a semi-professional basis. His subject matter was individual, consisting almost exclusively of scenes of death, particularly the crucified Christ. The pictures were definitely dark, in more than one sense of the word, but he had his own eclectic following and held court among a coterie of admirers, particularly at exhibitions. I suspected that he had damaged part of the temporal lobes and/or their connections, but I never found out because I lost touch with David before brain scans were invented. Maybe I missed an opportunity to discover the surgical cure for schizophrenia.

**'WOULD YOU MIND HAVING A LOOK** at Scott Stokes next?' asked the charge nurse, returning to join our ward round after having been interrupted by a serious-looking junior nurse.

'What's the matter with him?' I enquired, feeling slightly irritated at having the routine ritual of our ward round interrupted.

I had just finished seeing a 60-year-old woman who had suffered a transient ischaemic attack that had caused paralysis of the right side of her face and her right arm, and the inability to speak. Fortunately, the symptoms had cleared spontaneously within an hour of her admission to hospital. She had a bruit, a hissing sound that was synchronous with her pulse, which could be heard through a stethoscope placed over the left carotid artery in her neck. This suggested that the artery had narrowed due to a build-up of atheroma and that a piece of this or an associated clot had broken loose and been swept up into the left side of her brain. There it would have caused temporary obstruction to the blood supply before breaking up and being swept on. She had been lucky to have this minor event as it was a warning that a permanent stroke could occur and now it would enable us to take preventive measures. If tests confirmed my suspicion she could have an endarterectomy, an operation to clean out the atheroma, before it did further mischief. I had my registrar and house officer in tow, and we were busy discussing the details of the case and the best course of action when the charge nurse rejoined us. I thought that there were more urgent inpatients to be seen than Scott.

'He had an epileptic seizure earlier this morning and he hasn't regained consciousness,' the charge nurse told me. 'The nurse who is specialing him is worried. He is still deeply unconscious and his breathing seems very laboured. I have just seen him and he looks in a bad way.' She went on, 'It seems strange, because it was only one of Scott's usual epileptic attacks and the nurse who saw it said that the seizure seemed quite short, perhaps no more than five or 10 seconds.'

'Okay, we'll see him next,' I said, and we headed in the direction of Scott's bed.

The 25-year-old was lying immobile on his side in the recovery position with his special nurse and one of her colleagues anxiously hovering over him. His breathing was noisy and rather rapid, but his airway did not seem to be obstructed. I called to him loudly, shaking him at the same time. He was floppy and there was absolutely no response. Was there a flicker of resistance when I lifted an eyelid to examine the pupil? When I touched the cornea with a piece of cotton wool there was the usual blink reflex, suggesting that he was not deeply unconscious. A person who is only lightly unconscious will often groan and move in response to a painful stimulus. This is traditionally applied by squeezing an earlobe, but there are multiple other techniques, some of which would undoubtedly excite the Marquis de Sade. Perhaps I erred on the side of the conservative but I could obtain absolutely no response. Otherwise, neurological examination was completely normal.

A week earlier I had been asked to review the patient by a colleague who had found Scott's case perplexing. Scott was the son of a family doctor, who had made the diagnosis of epilepsy himself. At 10 years of age Scott had started to have bouts of strange behaviour, which his father concluded were complex partial seizures due to temporal lobe epilepsy. He had been referred to a paediatrician who had concurred with the probable diagnosis and started the lad on antiepileptic medication. The episodes of strange behaviour largely disappeared within a few months, only to be replaced by *grand mal* seizures. Without warning, Scott would lose consciousness, collapse and shake all over for about half a minute. Later he would feel groggy but he would usually recover and be back to normal within 10 to 15 minutes. He had been tried on many different medications and drug combinations, each of which would seem to work well for several months and then lose its efficacy. The *grand mal* seizures would return with renewed vengeance. He might have several in a day and then be free of them for a week or so. They had ruined his education and his life. A kind employer had once given him a job for several months, but otherwise he had been unemployed and was living on the sickness benefit.

Scott had had multiple electroencephalograms, all of which had been normal, but this is not particularly uncommon in patients with epilepsy, particularly when the seizures start from deeply within a temporal lobe where the abnormal electrical activity is a long way from the recording electrodes that are on the scalp. It is difficult to obtain an electroencephalogram taken during *grand mal* due to the unpredictability of the occurrence of attacks. Even if you are able to get such a recording it is generally useless, because the electrical interference caused by the shaking of the head obscures the electrical activity produced by the brain itself. Scott's other tests, including a brain scan, had all been normal. It all seemed kosher enough, but I was left with a sense of unease for reasons that I could not quite explain. Was it Scott's affect — his sense of martyrdom — at the same time coupled with a fierce type of pride in his illness?

I turned him over and held up his limp arm with his hand suspended well above his face, and then I let the hand go. As it fell it curved in a slight arc so that it avoided hitting him directly in the face. I did this again and again and again, with the same result each time. It strongly suggested that he was not unconscious.

'Scott! Scott! Scott!' I shouted again, shaking him vigorously.

There was still no response. I then produced my secret weapon from inside the little black bag of tricks that I was carrying: a small, tightly sealed bottle.

In Victorian times it was fashionable for young ladies to swoon. If they found anything particularly disagreeable then they would simply collapse in what appeared to be a faint. It was not seemly to crash over, rather they would fall against someone, lower themselves gently or subside onto an adjacent sofa or chair. Any gallant Victorian male knew exactly what to do. He would call for a bottle of smelling salts and waft it gently under milady's nose. Her eyes would flutter charmingly and, amazingly, she would revive.

My little bottle contained a ball of cotton wool that had been soaked in strong liquid ammonia many years earlier. In spite of its age it had lost none of its pungent power and it could assail and break through the walls of the strongest fortress. It was a civilised and refined version of teargas. I held the bottle a little distance from Scott's nose and the result was almost immediate. He coughed and a little tear trickled from the corner of his eye. He turned his head to try and remove his nose from the offending object. He next opened one eye and reached up to push the bottle away. He had miraculously and abruptly regained consciousness.

An Australian neurologist whom I trained with once told me that he thought my little coma-breaking bottle was just pussyfooting around. He had been taught that in cases of feigned unconsciousness the best diagnostic tool was a little needle-prick up the inside of the nose. I guess I am something of a sissy because I have never been brave enough to take up his recommendation, but then they breed them tough in Oz!

The fact that Scott appeared to have been feigning unconsciousness did not prove that he did not have genuine seizures, but it did add to my suspicions that he really might not have epilepsy.

One of my neurological colleagues had a middle-aged male patient, Mr X, who had been admitted to several major hospitals in New Zealand with *grand mal* status epilepticus. This condition is not just one of having frequent epileptic seizures but is a state of having a prolonged continuous convulsion or very frequent convulsions without regaining consciousness in between them. Like Scott, he had been tried on just about every known antiepileptic therapy and every combination of anticonvulsant medications possible. Because *grand mal* status epilepticus is a life-threatening condition if the seizures are not controlled, he had even been admitted in status to an intensive-care unit at

St Elsewhere and put into a drug-induced coma for a number of days. Like Scott, all of his 'interictal' tests, those carried out between the seizures or 'icti', had been normal.

By the time Mr X was investigated we had facilities for long-term monitoring of the electroencephalogram combined with simultaneous video of the patient. By this means the precise clinical picture of a seizure could be correlated with the electrical activity in the brain. Even though the electroencephalographic artefact renders the electrical recording useless once the shaking has started, in genuine *grand mal* epilepsy abnormal brain-wave activity can usually be seen during the second or so before this. Frustratingly, as soon as Mr X was put onto such monitoring his previously frequent seizures stopped. This can occur in genuine epilepsy, but my colleague was suspicious. Eventually Mr X had to be discharged because there is a limit to people's patience and hospital budgets.

My long-suffering colleague left instructions that he was to be called the next time Mr X presented to Christchurch Hospital with epileptic seizures and that medication was to be withheld until he got there. He did not have long to wait and, as Murphy's Law ensured, the telephone call came in the middle of the night. He found the unconscious Mr X having a typical *grand mal* attack, one that was so convincing that it would have fooled all but the savviest of the neurological fraternity. Mr X had rhythmical jerking of his whole body, laboured breathing and frothing from the mouth. In spite of this, my colleague sat and talked to the patient, explaining that he was not really having an epileptic attack and encouraging him to relax. The vigorous shaking associated with such an attack burns up a lot of energy and it is very exhausting. It is probably akin to running. Although it was the middle of the night the doctor knew he had time on his side and that Mr X must tire before he did. My colleague sat there for several hours, intermittently repeating what he had said earlier.

Eventually his patient stopped shaking, opened his eyes and hissed vehemently, 'Bugger you, Dr … You're just too bloody smart!'

I never discovered whether Scott's attacks were genuine or what we call 'pseudo-seizures'. They became too infrequent for it to be worth performing electroencephalographic and video monitoring. He seemed firmly wedded to them and his life as an invalid. He resisted all attempts at further investigation and would not countenance a trial of gradually reducing his medication to see if it could be completely withdrawn without deterioration in his condition. He re-presented occasionally when he was having 'a bad patch' and wanted his medication tweaked. These usually coincided with periods when he was under psychological pressure, but then bona fide epilepsy can also deteriorate at such times.

**A STROKE IS ALWAYS WORRYING** and it is particularly distressing when it occurs in a young person. Elizabeth Bradford was one such: a glamorous 23-year-old philosophy student who had a bright professional and social future in front of her when she was struck down by paralysis and numbness of her right arm and leg. She had been walking home from her boyfriend's flat and had only managed to get through the front gate of her shared student digs when her leg gave way and she tumbled onto the long grass of the unmown lawn. Fortunately, she managed to avoid landing on a neighbouring rose-bush. A couple of her flatmates happened to be lounging on a sofa on the veranda having a beer and they were able to rush to her immediate aid. She had been brought straight to hospital in an ambulance.

I was on call that Saturday afternoon, and when my registrar telephoned to say that Elizabeth had been admitted I was able to drop what I was doing to go to see her. She seemed to be bearing up very well for someone who had been so disastrously stricken in her prime, but then she probably did not realise the seriousness of her disability and was merely exhibiting the boundless optimism of youth. Her distraught boyfriend, a theology student with a mutinous mop of curly hair the same shade of red as Elizabeth's, was clearly not made of the same stern stuff. He had a downcast and furtive mien that seemed to encompass a plethora of possible emotional states, including guilt.

'Nothing unusual happened during Elizabeth's visit,' he volunteered.

I tactfully refrained from enquiring what was usual during such trysts.

A neurological examination was normal apart from the fact that Elizabeth could not move her right limbs. In spite of straining every other muscle in the body and grimacing and grunting with the evident effort, there was not a flicker of voluntary movement to be seen in her right arm or leg. In addition, she had lost absolutely all sensation in the paralysed parts. She could feel nothing from the tips of her toes and fingers to her groin and armpit. Her right leg did flex briskly in response to a sharp jab on the sole, withdrawing the foot from the offending object, but this could have been due to a reflex. Lower spinal reflexes persist following a lesion in the brain or higher spinal cord.

Neurologists are miserly individuals when it comes to doling out lesions and they never like to hypothesise multiple nervous system lesions when all of a patient's signs and symptoms can be explained by one. This was not the case with Elizabeth; the features could not have been due to a single lesion, which meant she had two lesions that had appeared simultaneously, or that she did not have any at all. I felt that the latter was by far the most likely. Giving her the benefit of the doubt, however, I arranged several tests while reassuring her that I felt she had not suffered a stroke or any other neurological nasty and that her symptoms would probably resolve.

But I was to be proved wrong. When I saw Elizabeth the following morning she had not improved, and rather ominously she had become completely blind in her right eye. She would have had to have had a separate and third nervous system lesion to explain this on an organic basis. Both her pupils constricted normally in response to a bright light. This reflex depends, among other things, on normal brainstem function, so it confirmed that the eye, the optic nerve and the brainstem were not the cause of the problem. Higher up in the brain, in the cerebral hemispheres, where vision is actually perceived, the fibres from the two eyes have merged so that a lesion on one side of the brain will cause loss of vision in the visual fields of both eyes on the side opposite the damage. Thus, a lesion in the visual pathways in the left cerebral hemisphere causes impairment of vision in the right side of the visual fields of both eyes. In other words, like the findings in her right limbs, the blindness seemed incapable of an organic neurological explanation.

As I expected, all of Elizabeth's tests were reported to be normal. In particular, it could be clearly demonstrated that nerve impulses from the totally anaesthetic limbs reached the appropriate sensory cortex in her left cerebral hemisphere, as did those caused by visual stimulation of her right eye. The muscles in her right limbs responded normally to electrical stimulation of the peripheral nerves and magnetic stimulation of the brain. By using a system of alternating mirrors an ophthalmologist colleague was able to get Elizabeth to unknowingly read with her 'blind' right eye and confirmed that it had 6/6 (20/20) vision.

Subsequently, a nurse reported that Elizabeth had been seen walking back from the toilet in the middle of the night. When asked about this Elizabeth had replied that her right leg sometimes seemed to inexplicably regain a surge of nocturnal strength but that the improvement never lasted longer than 10 or 15 minutes. Distressingly, she would become paralysed again shortly after she got back to bed.

'Jo and I have been worried sick,' Elizabeth's father Rob told me. 'Do you think it could be multiple sclerosis, Doctor?'

Their tired appearance confirmed the parents' hours of anxiety and insomnia. By contrast, Elizabeth seemed a picture of physical and mental well-being, bearing up bravely in the face of the possibility of spending the rest of her life as a cripple. Meanwhile a sea of emotions was evidently awash in the theology student, whose change of visage at the mention of multiple sclerosis suggested that inward calm was retreating before a storm of terror. His hair looked as though he had been tied to the mast while rounding Cape Horn in a tempest.

Rob and Jo had requested a family meeting after flying down from Wellington to be at their daughter's bedside, and I was only too glad to oblige.

'I don't think it's that,' I replied. 'All the tests have come back negative. I'm happy to be able to tell you that we have found no evidence of any nasty neurological disease. In fact, it is my opinion that Elizabeth does not have a neurological problem.'

'How could that be?' Jo exclaimed, looking amazed.

I proceeded to go through the details of Elizabeth's case and the results of her investigations. The fact that we had done these tests reassured them that we had taken the matter seriously and not just brushed Elizabeth's complaints aside. Although the results were all normal, I was sure that if I had not ordered them I would not have been believed.

'So you don't believe there is anything the matter with me!' Elizabeth interjected in a voice that sounded both hurt and angry. 'You can't think I enjoy being like this. I'm not putting it on, you know!'

'Yes,' added the theologian in a quavering voice, 'surely you can see that she is suffering; suffering dreadfully. Her whole life is being ruined before our eyes. What does the future hold for her?'

'I didn't say that there was nothing the matter, because clearly there is a problem, and I didn't say that Elizabeth was putting it on. What I said was that her difficulties were not being caused by a neurological disease and hence we need to look at other possibilities. The subconscious mind can produce all kinds of neurological symptoms and signs and this needs to be checked. Elizabeth, I think it would be helpful to get a specialist in this area of medicine to see you and give us an opinion.'

'What sort of specialist?' Rob chipped in.

'A specialist from the department of psychological medicine; one who has a lot of experience in the neurological effects of the mind and works very closely with our department,' I replied, trying to sound reassuring.

'So, you think I'm a nutcase!' said Elizabeth as her composure slipped and she began to sob.

'Not at all,' I consoled her, 'but you do have nervous system symptoms and signs that don't seem to have a neurological basis. People's psychological nerves and their nervous systems act together and one can easily affect the other without their being aware of it. Seeing my colleague is the next logical step and the one that I would recommend. Would you be prepared to do that?'

'I guess so,' Elizabeth agreed unenthusiastically, sniffing loudly.

Her boyfriend patted her hand while Rob and Jo nodded their consent.

I spent more time with them, explaining things in more detail and answering further questions. I did not fool myself that I had solved Elizabeth's problem or that her neurological symptoms, signs or disability would suddenly disappear. Like most neurologists, I had seen enough similar cases to be well aware of the chronic and recurrent nature of the problem. I also knew that there were as many different views on how best to deal with it as there were clinical presentations of this complex and multifaceted problem. Options included reassurance without investigation, confrontation, in-depth psychoanalysis, cognitive behavioural therapy and hypnosis, to mention but a few.

But the assumption that physical symptoms and signs do not have an organic cause, just because one cannot be demonstrated, may be highly dangerous. I was asked by a surgeon to give my opinion on Brian McMaster who, perhaps rather irritatingly and ungratefully, had not responded to my colleague's skills with the knife. I found a thin and rather baleful-looking Brian curled up in a semi-foetal position on his hospital bed. He looked at me suspiciously, as though I had come to accuse him of a crime. He appeared relieved when I assured him that I was not the council for the prosecution but rather an impartial judge. Brian asked me if I could help him sit up so that he could talk to me more easily; not an encouraging request. He then proceeded to confirm what I had already read in his somewhat sparse case notes.

Brian had been admitted to hospital with nasty abdominal pain that was diagnosed as acute appendicitis. An urgent appendicectomy had been performed that night but, rather inconsiderately, the pathologist had not confirmed the diagnosis; the appendix was normal. The gut-ache continued to be troublesome, and then Brian developed diarrhoea. The problem was thus solved; he had a simple dose of the 'trots'. This could easily be fixed by giving him a potion to 'bind' him up and sending him on his merry way. Unfortunately, Brian's beastly entrails did not see it this way. They continued to growl and grumble and he complained of being exhausted. He felt that he was not well enough to go home, and continued to inconveniently block up a surgical bed. True, he was running a bit of a fever from time to time, but nothing to get too excited about. The days passed quickly, as did Brian's persistently liquid stools, but the latter eventually started to settle and it was time for him to hit the road. When this was mentioned he complained that he was feeling weak and was having trouble getting out of bed. My long-suffering surgical colleague had had enough.

'He told me to stop acting up and to get a move on,' reported the now-doleful-looking Brian, almost in tears. 'He said there was no reason for me to have become weak and that I was just malingering. And then the nurses, who had previously been so kind, began to side with the consultant. I asked to be taken outside on a sunny day to sit beside the Avon River so that I could see the ducks and the people passing. A couple of nice nurses wheeled me out but then they had to go back inside to look after the other patients. As they left, one called out to me that when I had had enough I was just to come back inside. I yelled back that I did not have the strength but she just laughed and waved at me, saying "You'll manage." I couldn't move. I just sat there helplessly. After several hours the people had all gone and it began to get dark and cold. I could see the lights on in the ward and I was desperate to get inside but nobody answered my calls. Eventually, when I didn't show up, the nurses began to worry and came out to rescue me. I think that's when the surgeon had second thoughts about my weakness.'

When a person is feigning weakness an experienced examiner is usually alerted by a number of inconsistencies in the physical examination of strength and muscle tone. Brian had none such. He was severely weak throughout his limbs, so that he was unable to stand and needed to be fed. All his tendon reflexes had disappeared. The diagnosis was simple. He had Guillain-Barré syndrome, a type of temporary inflammation of the peripheral nerves that results from an immune response to something, most commonly an infection. In this condition, the immune system attacks the nerves, instead of just fighting the germs, and it starts to strip the fatty myelin sheath from around each microscopic nerve fibre. As these sheaths electrically insulate one nerve fibre from another and they are essential for normal conduction of electrical impulses along nerves, the brain's instructions to activate muscles are impaired and they may become completely blocked. Because motor nerves tend to be selectively affected this typically results in weakness or paralysis without much, if any, impairment of sensation.

Because the nerves involved in breathing and swallowing, and even those controlling the heart, can be involved, this disorder is highly dangerous; Brian had every reason to look down in the mouth. He needed to be transferred to an intensive-care area in order to be closely monitored and treated.

When I told him my opinion he looked like a pauper who had just won the fat prize in Lotto.

'Thank goodness you believe me, Doctor. I'm so happy to be given a diagnosis.'

'Don't get too excited, Brian,' I replied. 'This is a serious neurological problem and it could get worse before it gets better. The good news is that the inflammation of the nerves is temporary, and people with this disorder usually make a good recovery and get their strength back again.'

Back in the office, I was arranging for Brian to be transferred under my care to another ward when the guilt-stricken nurse who was in charge of the surgical patients handed me a slip of paper, saying, 'This has just come through, Doctor.'

It was the result of a culture for microorganisms that had been carried out on Brian's stools. Initial cultures had been reported as showing no abnormal organisms, and this was an amended report saying that after a considerable delay strange bacteria had started to grow. These had been identified as *Campylobacter*, due to the bend in each bacillus. The booby prize that Brian had won was the notoriety of being the first person in Christchurch, and possibly New Zealand, to be diagnosed as sheltering this kinky little bug.

Either because of or in spite of my treatment Brian did not get any worse, but my initial optimism proved to be ill-founded; improvement was very slow. Eventually he could walk with the aid of elbow crutches, and his arms improved so that he was fairly independent in his personal needs, but he was left with a marked disability. His muscles were thin and wasted and he remained quite weak. Sadly, he was a shadow of his former self.

Because Guillain-Barré syndrome typically damages the myelin sheath, which has a reasonable capacity to regenerate, most patients with this disorder make a good functional recovery. They may be left with some disability, but it is usually minor. However, it had been recognised for many years that sometimes the nerve fibres themselves could be injured or killed and that occasionally this could lead to serious persisting weakness. Unfortunately, this was the case for Brian. It was several years later that an article appeared in the *British Medical Journal* reporting several cases of Guillain-Barré that had been caused by *Campylobacter*. The authors suggested that when this misguided maelstrom of the autoimmune system was due to the presence of this dastardly bug, persistent damage to the peripheral nerves was perhaps particularly likely to occur. Time has proved that this hypothesis was correct. *Campylobacter* has now become a rather commonplace organism, being responsible for a fair proportion of Guillain-Barré cases and leaving a trail of disability in its wake.

It is easy to dismiss a patient's symptoms as being fictitious if you do not know the cause and, like my surgical colleague, I have been guilty of this, but it is important not to fall into this trap without strong supporting evidence; absence of obvious aetiology and mechanism are not sufficient.

**MEANWHILE, TO RETURN TO SCOTT,** Mr X and Elizabeth, what was it that they and the droves of similar cases that present to neurologists were suffering from? Such patients inhabit a dim hinterland, that murky world that lies between neurology and psychiatry. These two medical disciplines separated from each other in France, Britain and Western Europe in the latter half of the nineteenth century but remained undivided in many parts of Eastern Europe until well after the Second World War. Sigmund Freud (1856–1939) was both a neurologist and a psychiatrist, and in 1885 he worked with Jean-Martin Charcot, the father of French neurology, at La Salpêtrière hospital in Paris. Among other things, they studied a disorder, hysteria, in which patients had a variety of bizarre symptoms and signs without clear physical explanations. They considered it to be a psychological disorder and experimented with hypnosis to try to treat it.

The name *hysteria* comes from the Greek word meaning 'womb'. Hippocrates had postulated that the disorder was caused by the uterus wandering about the body. It was originally thought to be the exclusive province of women, but any lingering doubts as to that assumption were laid to rest during the First World War. Thousands of male soldiers suffering from shell shock had confusion, amnesia, blindness, deafness, loss of speech, paralysis and the like, for which there was no physical explanation. Some were treated in the basement of the National Hospital, Queen Square, with a variety of experimental therapies, including those of a noxious variety, in the hope that it would 'shock' the unfortunates out of it and show them that they had no real physical disability. Pat Barker's Booker Prize-winning novels, which form the *Regeneration* trilogy, outline their trials and tribulations.

The obvious association between psychological trauma and shell shock supported the notion that had been proposed by Freud, namely, that the condition is an attempt to deal with underlying psychological conflicts by converting them into physical symptoms. The psychoanalytical movement endorsed this by renaming the problem 'conversion disorder', but this term begs the question by assuming that all such patients must have a psychological basis for their neurological symptoms, even if it remains obscure.

The reports on Elizabeth that came from the psychiatrist and psychologist were quite clear. While she had experienced the usual psychological stresses and strains there was nothing exceptional about these, and she seemed to have handled them very well. In essence, they could find no psychiatric or psychological basis for her symptoms, although they accepted that they were not due to any organic abnormality in the nervous system. The assumption that they represented a conversion from some unresolved inner conflict remained quite unproven.

My experience with Elizabeth and her frustration on being told that there was no sign of an organic or psychological basis for her problem reflects my general experience and that of many of my neurological colleagues. Psychiatrists and psychologists can only explore these matters with the full cooperation of the patient. They depend on the patient's willingness and ability to share their innermost thoughts and emotions. For one reason or another, this interaction frequently proves fruitless.

'The doctors are completely baffled by my case and have no idea what is wrong with me,' I heard Elizabeth say to another patient.

Sadly, this is the inevitable view that such patients and their relatives are left with.

There have been a plethora of other names given to illnesses like Elizabeth's, including dissociative disorder, somatisation disorder, psychosomatic disorder and psychogenic syndrome, to mention but a few. Sometimes these are associated with other recognisable psychiatric illnesses, such as depression or bipolar disorder, but often they are not. Pseudo-seizures, such as those experienced by Scott and Mr X, may be seen as just another manifestation of the same problem, distinguished only by the specific nature of their symptoms. It is well recognised, however, that people with undoubtedly genuine epilepsy may at times have pseudo-seizures, which can muddy the waters and make treatment extremely difficult.

In Mr X's case it seemed unlikely that he had ever had a true epileptic attack and he could be considered as having Munchausen syndrome. This disorder is named after the eighteenth-century Baron Munchausen, who told many fantastic tales of his adventures. Patients with Munchausen syndrome repetitively seek medical attention for a variety of fictitious medical complaints, often ending up in hospitals where they may even have life-threatening procedures, including surgery. More distressing is the so-called 'Munchausen by proxy' syndrome, in which fictitious illnesses are created by someone other than the patient, commonly a parent on behalf of a child, who then suffers unnecessary investigations and treatment. And then there is malingering, the intentional feigning of illness for gain, often related to insurance, compensation, benefit or work claims. All these different and interrelated entities need to be considered by the doctor when confronted with physical symptoms and signs that may not have an organic basis.

In this hinterland between neurology and psychiatry everything is painted in grey, not just 50 shades but in a continuous spectrum that flows from one tint into another. There are extremes, with malingering and Munchausen by proxy syndrome being on the dark side, and stress-related fatigue or dizziness sitting diametrically opposed, but these disorders meld into one another, forming a continuum. We recognise the peaks and call them by different names, but they all represent a symptom or a disability that has been invented or elaborated by the mind.

The question arises as to how the brain has done this and to what extent the process is conscious and deliberate. With malingering there is no doubt; the conscious mind is fully complicit. It seems likely that Mr X knew what he was doing, but I suspect that Scott did not. What about Elizabeth and her hysteria, conversion reaction, or call it what you will? Freud thought that such symptoms and signs were the result of subconscious processes and that the affected individuals believed in the physical nature of their disabilities. But how could they believe this when all the neurological and neurophysiological evidence shows that the sensory and motor nerves, with their central nervous system connections, right up to and including the seat of consciousness itself, the cerebral cortex, are intact and functioning normally? How could Elizabeth truthfully say that she could not feel anything in her anaesthetic limbs or see anything in her blind eye when their stimulation produced normal responses over the appropriate sensory cortex in the cerebral hemispheres? The messages were clearly getting right through to their intended target. Surely, she must have experienced some sensation. Well, as the song goes, 'it ain't necessarily so'.

The concept that the cerebral cortex alone is the seat of consciousness is a simplistic one. Interpretation of the signals it receives can be modulated and altered by deeper structures, including those in the so called 'basement of the brain'. The brain can alter perception, and frequently does so to fit in with an individual's beliefs. Magnetic resonance imaging (MRI) scans can show up not only brain anatomy but also which parts become active in appreciation of sensations, thinking or doing tasks. One US study involved MRI scanning while subjects were sipping a series of wines through tubes after being told how much each one cost. Participants not only said they preferred the expensive wines, but when imbibing these their brains also became more active in regions that are thought to be involved in reward value or pleasure. In fact, these people were all drinking the same wine. It seemed that they did not just say they enjoyed the more expensive wine, but the brain also altered their experience so that this was actually the case.

Well, you might say, pleasure is a bit airy-fairy; what about something really definite, like pain. As a medico I am well aware that placebos are very effective in many patients. These not only include fake medications but sham manipulations and the like. In fact, it is generally accepted that at least a third of patients will report benefit from such treatments. Now, it turns out that people do not just say they are better, they actually are. People given fake pain-relieving cream before being given electric shocks in an MRI scanner not only say the shocks are less painful, but the activity of pain-sensitive brain regions is also decreased. The brain has modulated their experience of reality to fit their expectations. This is how hypnosis works, by convincing subjects that their brains are under the control of the hypnotist. If they believe they are in a trance and cannot feel anything, then a noxious stimulus, which would normally be very painful, can be tolerated without difficulty.

There is an increasing body of evidence that in hysterical conversion reaction unconscious psychological mechanisms modulate the activity of structures in the 'basement of the brain', including the limbic system, and alter the way in which they interact with the areas of the cerebral cortex that control the motor or sensory functions in the body parts affected. This has been reported not only with loss of motor and sensory function but also in patients in whom conversion disorder has produced involuntary movements, such as tremor. These studies generally support the hypothesis that the mechanisms underlying such neurological disturbance are subconscious.

Elizabeth was one of the lucky ones and her symptoms gradually settled over a month or two, and by three months she was back to normal. She had a minor recurrence of somewhat similar symptoms about three years later, in the early stages of her first pregnancy. Fortunately, this rapidly cleared under the watchful eye of her husband, the Reverend Donald MacPherson. Follow-up studies from internationally reputable psychiatric clinics suggest that the prognosis is generally not so bright, with a high proportion of patients still suffering from their symptoms many years later.

**THESE ARE THE TALES** of but a few of the fascinating patients that I have had the privilege of seeing and trying to help. Do not think that my experience has been in any way unusual. Most of my colleagues would be able to recount a host of similar experiences. They are all part of that richly coloured and complexly interwoven tapestry that makes up the neurosciences.

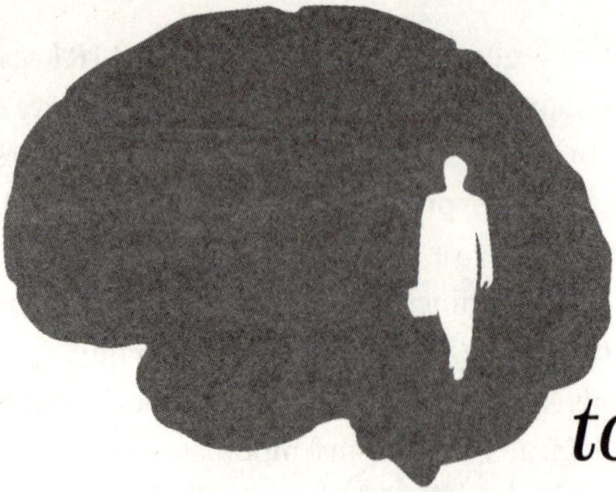

# CHAPTER 13
# *The* Path *to* Truancy
## 1994–2013

'**WHAT INTERESTING MOVEMENT** disorders have you seen recently?' I was back in David Marsden's office and this was his opening gambit, after we had exchanged greetings and he had settled back into his chair, lighting another cigarette.

'We seem to be having an epidemic of Creutzfeldt-Jakob disease, or Jakob-Creutzfeldt, as they used to call it. Why on earth they changed the name escapes me. Perhaps they didn't like the sound of JC disease, thinking that priority to those initials had been given to somebody else,' I replied, disappointed when my feeble attempt at flippancy fell on infertile soil.

'That's peculiar,' David said. 'I have never had a case of my own. Tell me what symptoms and signs your patients have shown.'

So I outlined the clinical features of the disease, which had become so familiar to me: the prominent involuntary jerking and dementia that progressed over months to a tragic bedridden, semi-conscious state, soon followed by inevitable death. These were accompanied by textbook laboratory findings.

We discussed possible causes for this mysterious outbreak, which was to continue for a decade or two before finally petering out. There was no inkling then that David would have ample opportunity to see for himself the devastation wrought by Creutzfeldt-Jakob disease, popularly known as mad cow disease, when an outbreak was to hit Britain several years later. This was the result of people eating beef infected by the smaller-than-virus-sized prion that causes bovine spongiform encephalopathy. The source of the Christchurch outbreak was never established.

This entire preamble, however, was skirting around the real reason for my visit, which was to re-kickstart the book that we were supposed to be writing together but which had stalled, at least at David's end. When we were together I could tie him down and it would progress well. We would work away at it and make good headway. Once I left, however, David would be diverted by all the other academic, clinical and teaching demands on his time. I knew the syndrome only too well. He also had many balls to juggle, and while he had a host of junior staff to help him twirl them, his professional balls were much bigger than mine and these very staff also demanded his attention. Each time I went back to New Zealand I simply dropped off the radar.

A fair proportion of the precious academic time that I had was devoted to writing the book, but this was not being matched by David. I had made a number of visits to London to work with him, not only using sabbatical leave for this purpose but also tacking such trips on to European conferences that I attended. True, Chris and I also combined these sojourns with little dalliances in European wine regions. The latter, however, were taken in my precious holidays, which were also being eroded by time spent in London.

I had earlier met with David and Stanley Fahn at a conference in Hawaii and we had discussed our various contributions. Without having contributed anything, Stanley had wisely withdrawn from the project when he realised he did not have sufficient time to devote to it.

'David,' I said now, 'we need to do something radical about *The Book*. It is progressing far too slowly and I can't spend all my time here in London prodding you into action. At the rate we are progressing we'll be dead and buried before it is published! Not only that, but all of the chapters that we have written are now in need of being updated. The field is moving so rapidly that this will be a big job in itself. We should update the first part of the book and publish it as a separate volume, which will leave us free to concentrate on the second part.'

'I really don't want to do that,' David replied; 'I think it would destroy the continuity of the book. Let's make a real effort to get it finished within the next year. We'll ask OUP to edit what we have done, and provide them with a firm timetable for delivery of the remaining chapters. That way we will have pressure put on us to meet deadlines and we will just have to make certain that we stick to them.'

Reluctantly I acquiesced, and after another of what had become rather repetitious and overly optimistic meetings with our tolerant publishers, all was agreed. The process would be completed within a year.

When age had forced retirement on the reluctant Roger Gilliatt, he had decided to fight back and took up a neurology post in the US, where he died of cancer of the pancreas several years later. Roger's former position as Professor of Clinical Neurology at the Institute of Neurology and consultant neurologist at the National Hospital was keenly sought after by two of my colleagues, who became the only ones to be shortlisted for the job. Ian McDonald, under whom I had nominally worked as a Commonwealth Medical Fellow and who had been my unofficial mentor while I was on The House at The Square, had become a close friend of mine. He had a personal chair but had long dreamt of filling Roger's shoes. Rivalry was fierce, and when David Marsden was appointed to the position Ian believed he had been disadvantaged by being gay.

While I commiserated with Ian and congratulated David, it was with very mixed feelings. The Chair of Clinical Neurology would further enhance David's reputation and allow him to expand his research programme, but at the same time it would put him under much more pressure. Would he be able to fulfil the agreed programme and meet the strict deadlines that we had agreed upon for the book? Time would tell, and tell quite quickly.

I had first met Anita Harding in David's new department at the Institute of Neurology. She was a vivacious, confident and very able younger neurologist who had made a name for herself sorting out the clinical features and genetics of the inherited cerebellar degenerations and peripheral neuropathies, a group of disorders that cause shrinkage of the cerebellum, or balance organ in the back of the head, and degeneration of the nerves in the limbs. Such patients develop clumsiness, unsteadiness, slurred speech and limb weakness. Anita was married to Professor Peter ('PK') Thomas, an expert in peripheral nerve disorders; she had earlier been his student, and there was a considerable age gap between them. PK was as reserved as Anita was outgoing. They were both very friendly with David, and at times they had holidayed together. She was David's protégée and second-in-charge. I got on well with Anita, who was also helpful to Chris. They sometimes met in the evenings when Chris was working on the manuscript of the book at the Institute.

Time proved that I had been correct in having my doubts about David's ability to meet deadlines. While I worked away writing new chapters and updating earlier text, he produced little when I was not there to prod him into action. There would be a flurry of activity when I was in London, but as soon as I left he would grind to a halt. It is not that he was unproductive; far from it. He was being incredibly productive, guiding and contributing to the substantial output of scientific papers coming from his junior staff and his colleagues. They were under his nose where they could grab his attention, while I was on the other side of the world. Every time I came to London a new and 'final' timetable would be set and agreed to by our long-suffering publishers, only to disappear eventually into the dim and distant past like all of the others.

Although I was frustrated, I felt that during this period David was perhaps at his happiest. It was not that I had ever seen him unhappy, but at that time he seemed to have a special energy and effervescence. Eventually, however, I found that he became diverted by clinical, research and administrative matters, even during my visits, and I had to protest loudly.

'Ivan, you are quite correct,' he said. 'These continual interruptions from other commitments have made our work together difficult. In future, should I not be free when you come to London, I will take time off and you can stay with me, Jenny and the girls at our home in Ash, down in Kent. We will be able to work down there each day without interruption.'

So we did this, and David and I would start as soon as breakfast was over and work steadily until about 1 p.m., when we would retire to the local pub for lunch and a pint. We would talk about our interests, hobbies and dreams. What would we do when we retired? My plans rotated around wine, our vineyard and the winery. I found it curious that David had a fascination with model steam trains, the type that are big enough to perch on and to take children for a ride. He belonged to a local club of enthusiasts and he intended to devote more time to this in the future. There were the inevitable discussions of family matters and tales of the local gypsies, whose children his daughters had befriended, hopefully giving his household immunity from any nocturnal property loss.

All too soon lunch would be over and we would toddle back to David's living room-cum-conservatory to put our noses to the grindstone once again. Although the house had a lovely garden attached, it was usually too cold to sit outdoors. We would beaver away until David's three lovely small daughters and his wife came home. I had met his first family and former wife, Jill, at their home many years earlier, but had not previously met the attractive Jenny. Although I felt I was intruding, she made me very welcome. After dinner we would all retire to our beds early so that we could be up and ready for action again as soon as the girls had gone off to school. My bedroom was in a part of the house that was close to the road and I tended to sleep fitfully from early morning, when trucks started to roll by. In spite of my being tired we made good progress, but there always seemed to be a daunting amount left to be done.

When I met Anita again less than a year after I had last seen her she seemed to have aged more than a decade. She had lost her attractive hair and had become gaunt. It had all started with a pain in the lower back, she told me. At first she had thought she must have twisted it and irritated a nerve. The pain became more persistent and spread from her buttock down into her leg. She was investigated for sciatica. It was only when the leg began to swell up that alarm bells started to ring. It was found that she had bowel cancer, which had spread to invade the nerves and then moved on to obstruct the blood flow from that limb. Surgery had been unable to remove the entire tumour and she had been started on chemotherapy.

Anita was plucky, positive and active but quite realistic. She had a lot that she wanted to get done and she was intent on finishing it. Her death at the age of 42 came as a great blow to David. Her entire illness had been quite brief. Anita had been the star of David's coterie, and she died shortly before she was due to succeed him as Professor of Clinical Neurology, a position for which he had groomed her. David was about to become Dean of the Institute of Neurology. Tragically, the music had stopped before she could sit in the chair. Ironically, it was taken by David's former rival, the gentle and gentlemanly Ian McDonald. Ian, a world-renowned figure in the field of multiple sclerosis, had got his dream at last and he held on to the post until he retired.

In the year or two after Anita's death David seemed to lose some of his sparkle and drive. We continued to work together but his mind never seemed to be wholly on the job. Then there came a time when I was back in New Zealand and I could get no reply from him. He did not respond to email, phone call or letter. I became very irritated and frustrated. At last, I got through to him at his home one Sunday evening. He was very subdued and apologetic. He had not been able to respond because he had been ill and had been in hospital. He had been unable to let me know. He hoped that I would understand.

I was stunned and I began to feel guilty that I had been annoyed with him. I told him that I appreciated his frankness and that I would continue to work away. In the meantime he should concentrate on getting better and not worry about the book. He finished the conversation with his usual 'Ciao'.

Little did I know that it would be the last time I heard his voice.

Not long after this, I was sitting inside, gazing out of the window onto our garden, lost in thought. There was a light drizzle and the tiny droplets, seen against the afternoon light, seemed to shimmer and float gently downwards, rather than simply fall. Gradually the path became wet and a puddle began to form, slowly making the vague outline of a head. It was nobody's in particular, just a head, but memories started to drift into my mind. They were only little snippets but they came floating in from different directions and times, coalescing to form a shape, a mosaic, a jigsaw of a person, and I felt that at last I was starting to see and understand what had eluded me before; what had helped fuse together such drive, energy, productivity and flair but what had, by its very nature, also imparted a brittle flaw.

A little later I received a letter that I opened with a mixture of impatient curiosity and foreboding. I had recognised the writing on the envelope. It contained a single handwritten page. The letter was short and to the point. David wrote that he was very sorry for having let me down. He was aware that he had messed me about and that he had not lived up to his part of the bargain. This may have affected my career and he was immensely regretful.

I did not disagree with any of this, but why now, I wondered? It seemed strangely inappropriate that he would send me this letter out of the blue and at this time. What had prompted his remorse? Perhaps he was going to turn over a new leaf. I put the letter away and forgot about it. I would take it up with him the next time we were in contact.

**'THIS IS FOR YOU, IVAN**. It's from Queen Square,' Chris said, handing me the telephone.

'Hello Ivan,' a voice said. 'This is Niall Quinn. I am just telephoning to let you know that David Marsden is dead. I thought you would want to know straight away. You two have been working together for so long.'

The genial Professor Niall Quinn had also worked closely with David for many years and had become his right-hand man.

'That's absolutely dreadful, Niall. What happened?'

'No one really knows at this point. David was found dead last evening in an apartment in which he was living in New York. I guess there will be an autopsy, which will no doubt show.'

For a long time it was hard to think of anything else. David had not told me he was moving to New York, so I would have had difficulty contacting him if I had tried. I had not looked at the postmark on the letter he had sent me not so long before. I wondered if it had been sent from New York.

I was desperate to go to London but pressure of work prevented this. I was determined to finish the book by myself but I needed material that was unavailable locally. David had a good personal library and an elaborate filing system on movement disorders, which served him as a reference centre and memory bank. These contained all sorts of old books and original articles that he had collected over the years and many that were generally unavailable. Much of this material came from the pre-digital era and it was not recoverable via the internet. I needed to have access to this to help me in my mission.

I had mentioned it to Niall and I now spoke to Beth Howell-Hughes, who had been David's devoted secretary, personal assistant, guard dog and mother confessor. Beth was able to help me join up many of the dots in the enigmatic picture of David. She told me that he had separated from Jenny and that he had died on the day the *decree nisi* was issued. She advised me to come as soon as I could, and meanwhile she would try to keep David's filing system intact.

It was nine months before I met Beth in David's former office area at the Institute of Neurology. She and Niall Quinn had done their best, but with the changing of the guard all of David's files had been relegated to the basement. I would have to seek out my gems there. It was with foreboding that I descended into the bowels of the Institute accompanied by a porter who resembled an elderly jailer. He appeared to have a movement disorder himself, walking with a stoop and a shuffle, while clanking a large bunch of keys. After close inspection he selected one from the ring and proceeded to open a door for me. As I stepped into the gloom there was a click behind me and the room went black. I realised that my jailer had not followed me in but had just closed the door on me. Fortunately I had brought a torch, and I located a light switch without difficulty.

The sight that greeted me was one of chaos and it filled me with despair. The basement was a repository for all sorts of junk and unwanted material, which was scattered about and piled high at random. Everything was covered with dust. After a bit of hunting around I found David's filing system. Fortunately it was all contained within one area, but the sliding drawers, which once contained hanging manila files of precious papers, were largely empty. The files themselves and the papers that they had contained lay strewn across the floor in a higgledy-piggledy mess. It was with a heavy heart that I surveyed the scene. What would he, the collector and once-proud owner of this treasure trove, have thought of this jumble?

Without a doubt, David was the most gifted scientist and clinician that I had ever met. He had the rare talent of being extremely proficient in basic scientific, laboratory and clinical work as well as having an excellent rapport with patients. His scientific and medical output had been prodigious, and from the time he graduated from medical school until his death he had averaged one medical publication every nine days. Between 1975 and 1978 his output was one a week. He was hard-working and ambitious, and he had built up a team of very able people around him. Together they had carved out a worldwide reputation. He should have been at the pinnacle of his career and yet it had all slipped through his fingers. His castle had tumbled down.

All we who work in clinical medicine are daily confronted by evidence of our own frailty and transient nature, but we sometimes ignore it, conveniently thrusting it aside in pursuit of our goals. All, the great and the small, must end in dust. David, a man small in stature but a colossus by reputation and intellect, had died alone in an apartment in a foreign city at the relatively young age of 60. Here were the crumbled remnants of his empire. Suddenly, a vivid mental image came to me, that of van Gogh's tragic self-portrait with his head swathed in a bandage. I felt that I was now truly in the dim and dusty *basement of the basement of the brain*. I promised myself then and there that I would stick to an earlier promise I had made to Chris and that I would leave clinical practice when I was 60.

Shaking myself out of my lugubrious ruminations I set about the task at hand. It took me until the end of the day, but eventually I had all that could be gleaned from the apparent rubbish dump. It would have to do. It was with a sense of relief that I emerged into the cool evening and slowly strolled through the garden that enlivens the centre of Queen Square, breathing in the pure fresh air.

**ALTHOUGH I HAD REAFFIRMED** that long-standing vow about leaving clinical medicine, when the fateful time loomed large on the horizon I began to fight against it. I made up all sorts of excuses; I had taken on a new project that I needed to finish, I had another that I wanted to start, I would be leaving my colleagues in the lurch, there were patients who were relying on me ... Of course, both my colleagues and my patients might have been glad to see the back of me, and any vital project could still be undertaken. I did, however, intend to keep my promise; well, sort of. When I finally did resign, did I jump or was I pushed? As it turned out it was neither; I was pulled, and rather roughly.

'You promised many years ago that you would leave medicine when you were 60 and you have planned this for ages,' argued Chris. 'There is no point in carrying on until you have passed your use-by date, like some doctors do. What else do you want to do in medicine? Most doctors cling on because they have no other interests, but that is not you.

'You have this other half to your life that we have built up, and now it needs you. The boys and I cannot do everything. You need to make the swap for your benefit as well. If you leave it too long you will be too old to adjust to the change.'

'I don't really know how I found time for that neurology lark,' I commented to Chris one evening over dinner, a few months after I had left medicine. 'The amount of work there is to do at the winery and vineyard seems quite overwhelming.'

'It's Murphy's Law,' she replied. 'Being in the wine business is like being on a farm. You never really finish work. However much you do there is always more to be done.'

Two years after I resigned from my university and hospital posts an article appeared in the *Journal of Neurology, Neurosurgery, and Psychiatry*, which is published in Britain; it used to be affectionately called 'The Green Rag', in reference to the colour of its cover. The article, entitled 'Neurological Truant', explained that the term 'Medical Truant' had been coined many years earlier by Lord Moynihan. He used it for those who qualified in medicine but later hived off to carve themselves a career in some unrelated field, leaving their chosen profession abandoned. It was a vignette about me and it sported a reproduction of a postage stamp that featured our vineyard. In 1997 New Zealand Post had put out a series of stamps celebrating New Zealand wine industry, and these stamps featured six vineyards from around the country. A well-known Kiwi artist, Nancy Tichborne, had been commissioned to paint a picture of each vineyard. That is how the image of our son Paul, frozen forever in the act of picking grapes, happened to grace the front of many a letter and parcel sent nationally and internationally.

The article went on to say that as numerous scientific studies suggested mild to moderate intake of wine had beneficial effects on brain function and vascular disorders, then I may have done more to help patients than any other neurologist. It was written by none other than my neurologist friend Lindsay Haas, who had a keen interest in medical philately. In modesty I thought that I should protest, but who was I to argue with the views of my superior. In fact, after I had come out, so to speak, and nominally gone over to the dark side, I did not totally sever my ties with medicine or neurology, as I shall later elaborate. In addition, I continued to work on David's and my book, whenever my new full-time occupation allowed. Sadly, however, time ran out for Lindsay, who on many occasions had spoken to me longingly of retiring from medicine. He worked as a neurologist until shortly before he died from a metastatic malignant melanoma deposit in his brain.

After I returned to New Zealand from my disturbing visit to the basement of the Institute of Neurology, I had devoted all the spare time I had to writing the rest of the book by myself and within a month I had finished; all 52 chapters. Now I was faced with the daunting task of updating it. The chapters that I had written were reasonably up-to-date as I had inserted new material on the various topics as it had appeared in the scientific press. The chapters that David had been primarily responsible for, however, needed quite a lot of work, and I was not looking forward to this. My ever-faithful publishers, Oxford University Press, suggested that they get somebody from Queen Square, who was working in the movement disorder field, to review the manuscript to see exactly how much updating was required. That is how in June 2000 I came to meet Kailash Bhatia, one of David's protégés.

Kailash agreed to take over the job of updating the whole book, on condition that he became an acknowledged co-author. He estimated it would probably take him about six months to complete, but this proved to be unrealistic. A new and more generous timetable was agreed to and drawn up with OUP. The provisional publication date was now the end of 2001. This came and went without any end in sight, so new deadlines were set and then passed, only to be reset again. *Déjà vu* had well and truly set in. Then, in 2010, Kailash introduced me to Susanne Schneider, a bright and attractive young German neurologist who was doing a PhD at Queen Square. Kailash suggested that Susanne come aboard and take over the updating, on the condition that she also became a co-author. Her PhD was on the genetics of neurological disorders, a field that had advanced dramatically in the preceding decade. I found Susanne to be effective, efficient and very easy to work with. Within two years she had completed her task, and at long last the book was finally published in 2012.

When I started in neurology the functions of the 'basement of the brain', the basal ganglia, were largely surrounded in mystery and the field of movement disorders did not exist as such. Many, if not most, of the individual disorders were known but no one had really tied them together. For three decades David had laboured to carve out this subspecialty from the gigantic granite block of which general neurology is formed. With Stanley Fahn, he had started the *Journal of Movement Disorders*, and he had been closely involved in the establishment of the International Movement Disorder Society. I believe that he earned himself the title of The Father of Movement Disorders, but even should this paternity be debated there is no doubt that he was right at the centre of the delivery suite when the infant subspecialty was born.

In his sad absence, I and the book's other co-authors unanimously agreed on the title *Marsden's Book of Movement Disorders*, in his memory. Of his 1368 publications, this was to be the last.

# Epilogue

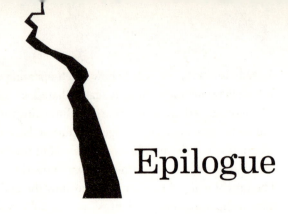

**BUT WHY DID I REALLY** choose to combine medicine with wine? Looking back at the words I have written I am not sure that they explain everything. There is a long history of the medical profession's involvement with wine, and I am not just referring to those who become too fond of the bottle. A look at the history books shows that doctors are disproportionately represented in the wine industry, and even in our small young vineyard community of Waipara Valley there are at least seven vineyards or wineries that have been started or are owned by doctors. Philip Norrie, an Australian medic, has written a series of booklets on some of the Australian doctors who have owned vineyards and/or wineries and there are quite a number, at least 150. A few have left their names on some of that country's most famous wine brands, including Penfolds, Lindemans and Hardys.

Is it that these medics have observed the health benefits of wines in their patients? Possibly, because there is plenty of evidence in the scientific literature to show that wine drinkers are healthier than those who drink other forms of alcoholic beverages or, for that matter, teetotallers. This is not, however, to say that wine-drinking is the cause of their better health. According to a number of epidemiological studies wine drinkers as a group smoke less, eat healthier diets, do more exercise, have higher socioeconomic status and even have greater IQs than other groups in the community. Mild to moderate intake of wine could be the cause of their better health, but the relationship is confounded by these other factors, hence the theorised cause and effect remains unproven.

Another possible explanation is that winemaking, like medicine itself, is a curious mixture of science and art. You can be overflowing with technical information and still make a lousy winemaker or doctor; scientific knowledge is indispensable but not sufficient. A good doctor or winemaker needs to be able to apply his or her knowledge skilfully and sensitively. Both jobs have more than just a touch of craft in them. There is a special type of satisfaction to be gained from the skilful application of knowledge to a craft, and perhaps this is the common link.

When I finally mustered the courage to cross the divide from medicine to wine my colleagues gave me a rousing send-off. It took place during a meeting of the New Zealand Neurological Association, which was held in the little Canterbury alpine village of Hanmer. The official dinner was in full swing when suddenly Malvina Major appeared out of the blue and, accompanied by Philip Parkin, who had followed me as head of the Neurology Department at Christchurch Hospital, launched into a recital of operatic arias. Phil is an excellent pianist, and the combination of his playing and Malvina's ethereal voice was magical. What a way to go! Or did I really go? Had I completely severed my ties with neurology and medicine?

Even before I resigned from my posts at the medical school and the hospital there had been the whiff of something very exciting in the neurological wind. Years earlier Tim Anderson had been a protégé of mine, and from an early stage it was apparent that he was an exceptional student. As he neared the end of his second year as a neurology registrar in Christchurch I began to look into ways for him to do further training with David Marsden at Queen Square. At about this time an Englishman, Mr Smithers, was admitted to Christchurch Hospital with severe headaches and personality change. Investigations showed that he had a highly malignant incurable brain tumour, and he needed to be flown back to Britain. His condition was such that he required a medical escort, and I suggested that Tim should accompany him.

While this was a tragic situation for the patient and his wife, it was a good opportunity for Tim. He would be able to meet David Marsden, which would allow them to discuss what type of job would best suit both their requirements. The insurance company would cover Tim's travel costs, and all he had to do was to be an attendant. With medication the patient's brain swelling had settled and he was virtually symptom-free, apart from being easily fatigued. Hopefully he would sleep for a lot of the trip.

They were over the Atlantic when, much to the alarm of his wife and the other business-class passengers, Mr Smithers became agitated and aggressive. He shouted, raged and took off down the aisle, threatening other passengers. Tim, roused from his somnolent state, had to wrestle the poor patient to the floor and inject him with a sedative. Much to the relief of all the passengers, and especially Tim, Mr Smithers slept soundly throughout the rest of the trip, although his medical attendant remained fully alert. Needless to say, David was enormously impressed with Tim, and immediately offered him a job.

That had been years earlier and now Tim was my colleague at Christchurch

Hospital. Although new jobs were thin on the ground, I had somehow managed to cobble one together for him. A representative of the College of Education, a speech therapist, the dean of the medical school and I had formed a quorum to explore the possibility of establishing a degree course in speech, language and communication disorders at Canterbury University. After long, hard negotiations we succeeded in getting the go-ahead. I had insisted that there be neurological input into the course, and this was to form a significant proportion of Tim's new job.

Tim's other special interest was in movement disorders and he had taken over the care of Cas Van der Veer, a former patient of mine, who had Parkinson's disease. Cas died tragically during a trip to Europe, and he bequeathed his not inconsiderable estate to be used for research into neurological disorders, and in particular the malady from which he had suffered. The trustees of his estate visited a number of overseas neurological centres to see where the funds could best be put to use before finally deciding on Christchurch, where they were entrusted to the Canterbury Medical Research Foundation.

'I have been consulted about the possibility of starting a Neurological Institute in Christchurch, concentrating on movement disorders,' I told Chris one evening over our preprandial nibble and glass of wine. 'It sounds exciting, doesn't it? Just think, if I was to become involved my clinical work would be reduced and it would be possible to focus principally on research. It's what we have always dreamt about.'

'You mean, it is what you have always dreamt about; not me,' Chris responded firmly. 'Don't think that you're going to wriggle out of that promise you made me. You are definitely going to quit neurology when the time comes, not just change one job for another! Don't forget, we need your help!'

That is how we left it, and that is how it was. But I did not entirely play truant. I joined the board of directors of the new institute, which morphed into the New Zealand Brain Research Institute Ltd, and I have had the pleasure of helping guide its development. It was especially pleasing for me to see that the institute formed a close working relationship with the New Zealand Institute of Language, Brain and Behaviour, which had developed out of the degree course that I had helped establish at Canterbury University. I was thrilled when Tim, now Professor Tim Anderson, became the clinical director of the New Zealand Brain Research Institute.

**AS I HAVE MENTIONED PREVIOUSLY,** the brain does not treat all events equally, and those that are associated with strong emotions form deep and lasting memories. One such memory of mine, which I still recall vividly, is a couple of young men conversing in a language that I did not understand.

'There is nothing exceptional about that,' you may say. 'It happens all the time.'

It was not the lack of comprehension, however, but the circumstances that amazed me.I had recently turned 18, and a few weeks earlier the school gates had closed behind me for the last time. It was essential that I earned sufficient money during the summer vacation to support myself during my first year at university and I had been lucky enough to get a well-paid job in an abattoir, the Makarewa Freezing Works. The downside was that the abattoir was 175 kilometres from home and I had to live in a camp with all the other itinerant workers. They were a fairly rough and tough bunch, spending most of their spare time smoking, boozing, gambling and whoring; as far as I could see, in roughly equal proportions. One evening, shortly after I arrived, I was in the rudimentary ablutions block cleaning my teeth when in walked two muscle-bound young Maori engrossed in a loud conversation. It was then that I was amazed, no, shocked, to realise that they must be speaking their native tongue.

It will no doubt seem strange to any younger person living in modern New Zealand that I had never heard Maori, but that is how it was. Almost the only Maori words that were heard were place names, at least in the South Island, where the Maori population was small. I had not been to the North Island but I had not led a particularly sheltered life. I suspect that my father could speak Maori but I never heard him utter a word. Perhaps my mother would not allow it in case their children became infected with the tongue. There had been a general feeling, and possibly a hope among Pakeha, that the language would die out — children had been discouraged from speaking Maori at school — and I had imagined that it was already extinct.

These days Maori can be heard almost anywhere; there is a Maori television channel and it is common for elements of the language and culture to be taught in schools throughout the land, but in the 1950s ... ! Like many, I now regret that I was sanitised by my well-meaning parents and by the community at large, but that is how it was.

When I was asked to join the board of directors of He Waka Tapu (The Sacred Canoe) it did not take me long to make up my mind. This non-government charitable organisation is the largest Maori provider of health and social services in the South Island. In spite of my woeful ignorance of the language and culture I hoped that my medical background would be of assistance, and I was keen to help reduce the sad gap in health and social statistics that has developed between Maori and Pakeha.

**SIR DON BEAVEN'S DEATH** came as a great shock but he died as he had lived, on his feet and fighting. A few years earlier he had been knighted for his numerous medical good works and in particular for his struggle to improve diabetic services. In his time he had taken on all sorts of causes and fought hard for each one of them. After Pleurisy Point had been sold and turned into real estate he retained a lively interest in the product of the vine but did not continue grape-growing or winemaking. Instead, he and his wife Gillian became passionate about olives and olive oil, establishing a small grove in the tiny seaside settlement of Little Akaloa on Banks Peninsula, where they had a holiday house. For many years we had gone there with friends on New Year's Day to have *lonuch*, a long lunch to which we all contributed. It started at midday and continued in leisurely fashion, via multiple dishes and matching wines, until about 7 p.m.

On the fateful day of his death, Don had gone to the property to work in the garden and olive grove, leaving Gillian in Christchurch. Somehow a fire started, and by the time the neighbours got there the house was an inferno. A garden hose, trailing through the front door and still squirting water, bore mute witness to Don's plucky attempt to save his beloved retreat. He was 85.

**ONE BITTERLY COLD SEPTEMBER** night, Chris and I had gone to Akaroa to attend a dinner put on by a local restaurant, featuring the wines of a neighbouring Waipara Valley producer. A southerly storm had been raging and there were small drifts of hail lying on the ground.

It was well after midnight by the time Chris and I retired to bed at our Akaroa holiday house. Several hours later I felt her shaking me, and then she shouted my name. She shook me more violently and began to scream.

'Ivan! Ivan! Wake up! It's an earthquake!'

As I came to groggily I realised that it had not been Chris shaking me. It felt as though we were being tossed about by a giant's hand. Terrible thrusting made it difficult even to get out of bed, let alone cross the room. We both fell before we got to the door. It was pitch-black and none of the lights worked. We were thrown from one side of the corridor to the other as we stumbled and groped our way towards the front door. Once outside we moved well away from the house, as it seemed that it might collapse. A clear moon rode on high, while torn little shreds of clouds fled before the vicious southerly wind.

The shaking finally stopped and after a few moments we became aware of barking. We had been dog-sitting for Matthew and Lynnette who were overseas, and we had forgotten that their little darlings were now trapped inside the house. Chris rushed back in to open the door of the room they were in, and emerged a few seconds later carrying a pullover.

'Put this on,' she instructed; 'you'll die of the cold standing there in the nick.'

It was only then that I realised I was freezing.

'Where did the dogs go?' Chris asked.

'They fled into the bush in terror. No doubt they'll come back before long.'

'What do we do now?'

'Go back to bed, I guess. It must have been around 25 minutes since the last shake and we can't stand out here forever. It's probably no more than one or two degrees.'

You cannot live in New Zealand for very long without feeling a tremble. Our little country is not known as the 'Shaky Isles' for nothing. It owes its existence to the fact that it is the meeting point of the great Pacific and Australian plates of the earth's crust. Here they continually jostle and thrust up above the surface of the ocean, with the inevitable earth tremors that this tussle involves. But neither Chris nor I had felt anything like the earthquake that we had just experienced. It had to be a massive one.

As soon as we were back inside we telephoned Edward and Paul to make sure they and their families were all safe. We went back to bed by torchlight, the power still being out. Not surprisingly sleep evaded us as intermittent jolts and thrusts continued. About 20 minutes later we were startled when my mobile phone rang. I recognised the ringtone — it was Matthew, calling from a seaside resort in Thailand.

'Hello, Dad. I hear you had a bit of a rumble.'

'Yes, Matthew, you could say that. But how do you know?'

'I've just been called by a friend in Christchurch. Are you all right?'

'Yes, we're fine, but aftershocks are continuing every few minutes.'

'We have to get somebody into the winery to see what damage has been done.'

'There is absolutely no chance of that, Matthew. It's still completely black here and with these continuing aftershocks it would be far too dangerous.'

It was about an hour later when I received a phone call from Michael. He had been paying for petrol in an Irish garage when he saw a news flash about the terrible earthquake that had occurred in Christchurch.

'Yes,' I assured him, 'we are all safe and well here.'

The ease and efficacy of modern communication never cease to amaze me.

A type of uneasy peace came with the daylight; intermittent shocks continued but they were less severe. A scene of total chaos greeted us in the kitchen. The cupboard doors had flown open and discharged their contents all over the floor. There were broken jars of preserved fruit mixed with nuts, sugar, salt, pesto, flour, biscuits, wine, cereals, recipe books and all manner of other kitchen staples and utensils. Pictures had crashed off the walls and ornaments had been thrown on the floor. Cracks and fissures had appeared in the walls. But at least none of us had been hurt or worse. Chris and I set to and cleaned up the sticky mess, which was laced with dangerously sharp shards of glass.

It was 4 p.m. by the time we and our grand-dogs turned into the drive of our home in Christchurch. The pattern of damage there was similar but more severe as it was closer to the epicentre of the quake. There were cracks in the walls and ceilings, the floor was buckled and two chimneys had fallen down, but at least the house was still standing. Again, the kitchen cupboards had disgorged their contents to form a vast sticky heap, but we were saved the unenviable task of cleaning up that mess as Paul and his wife Rachel had kindly done that for us.

In spite of all our fears, damage at the winery was minor; two broken glasses, one bottle of wine, and a bent leg on a wine tank. My Christchurch wine cellar, however, proved to be more of a disaster!

It transpired that the magnitude of the earthquake on 4 September 2010, which was centred a short distance southwest of Christchurch, was 7.2 on the Richter scale. It was of about the same magnitude as that which had destroyed Port au Prince in Haiti several years earlier. The inhabitants of Christchurch congratulated themselves. By comparison to Port au Prince, damage to their city was minor and there were no deaths directly attributable to the event. Christchurch had never been regarded as particularly earthquake-prone, and the geologists said that the fault which had generated the earthquake must have lain undisturbed and undetected under the surface of the Canterbury Plains for at least 15,000 years. What rotten luck that it should choose to show its ugly scarred face once more. Although frequent aftershocks continued nobody dreamt that the worst was yet to come.

The following 22 February, around lunchtime, I was sitting at home in Christchurch, having just dialled a telephone number, when suddenly there was the most violent shaking imaginable. I really felt that the house was in danger of falling down. I managed to make my way down the stairs, being shot from side to side like a tennis ball at a Wimbledon final. When I eventually made it outside I realised that I was still holding the telephone in my hand

and that my cursing and semi-religious expletives had been recorded for posterity on an answer machine somewhere or other; I could not remember who I had been calling.

Although severe, the earthquake had been quite brief, and now that it had stopped I tried to telephone Chris, thinking at the same time of our children and their families, and other relatives and friends I needed to check on. It was to no avail, as the landlines and mobile network had failed.

Chris and Paul had gone to the vineyard that morning, so my first thought was for the safety of my daughters-in-law and grandchildren who were in Christchurch. The street was flooded with rapidly flowing dirty water so that only its raised centre was visible. I incorrectly assumed that the water mains had burst. The water had actually come from within the earth and, along with silt, it had been jetted upwards in vast amounts as the ground liquefied. Fortunately, my old Nissan Mistral SUV was high enough to wallow through the water, but other cars had not been so lucky. There were dangerously tilted lamp-posts and the surface of the street had become buckled, twisted and fissured. Gaping holes had appeared and I passed a car that had nosedived into one, its front wheels and engine submerged. It looked like an expert springboard diver who had been snapped by a camera at the moment of entering the water, the angled body and legs stiffly extended while the head and arms were beneath the surface.

As I turned into the street where Paul and his family lived I was alarmed by the sight of water lapping well up the wheels of several parked cars. However, Rachel was fine, as were her two youngest children, Clark and Olivia, but George was at school and she was desperate to go and collect him. Granddad was glad to help out by babysitting.

It was not all that long before an anxious Chris and Paul arrived, having braved the damaged roads to drive back into the city. Yet again, the winery and restaurant had emerged relatively unscathed. Diners in the restaurant had gripped the tables while their meals slid back and forwards in front of them and the chandeliers swung wildly over their heads. Although Chris was gratified that they were eager to continue eating, she prised them away from their dishes and drove them outside.

But how were Belinda and her two sons? We had not been able to contact her. The answer came quite quickly as my mobile rang and I saw that it was Edward calling. He was on a marketing visit to Canada and he had heard a news flash about this new earthquake. Fortunately he was able to call his wife and us and hence relay messages, although all local communication had failed. Belinda had been in the centre of the city and had been forced to run for her life as masonry from collapsing buildings fell around her. Edward also phoned the preschool where their boys were and was able to let her know that they were safe.

Because there was no tap water or electricity in much of the city and aftershocks were continuing, we decided we would all go and stay at the winery. It was chaos. Some roads had been destroyed, many were impassable, and it was unclear which ones could still be used, although all were to a greater or lesser extent damaged. There were huge queues of slowly moving or immobile vehicles as people tried to flee the disaster-stricken city. It took Belinda nine hours to drive the 70 kilometres, but by 10 p.m. that evening we were all joyously reunited at the winery.

Three days later Chris and I ventured back home. The house had suffered more damage, and again the cupboards had spewed their revolting mess all over the kitchen. We were slow learners, but from that time onwards we tied our cupboard doors shut to prevent a repetition. There was the slightest trickle coming from our taps and we were forced to resort to the swimming pool for our water, but we were amongst the lucky ones. Many were without electricity for a very long time and some had no water or sewerage for very many months. Entire suburbs had been destroyed, and Edward and Belinda, like many hill-dwellers, were never allowed to return to their home because of the risk of huge loosened boulders raining down on them. One such rock had passed right through a neighbour's house, tearing large holes in the walls before exiting onto the street.

The locked-down centre of the city was a disaster zone, with a large number of collapsed or partially destroyed buildings and many others that would need to be demolished. When we were allowed to re-enter the city centre large parts of it were unrecognisable as there were no familiar landmarks. Entire city blocks had disappeared and there were gaping spaces in those that remained. The churches had been singled out for the most severe punishment by this so-called act of God, as many had been built of unreinforced masonry, which was the single most vulnerable type of construction.

And what was the toll on human life? One hundred and eighty-five people had been killed and two thousand injured, many whose lives were to be permanently marred by their physical injuries. More than a few of our friends were among them. In addition, a substantial proportion of the population suffered from ongoing psychological disturbances caused by the stress of the event and its prolonged after-effects. Everyone who lived through those experiences has their own special story to tell and ours is not exceptional, only personal.

I do not claim to have any special knowledge of or expertise in seismology.

As I understand it, however, the magnitude of an earthquake does not reflect its ability to destroy; this is perhaps best estimated by its intensity. While magnitude is a measure of the amount of energy released (the Richter scale), the intensity is an estimate of the destructive forces to which buildings or other structures are subjected. This can be measured by the subjective Mercalli scale, which qualitatively assesses the effect and damage on people and structures. More objectively, destructive potential can be assessed with reference to the peak acceleration to which objects are subjected. This is measured with respect to gravitational force (G). Although the magnitude of the February earthquake (Richter 6.3) was smaller than that of the September quake, the intensity was much greater because its epicentre was closer to the city centre and at a shallower depth. In fact, the peak acceleration of the February earthquake measured 2 Gs in both the vertical and horizontal directions, a combination that is greater than in any previously recorded earth tremor in the world.

In the midst of death there is life, and in spite of the dreadful tragedy life had to go on. Staff had to be paid and businesses had to be run. In 2008 New Zealand wineries and vineyards had been subjected to a so-called 'perfect storm'. A bumper harvest coincided with large areas of new vineyards producing their first crops and with the start of a global financial crisis. The result was a surplus of New Zealand wine, which drove down prices and put a number of producers out of business. We had two wine labels in the marketplace: Pegasus Bay, which came from our own vineyard, and Main Divide, which was made from contracted fruit. This enabled us to ride out the downturn reasonably well, although we did see a change in buying patterns with a swing towards the somewhat lower-priced Main Divide.

The February 2011 earthquake closed all of the restaurants and wine outlets in central Christchurch, which was a significant market for us. Our family thus had the potential for a super-duper perfect storm, but it only loomed on the horizon before beginning to retreat. We were supported by excellent staff and, in spite of an initial loss of population, people started to flood back into the city. Many businesses, including restaurants, either started up in the suburbs or relocated there while waiting for the central city to be rebuilt.

People are very resilient in times of shared hardship, which often bring out the best in societies. Long-standing next-door neighbours who might never have conversed now offered to help each other, and people rushed to support community projects. There was a degree of cooperation and a community spirit that had not existed since the Second World War. Goodness can arise out of tragedy and we counted ourselves fortunate to have seen this happen.

**'WHAT'S THAT LETTER?' ASKED CHRIS**, selecting an envelope out of a pile of correspondence that was awaiting us when we returned from a holiday.

'I don't know,' I replied. 'It's from Government House. I guess it's some local MP wanting free wine, or else I'm going to get a rap over the knuckles for something.'

'Open it!'

'I'll get to it later,' I said unenthusiastically, replacing it on the heap. I have always been a lily-livered coward when it comes to bad news or distasteful work and I try to procrastinate as long as possible.

'Give it to me then. I'll open it.'

'No, it's addressed to me. Oh, all right. I'll open it just to please you, but I don't know why this one fascinates you.'

There was a long silence as I stared at the letter in disbelief.

'Well, what does it say?' Chris asked expectantly.

'Good grief! It ... it ... it says that I have been invited to accept being named a Companion of the New Zealand Order of Merit in the New Year's Honours list.'

'What for?' asked Chris with a conspiratorial air.

'For services to neurology ... but I have only been doing my job. There is no reason why I should have been singled out for this. Do you know something about it?'

'Some months back I was asked to provide some details about your background, but I wasn't really certain what it was about, and I was sworn to secrecy!' Chris replied with a wide grin.

**WORKING IN MEDICINE** makes you particularly aware that nobody is bulletproof and that anyone's life can be completely altered in the twinkling of an eye. The earthquakes dramatically demonstrated this to everyone in Christchurch.

I only had a split second's warning of an impending personal catastrophe when I glanced at the mirror above my head. Immediately, there seemed to be an explosion, a tremendous blow and I was spinning through the air. The panel in front of me disintegrated and I felt a searing pain in my neck.

'What was that?' Chris asked, sounding perplexed rather than worried.

It was an immense relief to hear her voice.

'We have just been crashed into from behind,' I groaned.

'Are you all right?' she enquired.

'No, I've hurt my neck.'

'I'm okay,' Chris said almost perkily as she opened the front passenger's door. 'I'll go and see if I can help those children.'

I suddenly became aware of the young children in the other car, who were screaming loudly.

'I'm not moving my neck until an ambulance comes,' I said rather selfishly. 'I'm worried that I might have fractured a cervical vertebra.'

Chris and I had been on our way to meet the Japanese distributors of our wine, who had brought a party of restaurateurs and sommeliers to the winery. We had been about to enter the northern motorway from Christchurch via a slip road but had been forced to slow to a virtual standstill because the lanes were full of traffic. I had suddenly had a glimpse of another vehicle that had appeared out of nowhere and was hurtling towards us at breakneck speed. It spun us around through 180° so that we ended up facing back in the direction we had come. Mercifully, we had not been shunted out into the busy lanes of traffic.

About 10 minutes later I heard Chris slip back into the front seat beside me.

'I might as well sit here and wait but I don't need to go to hospital,' she said. 'I'm fine.'

I was relieved to hear the friendly and reassuring voice of an ambulance officer, even before he poked his head through Chris's door to enquire how we were.

'It's my husband that you need to see,' she told him. 'He thinks he's hurt his neck, and he should know because he's a neurologist.'

The officer came round to me to make certain that my neck was supported.

'Be careful with his neck,' Chris said; 'he says that he needs to go to hospital, and he should know, because he's a neurologist.'

'You just said that,' I told her.

'Said what?'

'Said that I was a neurologist.'

'Did I?'

And that is when I had an inkling that we were in real trouble. We seemed to be at the accident scene for an interminable length of time but in reality it may not have been more than about 45 minutes. It was during that time that Chris happily informed the same ambulance officer up to a dozen times that he should take notice of what I was saying because I was a neurologist, and the repetitions were becoming more frequent, in spite of my pedantically continuing to correct her. I agreed that she had been 'fine' immediately after the accident, but now she was showing problems with her memory. To my mind this was highly suggestive of a subdural or extradural haemorrhage. I explained this to the now multiple ambulance officers who had arrived on the scene. I begged for Chris to be the first to be taken to hospital but to no avail. The crying children and their mother, who was the driver of the other car, were carted off while Chris languished at the roadside. At this stage I was starting to panic, but at least she left in the second ambulance.

By the time I arrived in the hospital's Emergency Department the mother and her frightened kids had been sent home. A normal cervical scan proved to be very therapeutic for my whiplash and my neck pains rapidly settled. Chris could remember nothing of the accident or her trip to the hospital and continued to tell the medical staff that I was a neurologist, and to ask questions to which she had been told the answers. Like my colleague Will, she had amnesia. Her brain scan showed a small sliver of subdural blood along the inner aspect of the right occipital and posterior temporal lobes, which was in keeping with her symptoms. She was admitted to hospital under the care of a neurosurgeon for observation as a 'precaution', but the amount of bleeding was minor. It all seemed rather surreal, she was a patient on the ward where I had been a consultant for 25 years and I had a strong sense of *déjà vu*.

That evening Chris held court surrounded by her adoring family. She had improved dramatically. The following morning she was not so well, but this was put down to a disturbed night in the intensive-care area of the ward and to her medication. I became increasingly concerned during the afternoon, and by evening there was no doubt; she was deteriorating and slipping into a semi-conscious state. An urgent scan showed that the bleeding had markedly deteriorated. There was now a large collection of blood over the outer surface of her right cerebral hemisphere and it was squeezing her brain across the midline towards the left. My morbid premonitions had come true and I now feared for my wife's life.

A terrifying spectre leered at me, its gaping maw a steadily growing black hole of emptiness, of dreadful all-consuming nothingness, and a tight grip seemed to be squeezing my chest. As a doctor, how many times had I had to deal with this type of situation; how many times had I needed to warn of imminent dangers; how many times had I been forced to console grieving relatives? Many, very many; but as a doctor you need to have a defence mechanism to protect you from the tragedies that are part of your daily life. You have to have sympathy and empathy but you also have to distance yourself to some extent from others' tragedies or you would not be able to cope. Now this was happening to me, and no sham barrier would suffice to offer protection, nor should it.

As I waited for what seemed like an eternity I uncontrollably shed hot, stinging tears of grief and fear. Would Chris survive, and if she did would she be left with brain damage? These thoughts kept going through my head, even as Matthew, Paul, Edward, Belinda and I sat in the small waiting room outside the operating theatre. We talked artificially about more jolly subjects and happier times in order to distract ourselves from the image of Chris's head being opened by the surgeon's saw. It was 1 a.m. on 28 March 2014 when the neurosurgeon emerged from the theatre and told me that the operation had gone well and that he had removed a thick layer of clot from the brain's surface. Chris had woken from the anaesthetic and seemed well.

We were allowed to talk to her briefly in the recovery room and we were all reassured. She was extremely drowsy for the following 36 hours and I was again beset by morbid anxieties, but I need not have worried. I think Chris recovered from our little adventure more rapidly than I did. Within days she was cheerfully up and about while I fussed over her every footstep as though it might be the last. Then another tragedy struck.

On that fateful day when Chris was admitted to hospital she had struck up a special relationship with a second-year student nurse, Sharla Haerewa. Sharla had been assigned to Chris when she was admitted, and she was with Chris when she deteriorated the following day. Sharla had been in the operating theatre to observe Chris's surgery and was there in recovery when the tearful and worried relatives had shuffled in during the small hours. Although no longer officially assigned to her, Sharla continued to visit and to write up Chris's case as part of her study requirements. She sat at Chris's bedside asking questions and making up her notes.

Sharla was a slim, attractive 22-year-old brunette, friendly, sympathetic and helpful. She seemed the epitome of the perfect nurse. One day she did not appear at the bedside, although she still had not finished her interviewing, but we thought nothing of it; Sharla was too busy, she had been rostered to another ward or perhaps she had a day off. When we read the newspaper headline the next morning Chris and I broke down in tears. Sharla was dead; her young life, so promising and full of hope, had been snuffed out in the twinkling of an eye. She had been cycling to Christchurch Hospital to start work, wearing a high-visibility vest and with lights on her bike, when a large articulated truck had turned in front of her, striking Sharla and dragging her a considerable distance along the road.

I never cease to marvel at the human body's capacity to mend itself and to recover from terrible insults, both physical and psychological. Chris's discharge was delayed by medical complications, but nonetheless it was with an immense sense of gratitude, relief and sadness that we returned home nine days after we had left for the ill-fated meeting with our Japanese distributors. Chris still has total amnesia for the accident and the events prior to waking after her surgery but, from her husband's point of view and from that of the neurologist who still lives inside of him, she is perfect! We will forever remain grateful to the Christchurch Hospital neurology and neurosurgical services that I helped establish so many years ago. I am doubtful that Chris would have survived the night or, at the very least, survived without a permanent neurological handicap if we had not had these neuroscience skills available in our city.

**BUT THERE ARE SOME THINGS** that are more unstoppable than people, and these are the mysterious forces that control our universe. Even as we were licking the wounds from multiple tribulations, consoling one another and preparing to battle on, Mother Nature was marching forward. The fateful spring of the 2010 earthquake rolled into summer as though nothing had happened; and what a summer was delivered up to us. It was as though nature was trying to make amends for the cruel card that she had dealt in the spring and the more deadly one that she had up her sleeve. As the lazy hot days of January and February passed into the golden glow of autumn it was clear that our vineyard had never seen a similar season. The fruit readily swelled, softened and ripened, so that the crop was ready to pick earlier than ever before. We had little time to lament the devastating February earthquake before the *vendange* of 2011 bore down on us.

Our motor vehicle accident and Chris's terrifying subdural haemorrhage occurred during the 2014 vintage at Pegasus Bay. While Chris and I were able to cocoon ourselves in hospital, the harvesting of grapes and the making of wine continued to flow around our personal problems. The rhythm of the seasons carries on regardless of what we mere mortals think or do, oblivious to our joy and grief. When you live off the land your life is governed by the inscrutable and unfeeling yearly cycle. In the icy days of winter the dormant vines demand to be pruned. Spring is the time of rebirth, when the leaves and flowers appear. The heat of summer produces growth and consolidation, while the golden days of autumn reward the vigneron with ripe fruits. Nature demands a huge amount of work in a vineyard throughout the year, but for a brief few weeks in autumn it yields its bounty.

If this treasure is treated with care and integrity it is capable of providing incalculable pleasure and joy, and soothing the hurts and wounds that are the inevitable part of the human condition. But in spite of the tightly controlled and predictable parameters of our days, weeks, months and years, each growing season and the wine it produces are different and individual.

That, of course, is one of the fascinations of wine. It is a product of the vagaries of nature and the craft of the human hand rather than just being an easily replicated factory-made product. This is surely the essence of what lured me over onto the dark side.

# Acknowledgements

**I WOULD LIKE TO ACKNOWLEDGE** the invaluable help of my wife, Chris, in writing this book. Her encouragement, suggestions and critical review of the text has been vital, not to mention her role as a colourful character throughout its pages. The exceptional tolerance of our four sons, Matthew, Michael, Edward and Paul, allowed us to explore the wine regions of Europe and to have adventures and fun that we could not otherwise have enjoyed as a family. Without our children's enthusiastic interest and participation our dream would have doubtless faded by now but they have infused it with new excitement and vigour.

I am indebted to my friend and neurological colleague, Dr Philip Parkin, for reading and commenting on chapter 12 and for his invaluable assistance in creating some of the illustrations and resurrecting some of the old photographs.

I am grateful to the editorial and publishing team at Random House for their expert assistance and in particular for the wonderfully professional guidance and help of Random House's publishing director Nicola Legat.